Quality Assurance in Haematology

Quality Assurance in Haematology

Edited by

S M Lewis, BSc, MD, FRCPath

Reader in Haematology, Royal Postgraduate Medical School, Consultant Haematologist, Hammersmith Hospital, London and Chairman International Committee for Standardization in Haematology

and

R L Verwilghen, MD

*Professor of Haematology, University Hospital, Leuven, Belgium
and Executive Secretary International Committee for Standardization in Haematology*

Baillière Tindall

London   Philadelphia   Toronto   Sydney   Tokyo

Baillière Tindall   24–28 Oval Road
W B Saunders   London NW1 7DX

West Washington Square
Philadelphia, PA 19105, USA

1 Goldthorne Avenue
Toronto, Ontario M8Z 5T9, Canada

ABP Australia Ltd
44–50 Waterloo Road
North Ryde, NSW 2113, Australia

Harcourt Brace Jovanovich Japan Inc.
Ichibancho Central Building, 22–1 Ichibancho
Chiyoda-ku, Tokyo 102, Japan

© 1988 Baillière Tindall

First published 1988

British Library Cataloguing in Publication Data

Lewis, S. M. (Shirley Mitchell)
  Quality assessment in haematology
  1. Man. Blood. Testing. Laboratory
  techniques. Quality control
  I. Title   II. Verwilghen, R. L.
  616.07'561

  ISBN 0–7020–1322–6

Typeset by Latimer Trend & Company Ltd
Printed in Great Britain by
T. J. Press (Padstow) Ltd, Padstow, Cornwall

Contents

Preface

It has always been necessary to try to ensure reliable results of the tests which are performed in the haematology laboratory, but never more so than today because of the special problems resulting from the use of complex automated instrument systems which function with little direct human control and also from the ever increasing workload which makes it virtually impossible for the laboratory staff to give close attention to every blood sample that enters the laboratory. On the other hand, many laboratories throughout the world are restricted to simple methods, perhaps confined to counting–chamber haemocytometry, haemoglobinometry and blood film microscopy. These laboratories, too, require the assurance of reliability. The quality of reagents, kits, pipettes and autodiluters, simple apparatus as well as complex equipment, must be scrutinized. Failure to standardize and harmonize the results of laboratory tests will lead to misleading data, especially when the tests are performed on a patient in different laboratories on successive occasions. In some circumstances even minor differences in measurement or a qualitative error will lead to wrong diagnosis or to incorrect treatment which may have a profound effect on the management of the patient.

The International Committee for Standardization in Haematology has been active in the field of standardization, and the complementary practice of quality assurance for 25 years. According to its constitution, ICSH is organized 'to promote the development of international standards that are needed to achieve international comparability of results of haematological analysis'. The importance of quality assurance in this context was reiterated by the ICSH Board in 1974 when this subject was taken as the theme for the ICSH symposium at the biannual International Congress of Haematology in Jerusalem. A book based on this symposium was subsequently published under the title 'Quality Control in Haematology', published by Academic Press. Increasing recognition of the importance of quality assurance by those who work in haematology laboratories and the remarkable developments in its practice during the past decade has encouraged the ICSH Secretariat to publish a new monograph. The contributors are eminent haematologists who are authorities on the scientific and technical aspects of the subject. The book is intended primarily for haematologists and the technical staff of haematology laboratories. It will be of value to students and to teachers, especially as there is a chapter which provides a series of exercises for a training programme in quality assurance based on workshops which have been organized by World Health Organization. The book will also be of interest to administrators, to laboratory workers in disciplines other than haematology and to public health authorities.

S M Lewis
R L Verwilghen
London and Leuven

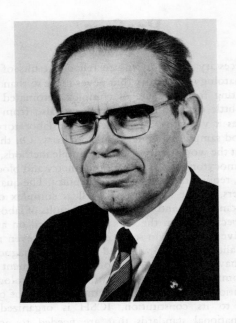

Dedicated to the memory of

Dr J Spaander

1914–1988

Foundation Board Member of the
International Committee for Standardization in Haematology 1963

President of the ICSH Board   1970–1972

Chairman of Secretariat   1964–1982

Emeritus Board Member   1982–1988

Contributors

R M BERTINA, PhD, Head of Coagulation Research Laboratory, University Hospital, Leiden, The Netherlands.

K C CARSTAIRS, MB, BS, MRCS, FRCPath, Associate Professor, Toronto General Hospital, Toronto, Canada.

I CAVILL, PhD, FRCPath, Senior Lecturer in Haematology, Department of Haematology, University of Wales College of Medicine, Cardiff, UK.

J M ENGLAND, MB, BS, BSc, PhD, MRCPath, Consultant Haematologist, Watford General Hospital, Honorary Senior Lecturer and Consultant, St Mary's Hospital, London W2, UK.

J A KOEPKE, MD, Professor of Pathology, Associate Professor of Medicine, Duke University Medical Center, Durham, North Carolina, NC 27710, USA.

S M LEWIS, BSc, MD, FRCPath, Reader in Haematology, Royal Postgraduate Medical School, Consultant Haematologist, Hammersmith Hospital, London, UK.

R M PARVIN, BS, MT(ASCP), SBB, Head of Serum Bank, Clinical Medicine Branch, US Public Health Service, Centers for Disease Control, Atlanta, GA 30333, USA.

R M ROWAN, MB, ChB, FRCP(Glas), FRCP(Edin), Senior Lecturer in Haematology, University of Glasgow, Honorary Consultant Haematologist, Department of Haematology, Western Infirmary, Glasgow, Scotland, UK.

N K SHINTON, MD, FRCP, FRCPath, Professor and Consultant Haematologist, Coventry and Warwickshire Hospital, Coventry, England, UK.

O W VAN ASSENDELFT, MD, PhD, Chief of Clinical Medicine Branch, Division of Host Factors, US Public Health Service, Centers for Disease Control, Atlanta, GA 30333, USA.

A M H P VAN DEN BESSELAAR, PhD, Deputy Director of Reference Laboratory for Anticoagulant Control, University Hospital, Leiden, The Netherlands.

R L VERWILGHEN, MD, Professor of Haematology, University Hospital, Herestraat 49, Leuven, Belgium.

Abbreviations

ACD	Acid citrate dextrose
AIDS	Acquired immune deficiency syndrome
ALL	Acute lymphoblastic leukaemia
AML	Acute myeloblastic leukaemia
APTT	Activated partial thromboplastin time
CMV	Cytomegalovirus
CPD	Citrate phosphate dextrose
CTAD	Citrate, theophylline, adenosine and dipyridamole
CV	Coefficient of variation
DI	Decision interval or deviation index
EDTA	Ethylenediaminetetraacetic acid
EQA	External quality assessment
ESR	Erythrocyte sedimentation rate
HEPES	N-2-Hydroxyethylpiperazine N'-2-ethane sulphonic acid
HIV	Human immunodeficiency virus
INR	International normalized ratio
IQC	Internal quality control
IRP	International reference preparation
ISI	International sensitivity index
IU	International unit

LRV	Lower reference value
MCH	Mean corpuscular haemoglobin
MCHC	Mean corpuscular haemoglobin concentration
MCV	Mean cell volume
MPV	Mean platelet volume
NA	Numerical aperture
NEQAS	National External Quality Assessment Scheme
PCV	Packed cell volume
PRP	Platelet–rich plasma
PT	Prothrombin time
RBC	Red blood count
RPA	Radiation protection advisor
RPS	Radiation protection supervisor
SD	Standard deviation
SEM	Standard error of the mean
WBC	White blood count

1

Introduction

S M Lewis and R L Verwilghen

In industry and commerce everybody recognizes the importance of having a procedure to ensure that the quality of the services which are provided and the goods and materials which are sold to the public are satisfactory, and reach a defined standard. This is no less important in medical practice. In the medical laboratory it is necessary to ensure that tests are carried out reliably and that the results can be used with confidence by the doctors, who require them for diagnosing and controlling treatment of patients. Reliable data are also necessary for individual health screening, for community health care, and for epidemiological surveys, studies of disease prevalence and establishing the reference values of various laboratory tests in health.

Such studies may be conducted at local, national or international level. In all these circumstances it is essential that results from the different laboratories are comparable and in harmony. Furthermore, there is an increasing enthusiasm for inter-laboratory collaboration for various reasons, notably for therapeutic trials, especially in diseases which are relatively uncommon and which require co-operative effort in order to accumulate sufficiently adequate data for analysis. Clearly, if the data from several laboratories are to be pooled, it is essential that the tests from which the data are derived must be strictly comparable. Similarly, the individual patient who requires therapeutic control based on the results of a laboratory test must be assured that the same reliance can always be placed on the results wherever and whenever the test is performed.

There are a number of procedures which should be used in all laboratories not only to avoid errors but also to recognize as early as possible when errors do occur, and correction becomes necessary. These procedures fall into two main categories—standardization and quality assurance.

Standardization refers to both the use of reference preparations (materials standards) and reference methods. A reference standard is a substance or device with a specification which is sufficiently well established for it to be used to calibrate an instrument or apparatus and to assign a numerical value for quantitative assays. If possible it must be based on or traceable to exactly defined physical or chemical measurement, ideally one of the base metrological units of length (metre), mass (kilogram), time (second), electric current (ampere), thermodynamic temperature (kelvin), luminous intensity (candela) and amount of substance (mole). A reference method is a clearly and exactly described technique for a particular determination which provides sufficiently accurate and precise data for it to be used to assess the validity of other laboratory methods for this determination. It is customary to use, with the reference method, a reference reagent with clearly defined reaction characteristics and level of analytic purity.

Quality assurance is the term used to encompass all steps which are taken by a laboratory to ensure the reliability of results, to improve intra-laboratory performance generally and inter-laboratory comparability. Thus, these activities would include internal quality control, participation in external assessment schemes, the introduction of standardized method, the use of material standards and participation in training courses, conferences and collaborative studies of instruments and laboratory methods, in order to achieve inter-laboratory reproducibility. A quality assurance programme in haematology should also be concerned with clinical aspects of haematology and should recognize the importance of professional audit.

Internal quality control (IQC) is the set of procedures undertaken by the staff of the laboratory for the continual evaluation of the reliability of the work of the laboratory and the results which are obtained for various tests, in order to decide whether the latter are reliable enough to be released to the requesting clinicians. The procedures should include tests on control material and statistical analysis of patients' data. The main object is to ensure day-to-day consistency of measurement of observation, if possible in agreement with some indicator of truth such as control material with assigned values.

External quality assessment (EQA) refers to a system of retrospectively and objectively comparing results from different laboratories by means of surveys organized by an external agency. The main object is to establish between-laboratory and between-instrument comparability, if possible in agreement with a reference standard where one exists. The organization and procedure of such a scheme is described in Chapter 7. The term 'inter-laboratory trial' is used to describe a collaborative exercise in which the performance of a test by a group of laboratories is used in order to assess aspects of the test or reagents used in the test, including the quality of the specimen. Its main purpose is to determine whether the tests might justifiably be incorporated in EQA surveys. The data obtained from an EQA scheme are intended primarily to assess individual laboratory performance. However, the data can also be analysed in terms of the test procedure, instrumentation and materials in order to assess the state of the art and to identify faulty types of instrument or kit or a poor method rather than poor performance.

Both internal quality control and external quality assessment are directed to specific test procedures, the starting point being the specimen at the laboratory bench. It is, however, equally important to ensure proficiency in specimen collection and labelling, delivery of specimens to the laboratory, record keeping and reporting, environmental and storage effects on specimens, interpretation of test results and relevance of various tests for the clinical information required. It also includes maintenance and control of equipment and apparatus, staff training and protection of staff, health and safety. These might be termed proficiency surveillance; they are essential components of good laboratory practice.

The reliability of test results requires consideration of four components: accuracy, precision, sensitivity and specificity.

(1) **Accuracy** is a measure of agreement between the estimates of a value and the true value. It requires a defined standard as described above. In order to obtain accurate measurement in practice, it is necessary to establish accuracy over the operating range of an instrument by appropriate use of reference methods, reference materials and/or calibrators. These are described in Chapter 9.

(2) **Precision** is the strength of agreement between replicate measurements. It has no numerical value but it is recognized in terms of imprecision, as defined by standard deviation or coefficient of variation of the results in the set of replicate measurements.

(3) **Specificity** is particularly important in clinical analysis. When a substance is analysed either by physical or chemical methods, the property of the substance being examined should be uniquely possessed by that substance. If the property is affected by the presence of other substances, specificity will not be possible and the interfering substances may suppress or enhance the reaction, leading to an incorrect result. This is a serious problem with blood samples as the matrix (i.e. cellular or plasma component) contains many analytes in addition to the one which is being measured. Thus lipidaemia and raised plasma proteins or an excessively high leucocyte count may cause an erroneously high haemoglobin measurement, microcytes may, in a cell counter, be registered as platelets and aggregated platelets as leucocytes. Hyperglycaemic blood may give a falsely high MCV. Recovery experiments are useful for assessing the extent of interference.

(4) **Sensitivity** is the ability of the procedure to detect the analyte and to measure it within narrow limits of imprecision. In practice, it is necessary to establish the instrument settings and/or range of analyte concentration which can be measured reliably. In this context sensitivity does not mean the *lowest* concentration at which an analyte can be detected. Essentially, sensitivity is the ability to detect an abnormal state by a particular test whereas specificity is the ability to obtain normal results in a normal situation.

The International Committee for Standardization in Haematology (ICSH) is active in the development of international standards which are used for haematological analysis and also in various aspects of quality assurance. There are also other international, regional and national organizations with similar interests. They co-operate with one another and in their work they share common technical and scientific problems. They also share the burden of lengthy titles which, for convenience, are abbreviated to acronyms. As they are frequently referred to throughout the text, their identification is listed below:

ACDP	Advisory Committee on Dangerous Pathogens
AABB	American Association of Blood Banks
BCR	European Community Bureau of Reference

BSH   British Society for Haematology
DHSS   Department of Health and Social Security (UK)
ECCLS   European Committee for Clinical Laboratory Standards
ICSH   International Committee for Standardization in Haematology
ICTH   International Committee on Thrombosis and Haemostasis
IFCC   International Federation of Clinical Chemistry
ISO   International Organization for Standardization
NCCLS   National Committee for Clinical Laboratory Standards
WHO   World Health Organization

2

Specimen Collection, Handling and Storage

O W van Assendelft and R M Parvin

The necessity for accurate and precise methodology in the clinical laboratory is repeatedly stressed. Quality-control monitoring of the analytical process has become a way of life, yet, in general, little attention has been devoted to establishing quality-control measures for collecting, handling, processing and storing blood specimens. Highly controlled, sophisticated laboratory technology is of no avail if the specimens are error-ridden due to faulty identification or poor collection techniques. Proper specimen collection and handling are, therefore, of the utmost importance; the likelihood for error in these areas is probably greater than the likelihood of errors that may occur during the laboratory determinations themselves.

Collection errors range from incorrect identification of the patient specimen to haemolysed specimens or the use of inappropriate anticoagulants. Studies have indicated that as many as 8% of errors in patient name, age, sex and identification numbers go undetected, even with extensive manual checking procedures (117). Standards and guidelines for proper specimen collection and handling can, and have, reduced or alleviated many of these problems. The International Committee for Standardization in Haematology has published guidelines for standardization of blood specimen collection for establishing reference values (42). This chapter reviews these and other guidelines and recommendations for specimen collection, handling and storage, primarily oriented towards specimens for the haematology and immunohaematology laboratory. The recommendations and guidelines are equally valid for collection and processing in a blood-banking environment (1, 2).

Intra-individual variability

Variations in analyte concentration within one and the same individual can be divided into three major components: analytical variation, variation related to the subject, and variations related to the time of specimen collection. Analytical variation will not be considered in this chapter.

Subject variation

Subject variation includes all sources of variation that are not analytical and not related to the biological problem for which the laboratory test was ordered. Factors causing subject variation include use of drugs, caffeine, alcohol; intake of food; physical activity; emotional stress; patient posture; and tourniquet application time. Only some of these factors are known to influence haematological test results. For example, a 48-h fast increases the total serum bilirubin concentration by 240% (5), and there has been much controversy regarding the effect of a meal on leucocyte counts (24, 101, 107, 116). Smoking causes erythrocytosis, leucocytosis and eosinopenia (125), as well as a doubling of carboxyhaemoglobin concentration between 10:00 and 14:00 h (33, 123). Significant changes in the red cell count and in haemoglobin and haptoglobin concentration have been described after strenuous exercise (36, 97, 98, 122). Brief, severe exercise is generally accompanied by lymphocytosis; prolonged exercise causes neutrophilia (116); heavy manual work can result in neutrophilic leucocytosis, lymphopenia and eosinopenia (39, 49, 50). Leucocytosis has also been reported following emotional stress (70). Exercise and stress influence coagulation and fibrinolysis (4). Position, standing or supine, can affect serum iron (109, 110), packed cell volume and haemoglobin concentration (19, 20, 59, 119), and is probably related to a shift of body water from the vascular to the interstitial compartment. A significant drop (-24%) in serum iron and an increase ($+6\%$) in iron-binding capacity has been found in subjects after donation of a unit of blood (61).

Variations related to the time of specimen collection

These are often difficult to document accurately (107). Substantial physiological day-to-day and within-day variation has been reported for serum iron concentration (6, 108, 110) and, to a lesser degree for iron-binding capacity (108). Intra-individual variations of haptoglobin and transferrin are relatively small when compared with the inter-individual variation (111). A 10% day-to-day variation has been reported for plasma fibrinogen (29), as well as a 'diurnal fibrinolytic rhythm' (9, 22). Numerous reports have appeared (21, 67, 72, 114), which indicate that haemoglobin concentration and packed cell volume exhibit a diurnal variation: lower values in the afternoon and evening as compared to morning values. Significant diurnal variation has also been reported for total white cell counts (52) and for the five main subsets of leucocytes (107, 112, 126).

   It is thus important that the time of blood collection and relevant particulars of the patient are reported to the laboratory and to the physician requesting a test.

Specimen collection

Specimens for the haematology laboratory may be whole blood, collected by venepuncture or skin puncture, peripheral blood smears or bone marrow, obtained by aspiration or biopsy. Specimen collection by arterial puncture is generally reserved for blood gas tension and blood pH measurement (80).

Specimen labelling

Organization is essential in areas where blood specimens are collected so that records of patients seen and specimens drawn may be accurately maintained. Record, in order of acquisition, each request for a blood specimen. This accessioning provides a means of identifying all paperwork and supplies associated with each patient. Use the assigned accession number on all specimens taken from a patient at one time. Record on labels the information given on the specimen request form. Always include: (1) patient's full name, (2) identification number, (3) accessioning number, (4) date, and (5) time of collection. Other information may be added, e.g. the physician, room number, name of test, initials of person drawing the specimen and relevant patient information. Print labels in ink, indelible pencil or by computer print-out.

Patient identification

Before drawing any specimens, positively identify the patient to ensure that the specimen is being taken from the individual designated on the request form: ask the patient to give her or his full name. If the request form includes a home address, ask for this information and compare it with the information given on the request form and labels. Also check the bracelet information usually issued by hospitals. If the patient is unable to speak, ask a family member, a doctor, or a nurse for assistance in identification. If there is any discrepancy whatsoever, such as a slight misspelling of the name or reversal of identifying numbers, ask the nurse in charge to identify that patient by name and number. Label all specimen tubes immediately before or after drawing the specimen.

Collecting a venous blood specimen

After positively identifying the patient, verify diet restrictions, position the patient comfortably, verify the collection tubes, assemble necessary supplies, and select the appropriate system for drawing the specimen. Two systems are used in drawing venous blood specimens: the syringe and needle or the evacuated tube system. A syringe and needle is preferable when difficulty in drawing the specimen is anticipated, e.g. patients with fragile or hardened vein walls, but in general the evacuated tube system is a popular method for specimen collection. Evacuated tube systems are composed of three basic elements: a sterile needle, a holder securing both the needle and the evacuated

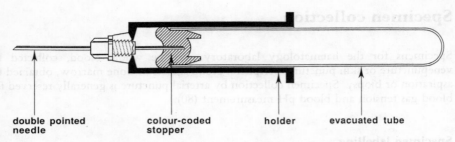

**double pointed   colour-coded   holder   evacuated tube
needle   stopper**

Fig. 2.1   Components of an evacuated tube system. (From NCCLS, (73), with permission.)

tube, and an evacuated tube containing a pre-measured vacuum and with or without a pre-measured additive (Fig. 2.1).

Performing a venepuncture involves several simultaneous steps: applying a tourniquet, closing the patient's hand, selecting and cleaning the vein site, inspecting needle and container, grasping the patient's arm, performing the puncture, releasing the tourniquet and opening the patient's hand, placing gauze and removing the needle, applying pressure over the puncture site, and bandaging the arm.

(1) **Tourniquet.** Use a tourniquet to increase venous pressure to facilitate vein identification and entry. Apply the tourniquet 7–10 cm above the venepuncture site. Never apply the tourniquet for longer than 1 min, so as not to invalidate test results as a consequence of fluid shifts and altered metabolism due to prolonged stagnation. Venous occlusion causes haemoconcentration, increased fibrinolytic activity, platelet release and activation of some clotting factors. Gerbrandy *et al.* (26) found that in venous blood specimens taken before, during and after the upper arm was compressed for more than 7 min, the plasma protein concentration was increased by an average of 20%.

(2) **Closing the patient's hand.** This can accentuate the arm veins. Avoid vigorous hand exercise ('pumping').

(3) **Vein site.** The veins of a patient may be required as an avenue of entry for various therapeutic agents or blood transfusions. Therefore, the vein site must be selected carefully to preserve vein patency. Preferentially use the superficial veins of the anterior surface of the arm, e.g. the median cubital and the cephalic, for drawing blood specimens. Palpate the selected vein to identify its course and depth; avoid nearby arteries. Complete palpation before the sterile preparation of the puncture site.

(4) **Cleansing the site.** Cleanse the puncture site to prevent chemical or microbiological contamination. Satisfactory antiseptic agents are 70% isopropyl alcohol solutions and 0.5% chlorohexidine in 95% ethanol. With a circular motion, clean the puncture site with an antiseptic-soaked gauze pad from the centre to the periphery. Allow the area to dry to prevent haemolysis and/or a burning sensation when the venepuncture is performed. Do not palpate the vein after the site has been cleansed. If the venepuncture proves difficult and the vein must be palpated again to draw blood, cleanse the finger with alcohol before touching the site.

(5) **Inspect needle and container.** Make sure the needle is sharp with no barbs.

(6) **Grasping the patient's arm.** Grasp the patient's arm firmly and with the thumb draw the skin taut to anchor the vein; the thumb should be 2–5 cm below and to the side of the venepuncture site.

(7) **Performing the venepuncture.** (a) When syringe and needle are used: position the appropriate needle on the syringe. With the patient's arm in a downward position, align the needle and syringe with the vein from which the blood will be drawn. With the bevel side in an upward position, push the needle into the vein; a sensation of resistance will be felt, followed by ease of penetration as the vein is entered. Withdraw the desired amount of blood. Replace the first syringe with another if additional blood is needed; the needle should remain in the vein as long as this is being done. (b) With the evacuated tube system: thread the appropriate needle into the holder until it is secure and insert the appropriate tube into the holder up to the recessed guideline on the needle holder. With the patient's arm in a downward position to prevent the possibility of backflow, align the needle with the vein from which the blood will be drawn. With the bevel in an upward position, push the needle into the vein. Depress the tube to the end of the holder to puncture the diaphragm of the stopper. Remove the tube from the holder as soon as the blood flow ceases. If multiple samples are needed, other tubes are placed in the holder.

When transferring blood from a syringe to an evacuated tube, do not remove the rubber stopper from the tube. Blood must be transferred from the syringe by the action of the vacuum in the tube and it must not be injected into an evacuated tube. This technique is extremely important if the tube contains an anticoagulant or other additive. The vacuum ensures the correct proportion of blood to additive.

(8) **Release the tourniquet** before removing the needle from the vein.

(9) **Opening the patient's hand.** Ask the patient to open her or his hand to allow the blood circulation to return to normal and to reduce pressure in the vein and bleeding at the puncture site.

(10) **Withdrawing the needle.** Place a gauze pad above the venepuncture site and remove the needle slowly, keeping the bevel in an upward position. Then slip the gauze pad down over the puncture site and apply slight pressure.

(11) **Bandaging the arm.** Wrap a gauze bandage tightly around the arm over the gauze pad.

Special care must be taken when collecting specimens for coagulation testing. Factor VIII coagulant activity is known to be labile; the slightest trauma or delay can produce artefactual changes in fibrinopeptide A and β–thromboglobulin test results.

Prevention of haematoma and/or haemolysis

Fully penetrating, yet only puncturing the uppermost wall of the vein will prevent haematoma formation while performing a venepuncture. Partial penetration may allow blood to leak into the soft tissues surrounding the vein by way of the needle bevel. Use only major veins for a venepuncture and release the tourniquet before removing the needle.

Avoid drawing blood from a haematoma. Avoid using a needle with too small a bore size. When using a needle and syringe, make sure the needle is fitted securely on the syringe to avoid frothing and avoid drawing the plunger back too forcefully. Mix anticoagulated specimens gently but thoroughly; do not inject blood from a syringe into an evacuated tube.

Phlebotomists

Reducing errors during the blood collecting phase will result in biologically representative specimens, comparable from one institute to another. A standard procedure has been published by the European Committee for Clinical Laboratory Standards (18). Without question, a sound training programme is needed to develop efficient, well-trained phlebotomists. The National Committee for Clinical Laboratory Standards (NCCLS) has published guidelines for such a training programme (74).

Evacuated tubes

The containers which form part of the evacuated tube system are available in different sizes (Table 2.1) with and without additives. Colour-coding of the stoppers indicates the type of additive (Table 2.2).

The degree of vacuum in evacuated tubes is such that the tube generally will fill to within ±10% of the stated draw volume, thus ensuring a correct final blood/additive ratio. However, the tube vacuum may diminish with time, resulting in 'incomplete draws'. If so desired, laboratories can determine the degree of vacuum draw of an evacuated tube using a calibrated buret (45, 73).

Special precautions should be taken before implementing the evacuated tube system for collecting blood specimens for coagulation testing. Contact with glass activates certain clotting factors (2a, 103a, 103b). Activation appeared to have been circumvented with the introduction of siliconized evacuated tubes. However, various studies showed inconsistent test results when tubes of different brands, or different lots of the same brand, were used (34, 91, 118, 121). Further evidence is clearly required before

Table 2.1 Dimensional guide for evacuated tubes

Nominal size (mm)	Nominal draw (ml of blood)	Outside tube diameter (mm)
10 × 65	3	10 −11
13 × 75	5	11.5–13
13 × 100	7	11.5–13
16 × 100	10	15 −16
16 × 127	15	15 −16

Table 2.2 Letter and colour codes for specimen tubes

Additive	Use	Letter code[a]		Stopper colour	
		ISO	NCCLS	ISO	NCCLS
None	Serum	Z		Red	Red
EDTA					
K₂,K₃	Plasma or whole blood	KE	K3E	Lavender	Lavender
Na₂		NE	N2E	Lavender	Lavender
Heparin (Na, Li)	Plasma or whole blood	NH	NAH	Green	Green
		LH	LIH	Green	Green
Trisodium citrate					
1:9	Coag. studies	9NC	NC9	Light blue	Blue
1:4	ESR (Westergren)	4NC	NC4	Black	Blue
Acid citrate dextrose		ACD		Yellow	Yellow
Sterile interior of tube					
Fluoride/oxalate	Glycolysis inhibition	FX	NFX	Grey	Grey
Serum separation material	Serum	S		Red/black	
		S		Red/grey	

[a]Manufacturers of evacuated tubes are currently not using letter coding on the tube labels to indicate the type of additive.

indiscriminate use of evacuated tubes is justified and laboratories that wish to use these tubes for coagulation testing specimens will have to validate each particular brand or lot.

Needles for evacuated tube holders are available in different sizes. Generally, 19–22 gauge needles (20 SWG–23 SWG; 1.06–0.71 mm outside diameter) are preferred. The choice of a needle is usually a compromise between optimal flow rate for blood collection and minimal size to reduce tissue/vessel wall damage and pain. Small-bore needles require considerable suction pressure through the needle resulting in a strong possibility of red cell damage in the needle (88). If sufficient blood flow rate through the needle is not obtained, the time required for collecting the specimen may be unduly prolonged, coagulation is liable to occur, and the normal plasma/cell ratio may be upset.

Additives

Heparin

Heparin as anticoagulant is specifically recommended when determining carboxyhaemoglobin (100) and zinc (14). It is also valuable as anticoagulant when unhaemolysed, unaltered red cells are required for fragility studies and red cell enzyme determinations. The lithium salt of heparin has been particularly recommended for anticoagulation (82). Heparin anticoagulation is not recommended for blood cell counting because of its clumping effect on platelets and leucocytes. Blood films made from heparin-anticoagulated blood are difficult to stain clearly.

The quantity of heparin required for adequate anticoagulation depends on how it is introduced into the specimen and on the solubility characteristics of the particular salt. For evacuated tubes, a range of 15–30 IU/ml of blood is recommended (82). Certain plastic microcollection devices may require less than 15 IU of heparin salt per ml of blood (81).

To determine an upper limit of heparin as anticoagulant without increase in erythrocyte size, microhaematocrit capillaries (79) containing increasing amounts of heparin were tested at the Centers for Disease Control (CDC). The packed cell volume (PCV) remained constant in capillary tubes containing from 4 to 7.25 IU per tube and increased by 1.5% with 9.75 IU per tube. Thus, 7.5 IU of heparin per capillary tube may be considered a 'safe' upper limit for PCV determination. An amount of 7.5 IU heparin per capillary tube is equal to 125 IU per ml of blood.

Trisodium citrate

Trisodium citrate, $Na_3C_6H_5O_7$, is the usual anticoagulant for coagulation investigations. For coagulation studies either a 109 or a 129 mmol/l (32 or 38 g/l of the dihydrate form) solution is acceptable in a 1:9 anticoagulant/blood ratio (85). For determining Erythrocyte sedimentation rate (ESR), a 109 mmol/l solution is recommended in a 1:4 anticoagulant/blood ratio (41).

The 109 mmol/l solution has been recommended by the International Committee on Thrombosis and Haemostasis, ICTH (43, 44). If a patient's PCV is very high or very low, the results of the prothrombin time may be inaccurate when a 1:9 anticoagulant/ blood ratio is used (30a). Different anticoagulant/blood ratios have been advocated for specimens with PCV < 0.20 and > 0.60 (44, 53, 85).

EDTA

The most frequently used anticoagulant in the haematology laboratory is ethylenediaminetetraacetic acid, $C_{10}H_{16}N_2O_8$. EDTA acts as a sequestering or chelating agent and effectively chelates the calcium in blood. Because of its chelating properties, EDTA is unsuitable for specimens for calcium and iron analyses using colorimetric or titrimetric techniques. The lack of solubility of the free acid in aqueous solution makes the sodium and potassium salts preferable for use. The disodium and dipotassium salts are generally used in the dry form, the tripotassium salt usually in the liquid form.

The recommended range for adequate anticoagulation is 3.7–5.4 µmol/ml of blood of the free acid. Table 2.3 gives the mass amounts and the pH of aqueous solutions of the sodium and potassium salts of EDTA. Na_3-EDTA is not recommended because of its high pH; in liquid form it may adversely affect glass and plasma proteins.

EDTA is particularly useful in the haematology laboratory because it preserves the cellular components of blood. Reports indicate 24-h stability of red cell, white cell and platelet counts, packed cell volume, haemoglobin concentration, and mean cell haemoglobin (MCH) and mean cell haemoglobin concentration (MCHC) when EDTA is used in amounts of < 4 mg/ml of blood (103). Reticulocyte counts are reliable up to 48 h in blood stored at either 23°C or 4°C (58). Extended storage of over 6 h, however, is generally not recommended because the stability can vary to a considerable degree, depending on reagents and instrumentation. At CDC, K_3-EDTA-anticoagulated blood was followed for 24 h using a microhaematocrit centrifuge and an automated haematology analyser (Coulter, S-880), with specimen storage at 4°C and at 22°C. Table 2.4 summarizes the results. The specimen stored at 22°C demonstrated a gradual increase in mean cell volume (MCV) over the 24-h period (+ 1.5%) but no change in PCV. The platelet count of the specimen stored at 4°C showed a continuous decrease (− 34% in 24 h). Preliminary studies comparing K_2- and K_3-EDTA have shown a difference in MCV of nearly 3% when PCV is determined by the microhaematocrit method.

Table 2.3 pH of aqueous EDTA-salt solutions and required amounts for adequate anticoagulation

Compound	pH	Required amount per ml of blood	
		µmol	mg
Na_2-EDTA.2H_2O	4.5–5.3	3.7–5.4	1.4–2.0
K_2-EDTA.2H_2O	< 4.5	3.7–5.4	1.5–2.2
K_3-EDTA (anhydrous)	7–8	3.7–5.4	1.5–2.2

Table 2.4   Effect of storage at 4 and 22°C of a K$_3$-EDTA-anticoagulated blood specimen on selected haematology tests

Time (h)	PCV (microhaematocrit)		Haemoglobin (g/l)		MCV (fl)		RBC ($\times 10^{12}$ per litre)		WBC ($\times 10^9$ per litre)		Platelet count ($\times 10^9$ per litre)	
	4°C	22°C	4°C	22°C	4°C	22°C	4°C	22°C	4°C	22°C	4°C	22°C
0	0.381	0.386	130	130	93.8	93.8	4.08	4.08	7.9	7.9	294	294
3	0.384	0.389	131	132	94.1	94.4	4.02	4.02	8.3	8.0	268	285
6	0.395	0.395	132	131	93.7	94.7	4.04	3.99	8.2	8.25	243	286
12	0.400	0.400	130	132	94.6	95.3	3.99	4.01	8.3	8.2	246	292
24	0.384	0.384	131	130	93.9	95.2	4.02	4.03	8.2	8.2	195	280

PCV determined by the microhaematocrit method (79). Haemoglobin, MCV and cell counts determined with a Coulter S-880.

Sacker (103) reported that morphological changes in granulocytes, including loss of granulation, vacuolization, nuclear swelling, and changes in chromatin pattern, commence within 30 min of exposure of leucocytes to EDTA. An absence of significant changes in cell morphology for up to 5 h (51) and up to 6 h (62) has, however, also been reported. At CDC, slight vacuolization of monocytes was found after 1 h, progressing to moderate after 4 h, and slight vacuolization of neutrophilic granulocytes at 3–4 h, progressing to moderate after 6 h.

Acid citrate dextrose (ACD)

Acid citrate dextrose (63), is widely used in blood transfusion laboratories because of its anticoagulant and preservative properties. Its formula is given on p. 157. The storage life of red cells in ACD is 21 days.

Oxalate

Combined ammonium/potassium oxalate was extensively used in the haematology laboratory before the introduction of EDTA. Although this combination did not cause shrinkage of the erythrocytes, other oxalates cause cell shrinkage by drawing cell water into the plasma. The resultant reduction in PCV may be as much as 10%.

Capillary blood sampling

For small quantities of blood required for haematologic procedures or some chemical tests, adequate specimens can be collected by performing a skin puncture. Especially in premature infants, drawing large quantities of venous blood may result in anaemia. Thus, collection of skin-puncture blood is particularly important in paediatrics. Skin-puncture blood specimens from adults may be desirable from severely burned patients, extremely obese patients, patients with thrombotic tendencies, patients with malignancies where venepuncture is reserved for or limited to therapeutic purposes, and geriatric patients.

Some studies have shown no significant difference between an individual's capillary and venous blood values for PCV, red and white cell counts, mean cell volume (MCV), and platelet counts (115); others have reported significant discrepancies in PCV (87, 90). Discrepancies may, however, have been exaggerated by cold and resultant slow capillary blood flow (89).

Puncture sites

(1) the lateral or posterolateral portion of the heel, and (2) the big toe; (3) the palmar or dorsal surface of the last digit of the finger. The heel is used most often prior to 1 year of age. Care must be taken to prevent the point of the lancet from penetrating the bone in newborns. Puncturing deeper than 2.4 mm on the plantar surface of the heel of infants may risk bone damage (84). Puncture of the calcaneus can increase the risk of

osteomyelitis. The puncture site must be non-oedematous, since tissue fluids can cause abnormal results. The skin puncture must bleed freely.

Containers

Several types of containers are used to collect capillary blood (81):

(1) Capillary pipettes, most often used for collecting routine blood test specimens. The specimen is collected into several tubes and can be distributed easily. However, the pipettes are hard to label and must be broken after centrifugation to obtain serum or plasma.

(2) Microcontainers composed of small polypropylene tubes with a capillary tube in the lid. The specimen is collected by capillary action and then flows into the tube. Little haemolysis results with the use of these microcontainers (35).

(3) 'Unopettes', disposable diluting pipettes consisting of a capillary tube and a reservoir containing a pre-measured volume of diluent.

(4) Small conical glass or plastic tubes. To move blood to the bottom of the tube, the technologist must flick her or his wrist after each drop is collected. This drop-by-drop collection increases the chance of haemolysis of the specimen. Special precautions are required when collecting capillary blood for coagulation tests (31).

Puncture procedure

After positive identification of the patient (see p. 7), the following are involved in the performance of a skin puncture:

(1) The skin-puncture site should be warm. This can be achieved by gently massaging the area or applying a warm, wet washcloth to the site for about 3 min.

(2) Cleanse the site to be punctured very well with 70% alcohol, and dry it with a clean gauze pad. Alcohol left on the skin can cause haemolysis of the blood.

(3) Grasp the finger or heel firmly.

(4) Make a quick puncture with a sterile lancet. Remove the first drop of blood with a gauze pad: this blood is most likely contaminated with tissue fluid.

(5) Collect the specimen. After a drop of blood forms over the puncture site, place the tip of a capillary tube or other collection device against the side of the drop. The blood will flow readily into the tube by capillary action. Blood should not be collected by 'scooping' it from the skin. Rapid pipetting is necessary to collect the specimen before coagulation begins; 0.5–1 ml of blood may be collected if an adequate puncture has been performed.

(6) Hold the puncture site downward and gently apply pressure to the surrounding tissue to facilitate bleeding at the puncture site. Excessive squeezing will cause contamination of the specimen with tissue fluid.

(7) After collecting the required specimen, prevent further bleeding by applying slight pressure with a gauze pad. The puncture site may be bandaged for protection.

(8) If necessary, seal the capillary tubes with sealing material. If 'Unopettes' with diluent have been used for collection, wash the specimen completely into the diluent immediately after collection and before coagulation can occur. For coagulation testing, special diluents may be required (16).

Filter paper collection

Many neonatal screening programmes use capillary blood collected on filter paper. Specimens may be collected directly from the puncture site, or the preprinted circles on the filter paper may be saturated with blood previously collected into sterile, heparinized capillary tubes. Apply blood to one side of the filter paper only. Examine both sides to make sure that the specimen has penetrated and saturated the paper. Avoid touching or smearing the blood spots. Allow the specimen to air-dry in a suspended horizontal position for at least 3 h at ambient (15–22°C) temperature. Do not heat, stack, or allow the blood spots on the filter paper to touch other surfaces during the drying process. After drying, place each filter paper card into a separate mailing envelope and mail to the laboratory within 24 h of collection.

Suitable filter paper should conform to specifications and the absorption capacity, homogeneity and retention volume of the 3 mm paper punch should be measured for each lot (47, 83).

Blood films

The reliability of information obtained from blood films depends on the quality of the smears. Properly spread films are essential for accurate work. Slides and cover glasses must be scrupulously clean and free of grease and dust so that they will wet and allow uniform spreading of the blood.

Two methods to prepare adequate films are used:

(1) **The two-slide method.** Place a small drop of blood about 2 mm in diameter on a slide 2 cm from the end. Place the edge of another slide, from which a small corner has been broken off, on the surface of the first at an angle of 30–40°. Draw this slide back against the drop of blood until the specimen runs across the end of this slide. Push the slide forward at a moderate speed to spread the blood evenly on the first slide into a thin film. Air-dry rapidly by waving the slide or by using a fan.

(2) **The coverslip method.** Using 2 × 2 cm coverslips, place a small drop of blood on one coverslip. Place a second coverslip diagonally over the first and allow the blood to spread out evenly. Smoothly slide the coverslips apart, parallel to their surfaces, and air-dry the smears.

Expert morphological evaluation of peripheral blood cells is one of the most vital procedures in haematology laboratory diagnosis. It is essential, therefore, that blood films be of ideal thickness. An acceptable wedge blood film (Method 1) has the following characteristics (76):

(1) A gradual transition in thickness from the thick to thin areas, ending in a squared, straight edge.

(2) At minimum 2.5 cm long, terminating at least 1cm from the end of the slide.
(3) Narrower than the slide on which the film is spread, with smooth, continuous side margins that are accessible for oil immersion examination.
(4) No artefacts introduced by technique.
(5) A far end that becomes gradually thinner, without streaks, troughs or ridges.
(6) Granulocytes, monocytes and lymphocytes that appear evenly distributed in the 'usable' fields of the film.
(7) When the white cell count is within the normal range, the number of leucocytes per $10 - \times$ field at the tail area should not exceed 2–3 times the number per field in the body of the film; the film edges should contain less than 2–3 times the number of cells per field in the body of the smear.
(8) Less than 2% of cells should be disrupted or non–identifiable (except in certain pathologic states, e.g. chronic lymphocytic leukaemia).

Bone marrow aspiration and biopsy

In addition to a careful and complete patient history, physical examination, and a review of a patient's peripheral blood film, collecting and studying a bone marrow specimen is of prime importance in clinical and laboratory haematology. The routine site for marrow sampling was formerly the sternum where the marrow is easily aspirated. The sternum has, however, been almost completely abandoned in favour of other sites. With the increasing need for marrow tissue biopsies, the posterior iliac crest has become the location of choice for both aspiration and biopsy. The anterior iliac crest in adult patients is also sometimes biopsied. Other sites, such as the spinous process of a vertebra or a focal lesion localized by X-ray examination, are occasionally aspirated or biopsied. In infants up to 8 months old, the proximal anterior aspect of the tibia, 1–2 cm below the greater tuberosity, provides a convenient site for marrow sampling.

After choosing the site, it is scrubbed with a soapy wash, then swabbed with antiseptic and/or bacteriostatic solutions. A small sterile drape with a 5–8 cm central opening is carefully placed over the biopsy site. If no assistance is available and the operator is dependent upon her- or himself for the entire procedure, only the skin immediately surrounding the site and the tip of the marrow needle are kept sterile. No gloves are worn because of the subsequent preparation of the marrow films. If an assistant is helping, the entire biopsy area, as well as the instrument tray are kept sterile throughout the procedure.

Use a longer-acting local anaesthetic, e.g. 1% lidocaine hydrochloride, to infiltrate the biopsy site. After infiltration of the biopsy site is completed, a waiting period of 4–5 min is required for the anaesthetic to take effect. Prepare the aspirating needle by inserting a properly fitting obturator into the needle lumen and check for proper fit. Push the needle through the skin with a twisting motion. Keep the obturator in place as the needle is pushed through the relatively thin bone; use a twisting motion as the needle is slowly advanced to about 1 cm into the marrow cavity. After being assured of proper placement, remove the obturator and attach a 5 or 10 ml Luer lock glass syringe to the needle hub. The required amount of marrow (about 0.5 ml) is quickly aspirated by sharply withdrawing the plunger of the syringe. Do not aspirate larger quantities. Remove the syringe from the aspirating needle and give it to the assistant who will express a small quantity onto a glass slide to ascertain if marrow particles are present and will make the films before coagulation occurs.

If aspiration only is being done, the obturator is reinserted and the needle withdrawn. If a biopsy is also required, two options are available. (1) The biopsy device is inserted through the needle in the same site but advanced 1–3 cm deeper for the biopsy, or (2) the biopsy needle is placed at a second site, using the same skin incision. This avoids biopsy of the same location that has just been aspirated and that generally results in a biopsy of trabecular bone with large quantities of sinusoidal blood but few, if any, marrow particles. Biopsy needles are available which cut out a core of marrow up to 3 cm in length with minimal destruction of tissue (46). Withdraw the biopsy needle with a slight twisting motion and remove the material obtained gently from the needle and place in the proper fixative. Observe the wound for undue bleeding, then place a small butterfly bandage to approximate the cut surfaces and a larger dressing over it.

The aspirated marrow specimen is used to prepare films of marrow cells on glass slides. Cover glass 'squash' preparations have been very popular. A small particle of marrow is placed on an acid–cleaned, alcohol-rinsed, 2.5 × 2.5 cm coverslip and a second coverslip placed obliquely on top of the particle. The coverslips are gently squeezed together, then the opposing corners of the two coverslips are grasped and quickly pulled apart, being careful to keep them parallel to each other. Make several preparations and fix them with water-free (<3%) methanol (15).

Two 2.5 × 7.5 cm microscope slides can be used instead of coverslips. A marrow particle is placed in the centre of a slide and a second slide placed lengthwise covering about two-thirds of the lower slide.

The slides or coverslips can be stained in the usual way, manually or with a slide stainer. The resulting films characteristically contain marrow cells in the central portions with sinusoidal blood at the periphery. Thus, morphology of circulating blood cells can be evaluated alongside the marrow cells.

Specimen handling and processing

Specimen transport

Handling and transport of diagnostic specimens must adhere to procedures that maintain the viability and integrity of the specimen from the point of origin to the laboratory. Although delays of blood specimens in transit from a patient to the laboratory are usually short, the time elapsing from separation of cells and serum or plasma until analysis may be considerable. For some tests (e.g. ammonia, blood gas determinations) specimens must be kept at approximately 4°C from the time the blood is drawn until the specimens are analysed or until serum or plasma is separated from the cells. Transfer of such specimens to the laboratory must be done by placing the specimen container in ice water. For all analytes that are thermally labile, serum or plasma should be separated from the cells in a refrigerated centrifuge. For the haematology laboratory, it has been recommended that specimens for coagulation assays be placed in melting ice immediately after drawing the specimen, transported to the laboratory as quickly as possible and centrifuged, at 4°C, within 60 min of the venepuncture (85). It is, however, also advocated (118) that specimens for prothrombin time and Factor VIII assay should not be chilled, especially when evacuated tubes are used for specimen collection. If siliconized evacuated tubes are used, chilled specimens should be tested within 2 h of drawing (28, 92, 93, 118).

Specimen transfer from the patient to the laboratory is usually done by messenger. In some institutions, however, pneumatic tube systems may be used to move specimens more rapidly over longer distances. In such systems, haemolysis may occur unless tubes are completely filled and movement of the tubes inside the carrier is prevented (8, 30, 60, 94, 95, 113, 124). Pneumatic tube systems should be designed to eliminate sharp curves and sudden stops.

Occasionally specimens are sent to a referral laboratory. Before a referral laboratory is used, the quality of its work should be verified by the referring laboratory (77). Specimen handling requirements of the referral laboratory must be observed and test results reported by a referral laboratory should be reported as such in the patient's chart. It should be assumed that transport to a referral laboratory could take as long as 72 h. Referring laboratories should retain enough of the specimen, stored under optimal conditions, for re-testing should unanticipated problems arise during shipment.

Specimen shipping

Certain environmental factors incidental to the handling and shipment of specimens should be considered:

(1) Avoid any temperature above 35°C. Deterioration of components frequently is accelerated at elevated temperatures.

(2) Avoid exposure to light, especially direct sunlight, which may cause rapid decomposition of certain chemical components, e.g. bilirubin.

(3) Avoid temperatures below −70°C (serum). Unless properly packaged, whole-blood specimens cannot be subjected to environmental conditions below 0°C because freezing will haemolyze the specimen.

(4) A package must retain the specimen when the ambient pressure is reduced to 50 kPa (0.5 atmosphere).

(5) Packages must withstand any vibration normally encountered during handling and shipment.

(6) Some components of serum or plasma are very labile at room temperature, and the specimen must be kept frozen before analysis. In some instances, temperature is so critical (e.g. renin) that chilled tubes and refrigerated centrifuges must be used when preparing the specimen. Dry ice (solid carbon dioxide) is the best way to maintain frozen specimens during shipment.

(7) Some specimens must be kept cold but not frozen. Pack such specimens in a polystyrene container with refrigerant packs. To avoid freezing, do not place the specimen directly on the refrigerant material. Wet ice is also suitable if packed in an individually sealed double bag to prevent leakage.

(8) Some specimens must be kept at 15–30°C to maintain stability. Use insulated packages to ship such specimens.

Packaging used for shipping specimens should be designed and constructed so that, when subjected to environmental conditions as described above, the contents of the package will not be released to the environment, and the effectiveness of the packaging will not be impaired.

(1) Polypropylene and polyethylene containers are suitable inside containers for most applications. Glass containers are not recommended unless extreme care is taken to prevent breakage.
(2) Do not place prepared glass slides face to face during shipment. Individually wrap the slides or place them in containers designed to keep slides separated during transit.
(3) Specimen containers must be leakproof.
(4) The specimen container must be equipped with a cap and/or stopper designed specially for the container. All components of the container that come into contact with the specimen should be free from any matter that might render a laboratory test misleading or useless.
(5) Containers should be free from manufacturing defects. The top of the container should have a smooth surface on which to seat the cap or stopper. The container opening should be symmetrical and round. Avoid using caps or stoppers that were not designed for the container.
(6) The filled and capped or stoppered container should not leak. Do not use mechanical devices to tighten the cap or stopper because the container, cap or stopper may crack or be bent out of shape. Shrink-wrap, tape or wire may be needed to ensure that the container cap or stopper does not loosen during shipment.

Shipping containers must be capable of withstanding weight and shock commonly associated with handling and shipment. Single specimens can be shipped by enclosing the sealed specimen container in a durable outer shipping container. When shipping more than one specimen in a shipping container, protect each specimen container individually to reduce shock and prevent breakage. Corrugated fibreboard, paperboard, polystyrene boxes or other materials with similar rigid characteristics are suitable if they securely enclose the specimen containers. Polystyrene or other materials with similar insulating qualities are suitable for shipping frozen and refrigerated specimens. The size and shape of the shipping container are critical. The container must permit the release of CO_2 gas and prevent the build-up of pressure that could rupture the package. Dry ice is the most convenient substance for maintaining a temperature of $-70°C$. The amount of dry ice needed depends on the insulating qualities of the shipping container and the length of time the specimen must be kept frozen. Excess air space or packaging material (e.g. newspaper, polystyrene chips) in the shipping container will cause dry ice to dissipate at a faster rate. A polystyrene container with a wall thickness of 2.5 cm and an interior capacity of 2 litres filled with a 5-lb block of dry ice will keep a specimen frozen for 48 h when the container is stored at room temperature (78).

Various laws and national postal regulations apply to the shipment of biological specimens. Airlines have rigid regulations covering the transport of specimens and deem dry ice to be a hazardous material. Thus, transporting most clinical specimens is affected by regulations (78).

Specimen processing

Multiple factors associated with handling and processing blood specimens can introduce test result imprecision or a systematic bias after the specimen has been collected but before the test is done. Several potential problem areas in handling and processing of blood specimens have been documented (10, 54–56, 65, 66, 104). Specific concerns may be related to prolonged contact of cells with serum or plasma, concentration changes due to evaporation or cell lysis, the use of serum separation devices, analyte deterioration because of improper storage, and the use of certain anticoagulants. Recognition and control of these variables will reduce error and contribute to medical usefulness of patient test results.

Pre-centrifugation phase

The pre-centrifugation phase is the interval after specimen collection and before specimen centrifugation. In general, blood specimens should be centrifuged within 60 min after collection. However, to obtain serum, allow the tube to stand a minimum of 20–30 min for clot formation to occur. Extend this minimum time to 30–60 min if the collected specimen has been chilled (2–8°C). When the collection device contains a clotting activator, the minimum waiting time before centrifuging the specimen can be as short as 5 min (thrombin) or 15 min (glass or silica particles) (10); anticoagulated specimens can be centrifuged within minutes after they are collected. If adequate time is not allowed for clotting to occur, latent fibrin formation may be a problem for many of the instrument systems used by laboratories.

Keep tubes of blood in a vertical, stopper-up position. This promotes complete clot formation and reduces agitation of the tube contents, which in turn reduces the potential for haemolysis. The stopper is also less likely to come off the tube by accident.

Chilling specimens inhibits the metabolism of blood cells and stabilizes some labile constituents. Do not chill whole-blood specimens unless there are documented recommendations for doing so. To chill specimens adequately, place them in either crushed ice or a mixture of ice and water. Good contact between the cooling medium and the specimen is essential. Large cubes of ice instead of water are not acceptable because of inadequate contact between coolant and specimen. Immerse the specimen completely in the cooling medium.

Exceptions to the recommended maximum time of 60 min between drawing a specimen and separating the cells from the serum or plasma are acceptable when an additive that prevents concentration changes within the specimen is used. Sodium fluoride, for example, is commonly used (2.5 mg/ml of blood) as an antiglycolytic agent to keep glucose stable in the presence of blood cells for 24 h at room temperature (22–25°C) or for 48 h at refrigerated temperatures (2–8°C).

Blood contact with tube stoppers may be a source of contamination. Current manufacturing practices are helping to eliminate problems of this type. Thus, for example, special tubes have been designed for trace element determinations to eliminate stopper interference for these assays (32, 37). Avoid vigorous handling of collected specimens to minimize haemolysis.

Explicitly label specimens from patients with hepatitis and other potentially transmissible diseases. Attach the label to the specimen container and the requisition to give high visibility to these particular specimens. Ensure that this identification also accompanies the specimen through successive handling and processing steps.

Avoid exposure to light, which causes breakdown of certain analytes, in particular bilirubin. This is especially important when the specimen is from an icteric newborn who is being monitored to decide on the necessity of an exchange transfusion. Protect specimens from light with, for example, aluminium foil wrap.

Under the following conditions blood specimens are not acceptable for testing purposes and should be rejected. Professional judgement at the laboratory supervisory level must be exercised in applying these criteria:

(1) Inadequate specimen identification, e.g. a tube is not labelled or is mislabelled.
(2) An inadequate volume of blood collected into an additive tube. The amount of additive placed in a tube is intended for a certain volume of blood; if there is less blood than is required, the excess amount of additive could negate the accuracy of the test result, e.g. prothrombin time (38) and MCV.
(3) Using the wrong collection tube when method-specific specimens are required. In particular, do not indiscriminately use tubes with additives. The wrong order of draw during multiple blood specimen collection can invalidate test results because of contamination by the additive (11). When drawing several specimens during a venepuncture, draw blood culture tubes first, non-additive tubes second, EDTA-containing tubes third, and oxalate/fluoride-containing tubes last (75).
(4) Excessive haemolysis can result from a difficult venepuncture or from improper handling of the collected blood. Certain tests should not be carried out on visually haemolysed specimens, e.g. plasma haemoglobin determination.
(5) Improper transportation, e.g. a specimen that should have been chilled is received by the laboratory unchilled.

When preparing specimens for centrifugation, never use a wooden applicator stick or similar device to release a clot stuck to or near the top of the collection tube. Clot/cell hang-up has been virtually eliminated by technical improvements in tube and stopper design and manufacture. 'Rimming' the tube is a potential source for laboratory-induced haemolysis. Keep all tubes closed until after centrifugation, either by leaving the tube stopper in place or by using a suitable tube closure.

Centrifugation phase

This is the interval when the specimen is inside the centrifuge. Do not begin to centrifuge blood specimens until adequate clotting has occurred within the recommended time limits.

Separating serum or plasma from cells is based on a time-honoured practice of empirical observation. Recommended time is 10 ± 5 min at $1000-1200 \times \mathbf{g}$ (75). However, consult the manufacturer's literature which makes specific recommendations for separating devices integrated into collection tubes or inserted into the blood before centrifugation. Relative centrifugal force (rcf) ('*g*-force') is a more meaningful term than revolutions per minute (rpm). The rpm is of limited use without an indication of the centrifuge model and its specific rotor, head, or effective radius:

$$rcf = 1.118 \times 10^{-5} \times r \times N^2$$

where r = rotating radius in cm, and N = speed of rotation (rpm).

Certain analytes require chilled conditions. Laboratories should have access to temperature-controlled centrifuges. Centrifuges often generate more internal heat than is appropriate for analyte stability. Unless documentation supports a specific temperature for a specific analyte, a centrifuge temperature setting of 20–25°C is adequate.

Do not centrifuge blood specimens, with or without serum separating devices, more than once. Harvesting additional serum or plasma by re-centrifugation of the original collection device can result in inaccurate test results. Do not use repeated centrifugation and decanting to obtain a cell-free serum or plasma. Centrifuge the tube once and carefully pipette the serum or plasma off the cells. Excessive handling increases the chances for sample identification error; repeated centrifugation generates heat build-up within the centrifuge, which may result in analyte deterioration.

Keep all tubes of blood closed until after centrifugation. Leave the tube stopper in place, or place a suitable tube closure on the tube. Inaccuracies in test results can occur when the tube stopper is removed because of a change in specimen pH. Keeping tubes closed also prevents evaporation and aerosol formation during centrifugation.

Post-centrifugation phase

The post-centrifugation phase is the interval between removal of an aliquot of plasma or serum for testing purposes and centrifugation of the specimen. The multiplicity of laboratory tests makes it mandatory that the laboratory staff consult specific references to determine exact handling and storage conditions necessary to ensure the stability of specific analytes (27, 48, 102).

Many analytes are stable for up to 48 h when serum is left in contact with the cell mass; many are not (e.g. glucose, chloride, potassium, iron). As a general rule, carefully separate serum or plasma from the clot or cells within 2 h after collecting the specimen. Pipetting is recommended to remove the sample. Separated plasma or serum should be visually free of erythrocytes.

If a test cannot be carried out within 5 h after the plasma or serum has been separated from the cells or the clot, storing plasma or serum at 2–8°C is acceptable for most analytes. For storage beyond 24 h, freeze (-20°C) the specimen. For certain labile analytes, e.g. folate, vitamin B_{12}, it may be necessary to refrigerate or freeze the specimen immediately after centrifugation. For coagulation specimens, cell-free plasma should be separated from the cells, after centrifugation, by means of plastic pipettes or pipettes having a non-wettable surface. Plasma should be stored in clean tubes with a non-wettable surface at 0–8°C or in melting ice. If testing cannot be completed within 4 h, freeze the plasma immediately at a temperature lower than -20°C in a non-frostfree freezer. Specimens that are rapidly frozen and kept at -70°C have a longer stability for coagulation testing (up to 14 days). Coagulation factor assays should not be performed on specimens stored for more than 4 h (85).

Keep plasma or serum specimens covered at all times to eliminate possible exogenous contamination and to prevent evaporation.

Serum separation devices

Basically, serum separation devices can be divided into two categories: (1) devices that function during centrifugation (e.g. gel devices, barrier devices), and (2) devices that are used after centrifugation (50a, 75). Regardless of the type of device used, careful reading of the manufacturer's directions is essential to identify potential problems, e.g. trace element contamination (17, 71, 96) or contamination with other substances that interfere with specific instrument analyses (7).

Serum separation devices are used extensively in the clinical chemistry laboratory (57) but have not been generally accepted in the haematology and immunohaematology laboratory. Interference of gel barrier devices with the direct and indirect antiglobulin test, and with compatibility testing has been described (25, 99). A density gradient system (SIMWASH™) has recently been described that does not cause false-positive antiglobulin tests and will, on some occasions, allow cell-bound IgG demonstration that may otherwise escape detection (120).

Storage of specimens

In recent years the value of well–characterized, properly stored biological fluid and tissue collections has become apparent as database for epidemiologic studies of newly recognized or emerging diseases, e.g. Legionnaire's disease, acquired immunodeficiency syndrome. Such collections can effectively be stored in a 'serum bank'. This section is limited to intermediate- and long-term storage of serum. Cryopreservation of cells and other biologic materials has been extensively documented by Hurn (40) and Ashwood-Smith and Farrant (3).

The eutectic point of human serum lies between -18 and $-22°C$. Therefore, to ensure a solid core of frozen material and to prevent cyclical freezing/thawing of core material, which is damaging to proteins, serum collections should be stored at temperatures well below $-20°C$. Although storage at -35 to $-45°C$ would be adequate, storage at $-70°C$ has become quite popular. This temperature seems to have evolved more from a question of availability than of necessity. Before the age of 'ultra-low temperature freezing', a choice had to be made between $-20°C$ freezers or the use of dry ice with a nominal temperature of $-70°C$. Industry then developed $-70°C$ freezer units to replace the cumbersome dry ice storage units (13).

Short- and intermediate-term storage

Specimens intended for testing and not part of an organized study specimen subset are stored at temperatures dictated by the stability of the specific analyte, e.g. 4–8°C, $-20°C$. Refrigerators and freezers must have continuous temperature monitoring and an alarm system. Temperature recorder sensors or the sensing end of thermometers be placed in no more than 250 ml of liquid (refrigerators) so that the heat transfer characteristics are similar to blood and blood component containers (86), or in a container of ice or antifreeze in water (freezers). The use of at least two temperature sensors is recommended for large refrigerators, freezers and walk-in units.

Long-term storage

If specimens are part of a long-range study where long-term storage is desirable or required, particular attention must be paid to sterile collection and processing techniques. Specimens should be aliquotted into several 0.25–1.0 ml separate portions to avoid repeated freezing and thawing when small amounts are retrieved for testing. Under no circumstances should storage take place in a so-called 'frost-free' environment. 'Frost-free' freezers are characterized by intermittent defrost cycles. These will cause specimens to become desiccated with resultant denaturation of protein material.

Specimen aliquots should be placed in suitable plastic cryovials equipped with a seal and an externally threaded cap. When −70°C storage is not available, lyophilization and storage at −20°C is an acceptable alternative.

Laboratory infection precautions

The increasing prevalence of, for example, hepatitis and human immunodeficiency virus (HIV) infections increases the risk that laboratory workers, phlebotomists and other health-care workers will be exposed to blood from patients infected with such agents (see Chapter 11). Health-care workers should, therefore, consider *all* patients as infected with HIV and/or other blood-borne pathogens and adhere rigorously to infection-control precautions minimizing the risk of exposure to blood and body fluids of all patients (12).

HIV has been isolated from blood, semen, vaginal secretions, saliva, tears, breast milk, cerebrospinal fluid, amniotic fluid and urine. Epidemiologic evidence has implicated only blood, semen, vaginal secretions and possibly breast milk in transmission. Standard sterilization and disinfection procedures for patient-care equipment currently recommended in a variety of health-care settings are adequate to sterilize or disinfect items contaminated with blood or other body fluids from persons infected with blood-borne pathogens, including HIV (23). Studies have shown that HIV is inactivated rapidly after being exposed to commonly used chemical germicides at concentrations that are much lower than used in practice (64, 68, 105, 106). In addition to commercially available germicides, a solution of sodium hypochlorite (household bleach) prepared daily is an inexpensive and effective germicide. Concentrations ranging from 1:100 to 1:10 of household bleach are effective, depending on the amount of organic material (e.g. blood, mucus) present on the surfaces to be cleaned and disinfected.

Since medical history and examination cannot reliably identify all patients infected with HIV or other blood-borne pathogens, precautions should be consistently used when collecting and handling material from *all* patients.

General precautions

(1) Appropriate barrier precautions should be used to prevent skin and mucous-membrane exposure when contact with blood or other body fluids of any patient is anticipated. Gloves should be worn when touching blood, other body fluids, mucous membranes or non-intact skin of any patient. Gloves should also be worn for handling items or surfaces soiled with blood or other body fluids and for performing venepuncture or other vascular access procedures. Gloves should be changed after contact with each patient. Masks and protective eyewear or face shields should be worn during procedures that are likely to generate droplets of blood or other body fluids to prevent exposure of mucous membranes of the mouth, nose, and eyes. Gowns or aprons should be worn during procedures that are likely to generate splashes of blood or other body fluids.

(2) Hands and other skin surfaces should be washed immediately and thoroughly if contaminated with blood or other body fluids. Hands should be washed immediately after gloves are removed.

(3) All health-care workers should take precautions to prevent injuries caused by needles, scalpels and other sharp instruments or devices during procedures. To prevent needlestick injuries, needles should not be recapped, purposely bent or broken by hand, removed from disposable syringes, or otherwise manipulated by hand. After use, disposable syringes and needles, scalpel blades, and other sharp items should be placed in puncture-resistant containers for disposal. Large-bore reusable needles should be placed in a puncture-resistant container for transport to the reprocessing area.

(4) Although saliva has not been implicated in HIV transmission, mouthpieces, resuscitation bags, or other ventilation devices should be available for use in areas in which need for resuscitation is predictable, to minimize the need for emergency mouth-to-mouth resuscitation.

(5) Health-care workers who have exudative lesions or weeping dermatitis should refrain from all direct patient care and from handling patient-care equipment until the condition resolves.

(6) Pregnant health-care workers are not known to be at a greater risk of contracting HIV infection than health-care workers who are not pregnant. Because of perinatal transmission risks, however, pregnant health-care workers should be especially familiar with and strictly adhere to precautions to minimize the risk of HIV transmission.

Similar precautions must be taken in the laboratory when handling specimens. Specific requirements for laboratories are described in Chapter 11.

References

1. AABB (1985). Quality assurance. In *Technical Manual* (9th edn), pp. 369–382. Washington, D.C.: AABB.
2. AABB (1987). *Standards for Blood Banks and Transfusion Services* (12th edn) pp. 8–14; 17–20. Washington, D.C.: AABB.
2a. Altman, R., and Hemker H. C. (1967). Contact activation in the extrinsic blood clotting system. *Thrombosis et Diathesis Haemorrhagica* **18**, 525–531.
3. Ashwood-Smith, M. J. and Farrant, J. (eds) (1980). *Low Temperature Preservation in Medicine and Biology.* Baltimore, MD: University Park Press; Tunbridge Wells, Kent, UK: Pitman Medical Ltd.
4. Astrup, T. (1973). The effect of physical activity on blood coagulation and fibrinolysis. In Naughton,

J. P., Hellerstein, H. K. and Mohler, I. C. (eds) *Exercise Testing and Exercise Training in Coronary Heart Disease*, p. 169. New York: Academic Press.

5.   Barrett, P. V. D. (1971). Hyperbilirubinemia of fasting. *Journal of the American Medical Association* **217:** 1349–1353.

6.   Bowie, E. J. W., Tauxe, W. N., Sjoberg, W. E. and Yamaguchi, M. Y. (1963). Daily variation in the concentration of iron in serum. *American Journal of Clinical Pathology* **40:** 491–494.

7.   Brown, H. H., Vanco, M. and Meola, J. M. (1974). Interference from serum separators in drug screening by gas chromatography. *Clinical Chemistry* **20:** 919.

8.   Bruner, K. W. and Kissling, C. W. (1980). Evaluation of a pneumatic-tube system for delivery of blood specimens to the blood bank. *American Journal of Clinical Pathology* **73:** 593–596.

9.   Buckell, M. and Elliott, F. A. (1959). Effect of butter lipaemia on the rate of clot lysis in normal males. *Lancet* **1:** 662–663.

10. Calam, R. R. (1977). Reviewing the importance of specimen collection. *Journal American Medical Technology* **39:** 297–302.

11. Calam, R. R. and Cooper, M. H. (1982). Recommended "order of draw" for collecting blood specimens into additive-containing tubes. *Clinical Chemistry* **28:** 1399.

12. Centers for Disease Control (1987). Recommendations for prevention of HIV transmission in health-care settings. *Morbidity and Mortality Weekly Report* **36** (Suppl. 2S): 3S–18S.

13. Cowley, C. W., Timson, W. J. and Sawdye, J. A. (1961). Ultra rapid cooling techniques in the freezing of biological materials. *Biodynamics* **8:** 317–29.

14. Dawson, J. B. and Walker, B. E. (1969). Direct determination of zinc in whole blood, plasma and urine by atomic absorption spectroscopy. *Clinica Chimica Acta* **26,** 465–475.

15. Diggs, L. W. and Bell, A. (1980). Bone marrow and morphology of bone marrow cells. In Schmidt, R. M. (ed.) *CRC Handbook Series in Clinical Laboratory Science, Section I: Hematology Volume II*, pp. 3–61. Boca Raton, FL: CRC Press.

16. Dormandy, K. M. and Hardisty, R. M. (1961). Coagulation tests on capillary blood. A screening procedure for use in small children. *Journal of Clinical Pathology* **14:** 543–547.

17. Ducsi, L. J. and Hackett, L. P. (1976). Interference in dilantin assays. *Clinical Chemistry* **22:** 1236.

18. ECCLS (1987). Standard for Specimen Collection. Part 2: Blood Specimen by Venepuncture. ECCLS Document, Vol. 4, No. 1. Berlin: Beuth Verlag.

19. Eisenberg, S. (1963). The effect of posture and position of the venous sampling site on the hematocrit and serum protein concentration. *Journal of Laboratory and Clinical Medicine* **61:** 755–760.

20. Ekelund, L.-G., Eklund, B. and Kauser, L. (1971). Time course for the change in hemoglobin concentration with change in posture. *Acta Medica Scandinavica* **190:** 335–336.

21. Elwood, P. D. (1962). Diurnal hemoglobin variation in normal male subjects. *Clinical Science* **23:** 379–382.

22. Fearnley, G. R., Balmforth, G. and Fearnley, E. (1957). Evidence of a diurnal fibrinolytic rhythm, with a simple method of measuring natural fibrinolysis. *Clinical Science* **16:** 645–650.

23. Garner, J. S. and Favero, M. S. (1985). Guideline for handwashing and hospital environmental control, 1985. Atlanta: Public Health Service, Centers for Disease Control, HHS Publication No. 99–1117.

24. Garrey, W. E. and Bryan, W. R. (1935). Variations in white blood cell counts. *Physiological Reviews* **15:** 597–638.

25. Geisland, J. R. and Milam, J. D. (1980). Spuriously positive direct antiglobulin test caused by use of silicone gel. *Transfusion* **20:** 711–713.

26. Gerbrandy, J., van Leeuwen, A. M., Hellendoorn, H. B. A., deVries, L. A. and van Daatselaar, J. J. (1960). The binding between electrolytes and serum proteins calculated from an in vivo filtration method. *Clinical Science* **19:** 181–193.

27. Gianpietro, O., Navalesi, R., Buzzigoll, G., Boni, C. and Benzi, L. (1980). Decrease in plasma glucose concentration during storage at −20°C. *Clinical Chemistry* **26:** 1710–1712.

28. Gralnick, H. R. and Palmer, R. (1981). Cold-induced contact surface activation of the prothrombin time in whole blood. Report of the Subcommittee on Standardisation of Prothrombin Time. Toronto: ICTH.

29. Grannis, G. F. (1970). Plasma fibrinogen: determination, normal values, physiopathologic shifts, and fluctuations. *Clinical Chemistry* **16:** 486–494.

30. Greendyke, R. M. and Banzhaf, J. C. (1977). Immunologic studies of blood samples transported by a pneumatic tube system. *American Journal of Clinical Pathology* **68:** 508–510

30a. Hardisty, R. M. and Ingram, G. I. C. (1965). *Bleeding Disorders, Investigation and Management*. Blackwell Scientific Publications, Oxford, U.K., p. 162.

31. Hathaway, W. E. and Bonnar, J. (1978). Technical aspects of blood coagulation. In Hathaway, W. E. and Bonnar, J. (eds) *Perinatal Coagulation*, p. 15. New York: Grune & Stratton.

32. Helman, E. Z., Wallick, D. K. and Reingold, I. M. (1971). Vacutainer contamination in trace element studies. *Clinical Chemistry* **17:** 61–62.

33. Helman, N. and Rubenstein, L. S. (1975). The effects of age, sex, and smoking on erythrocytes and leukocytes. *American Journal of Clinical Pathology* **63:** 35–44.

34. Heyns, A. du P., Berg, D. J. van der, Kleynhans, P. H. T. and du Toit, P. W. (1981). Unsuitability of evacuated tubes for monitoring heparin therapy by activated partial thromboplastin time. *Journal of Clinical Pathology* **34:** 63–68.

35. Hicks, J. R., Rowland, G. L. and Buffone, G. J. (1976). Evaluation on a new blood collection device (microtainer) that is suited for pediatric use. *Clinical Chemistry* **22:** 2034–2036.

36. Horder, K. and Klorder, M. (1970). Plasma haptoglobin and physical exercise: changes in healthy individuals concomitant with strenuous march. *Clinica Chimica Acta* **30:** 369–372.

37. Hughes, R. O., Wease, D. F. and Troxler, R. G. (1976). Collection of blood uncontaminated with Ca, Cu, Mg, or Zn, for trace metal analysis. *Clinical Chemistry* **22:** 691–692.

38. Humphreys, R. E. and McPhedran, P. (1970). False evaluation of partial thromboplastin time and prothrombin time. *Journal of the American Medical Association* **214:** 1702–1704.

39. Hurkat, P. C. and Jain, M. (1973). Some haematological changes during exercise. *Indian Journal of Physiology and Pharmacology* **17:** 71–74.

40. Hurn, B. A. L. (1968). *Storage of Blood*. London: Academic Press.

41. ICSH (1977). Recommendation for measurement of erythrocyte sedimentation rate of human blood. *American Journal of Clinical Pathology* **66:** 505–507.

42. ICSH (1982). Standardization of blood specimen collection procedure for reference values. *Clinical and Laboratory Haematology* **4:** 83–86.

43. Ingram, G. I. C. and Hills, M. (1976). Reference method for the one-stage prothrombin time test on human blood. ICSH. *Thrombosis and Haemostasis* **36:** 237–238.

44. Ingram, G. I. C., and Hills, M. (1976). The prothrombin time test. Effect of varying citrate concentration. *Thrombosis and Haemostasis* **36:** 230–236.

45. ISO (1987). Evacuated tubes for blood specimen collection. Draft International Standard ISO/DIS 6710. Geneva: ISO.

46. Jamshidi, K. and Swain, W. R. (1971). Bone marrow biopsy with unaltered architecture: A new biopsy device. *Journal of Laboratory and Clinical Medicine* **77:** 335–342.

47. Jensen, R. J., Adam, B., Turner, W. E. and Hannon, W. H. (1984). An evaluation of different filter paper lots used for blood spot collection during the last five years. In Ming, S. Chan (ed.) *National Newborn Screening Symposium*. Jacksonville, FL: Florida Department of Health and Rehabilitation Services.

48. Juul, P. (1967). Stability of plasma enzymes during storage. *Clinical Chemistry* **13:** 416–422.

49. Karvonen, M. J. and Kunnas, M. (1952). Erythrocyte and haemoglobin changes during protracted heavy muscular work. *Annales Medicinae Experimentalis et Biologiae Fennias* **30:** 180–185.

50. Karvonen, M. J. and Kunnas, M. (1953). Factor analysis of haematological changes in heavy manual work. *Acta Physiologica Scandinavica* **29:** 220–231.

50a. Keitges, P. W. and Mohrbacker, R. J. (1982). Reagents, specimen collection, calibrators, reference materials and standards. In Werner, M. (ed.) *Handbook of Clinical Chemistry*, Vol. 1, pp. 289–335. B Raton, FL: CRC Press.

51. Kennedy, J. B., Machara, K. T. and Baker, A. M. (1981). Cell and platelet stability in disodium and trisodium EDTA. *American Journal of Medical Technology* **47:** 89–93.

52. Kennon, B., Shipp, M. E. and Hetherington, D. C. (1937). A study of the white blood cell picture in six young men. *American Journal of Physiology* **118:** 690–696.

53. Koepke, J. A., Rodgers, J. L. and Ollivier, M. J. (1974). Pre-instrumental variables in coagulation testing. *American Journal of Clinical Pathology* **64:** 591–596.

54. Laessig, R. H., Indrikson, A. A., Hassemer, D. J., Paskey, T. A. and Schwartz, T. H. (1976). Changes in serum chemical values as a result of prolonged contact with the clot. *American Journal of Clinical Pathology* **66:** 598–604.

55. Laessig, R. H., Hassemer, D. J., Westgard, J. O., Carey, R. N., Feldbruegge, D. H. and Schwartz, T. H. (1976). Assessment of the serum separator tube as an intermediate storage device within the laboratory. *American Journal of Clinical Pathology* **66:** 653–657.

56. Laessig, R. H., Hassemer, D. J., Paskey, T. A. and Schwartz, T. H. (1976). The effect of 0.1 and 1.0

percent erythrocytes and hemolysis on serum chemistry values. *American Journal of Clinical Pathology* **66:** 639–644.

57.   Laessig, R. H., Westgard, J. O., Carey, R. N., Hassemer, D. J., Schwartz, T. H. and Feldbruegge, D. H. (1976). Assessment of serum separator devices for obtaining serum specimens suitable for clinical analysis. *Clinical Chemistry* **22:** 235–239.

58.   Lampasso, J. A. (1968). Changes in hematologic values induced by storage of ethylenediaminetetraacetate human blood for varying periods of time. *American Journal of Clinical Pathology* **49:** 443–447.

59.   Lange, H. F. (1946). The normal plasma protein values and their relative variations. *Acta Medica Scandinavica*, Suppl. 176: 1–202.

60.   Lapidus, B. M. and MacIndoe, R. C. (1978). A multi-station gravity delivery system. *American Journal of Clinical Pathology* **69:** 73–76.

61.   Lieden, G., Hoglund, S. and Ehn, L. (1975). Changes in certain iron metabolism variables after a single blood donation. *Acta Medica Scandinavica* **197:** 27–30.

62.   Lloyd, E. (1982). The determination of leukocyte morphology with time – its effect on the differential count. *Laboratory Perspectives* **1,** 13–16.

63.   Loutit, J. F. and Mollison, P. L. (1943). Advantages of a disodium-citrate–glucose mixture as a blood preservative. *British Medical Journal* **2:** 744–745.

64.   Martin, L. S., McDougal, J. S. and Loskoski, S. L. (1985). Disinfection and inactivation of the human T lymphotropic virus type III/lymphadenopathy-associated virus. *Journal of Infectious Diseases* **152:** 400–403.

65.   Martinek, R. G. (1966). Specimens for clinical laboratory analysis: collection and preservation. *Postgraduate Medicine* **39:** A46–56.

66.   Mathies, J. C. (1974). Evaluation of a new device for rapidly separating serum or plasma from blood. *Clinical Chemistry* **20:** 1573–1576.

67.   McCarthy, E. F. and Van Slyke, D. D. (1939). Diurnal variations of hemoglobin in the blood of normal men. *Journal of Biological Chemistry* **128:** 567–572.

68.   McDougal, J. S., Martin, L. S., Cort, S. P., Mozen, M., Heldebrant, C. M. and Evatt, B. L. (1985). Thermal inactivation of the acquired immunodeficiency syndrome virus-III/lymphadenopathy-associated virus, with special reference to antihemophilic factor. *Journal of Clinical Investigation* **76:** 875–877.

70.   Milhorat, A. T., Small, S. M. and Dietheim, O. (1942). Leukocytosis during various emotional states. *Archives of Neurology and Psychiatry* **47:** 779–792.

71.   Missen, A. W. and Dixon, S. J. (1974). Contamination of blood samples by plasticizer in evacuated tubes. *Clinical Chemistry* **20,** 1247.

72.   Mole, R. H. (1945). Diurnal and sampling variations in the determination of haemoglobin. *Journal of Physiology (London)* **104,** 1–5.

73.   NCCLS (1980). H1–A2. Standard for Evacuated Tubes for Blood Specimen Collection. Approved Standard. Villanova, PA: NCCLS.

74.   NCCLS (1984). H3–A2. Procedures for the Collection of Diagnostic Blood Specimens by Venipuncture. Approved Standard, Vol. 4, pp. 95–114. Villanova, PA: NCCLS.

75.   NCCLS (1984). H18–T. Procedures for the Handling and Processing of Blood Specimens. Tentative Standard, Vol. 4, pp. 219–233. Villanova, PA: NCCLS.

76.   NCCLS (1984). H20–T. Leukocyte Differential Counting. Tentative Standard, Vol. 4, pp. 257–309. Villanova, PA: NCCLS.

77.   NCCLS (1985). GP9–P. Selecting and Evaluating a Referral Laboratory. Proposed Guideline, Vol. 5, pp. 511–524. Villanova, PA: NCCLS.

78.   NCCLS (1985). H5–A2. Procedures for the Domestic Handling and Transport of Diagnostic Specimens and Etiologic Agents. Approved Standard, Vol. 5, pp. 1–20. Villanova, PA: NCCLS.

79.   NCCLS (1985). H7–A. Procedure for Determining Packed Cell Volume by the Microhematocrit Method. Approved Standard, Vol. 5, pp. 103–113. Villanova, PA: NCCLS.

80.   NCCLS (1985). H11–A. Percutaneous Collection of Arterial Blood for Laboratory Analysis. Approved Standard, Vol. 5, pp. 39–60. Villanova, PA: NCCLS.

81.   NCCLS (1985). H14–A. Use of Devices for Collection of Skin Puncture Blood Specimens. Approved Guideline, Vol. 5, pp. 193–219. Villanova, PA: NCCLS.

82.   NCCLS (1985). H24–P. Additives to Blood Collection Devices: Heparin. Proposed Standard, Vol. 5, pp. 365–389. Villanova, PA: NCCLS.

83.   NCCLS (1985). LA4–T. Blood Collection on Filter Paper for Neonatal Screening Programs. Tentative Standard, Vol. 5, pp. 395–406. Villanova, PA: NCCLS.

84.   NCCLS (1986). H4–A2. Procedures for the Collection of Diagnostic Blood Specimens by Skin Puncture. Approved Standard, Vol. 6, pp. 171–182. Villanova, PA: NCCLS.

85. NCCLS (1986b). H21-A. Collection, Transport, and Preparation of Blood Specimens for Coagulation Testing and Performance of Coagulation Assays. Approved Guideline, Vol. 6, pp. 595–609. Villanova, PA: NCCLS.

86. NCCLS (1986c). I16-T. Temperature Monitoring and Recording in Blood Banks. Tentative Guideline, Vol. 6, pp. 577–592. Villanova, PA: NCCLS.

87. Nelson, N. M. (1976). Respiration and circulation after birth. In Smith, C. A. and Nelson, N. M. (eds). *The Physiology of the Newborn Infants* (4th edn), p. 158. Springfield, Ill.: Charles C. Thomas.

88. Nevaril, C. G., Lynch, E. C., Alfrey, C. P. and Hellums (1968). Erythrocyte damage and destruction induced by shearing stress. *Journal of Laboratory and Clinical Medicine* **71**: 784–790.

89. Oh, W. and Lind, J. (1966). Venous and capillary hematocrit in newborn infants and placental transfusion. *Acta Paediatrica Scandinavica* **55**: 38–48.

90. Oski, F. A. and Naiman, J. L. (eds) (1982). *Hematologic Problems in the Newborn* (3rd edn), pp. 6–7. Philadelphia: W. B. Saunders.

91. Palmer, R. N. and Gralnick, H. R. (1981). Cold-induced contact surface activation of the prothrombin time in whole blood. *Blood* **59**: 38–42.

92. Palmer, R. N., Kessler, C. M. and Gralnick, H. R. (1981). Misinterpretation of prothrombin time in warfarin anticoagulation. *Annals of Internal Medicine* **95**: 393–394.

93. Palmer, R. N., Kessler, C. M. and Gralnick, H. R. (1982). Warfarin anticoagulation: Difficulties in interpretation of the prothrombin time. *Thrombosis Research* **25**: 125–130.

94. Poznanski, W., Smith, F. and Bodley, F. (1978). Implementation of a pneumatic tube system for transport of blood specimens. *American Journal of Clinical Pathology* **70**: 291–295.

95. Pragay, D. A. and Edwards, L. (1974). Evaluation of an improved pneumatic tube system suitable for transportation of blood specimens. *Clinical Chemistry* **20**: 57–60.

96. Pragay, D. A., Brinkley, S., Rejent, T. and Gotthelf, J. (1979). Vacutainer contamination revisited. *Clinical Chemistry* **25**: 2058.

97. Refsum, H. E., Treit, B., Meen, H. D. and Stromme, S. B. (1973). Serum electrolyte fluid and acid-base balance after prolonged heavy exercise and low environmental temperature. *Scandinavian Journal of Clinical and Laboratory Investigation* **32**: 117–122.

98. Refsum, H. E., Meen, H. D. and Stromme, S. B. (1973). Whole blood, serum and erythrocyte magnesium concentration after repeated heavy exercise of long duration. *Scandinavian Journal of Clinical and Laboratory Investigation* **32**: 123–127.

99. Renton, P. H. and Handcock, J. A. (1957). Antibody-like effects of colloidal silica. *Vox Sanguinis* **2**: 117–124.

100. Rodkey, F. L. and O'Neal, J. D. (1974). Effects of carboxyhemoglobin on determination of methemoglobin in blood. *Biochemical Medicine* **9**: 261–270.

101. Rorsman, H. (1962). Normal variation in the count of circulating basophil leukocytes in man. *Acta Allergologica* **17**: 49–65.

102. Rossing, R. H. and Foster, D. M. (1980). The stability of clinical chemistry specimens during refrigerated storage for 24 hours. *American Journal of Clinical Pathology* **73**: 91–95.

103. Sacker, L. S. (1975). Specimen collection. In Lewis, S. M. and Coster, J. F. (eds) *Quality Control in Haematology*, pp. 211–229. London: Academic Press.

103a. Shanberge, J. N., and Matsuoka, T. (1966). Studies regarding the effect of foreign surface contact on the one-stage prothrombin time determination. *Thrombosis et Diathesis Haemorrhagica* **15**, 442–450.

103b. Soulier, J. P., and Prou-Wartelle, O. (1960). New data on Hageman factor and plasma thromboplastin antecedent: the role of "contact" in the initial phase of blood conjulation. *British Journal of Haematology* **6**, 88–101.

104. Spencer, W. W., Nelson, G. H. and Konicke, K. (1976). Evaluation of a new system ("Corvac") for separating serum from blood for routine laboratory procedures. *Clinical Chemistry* **22**: 1012–1016.

105. Spire, B., Montagnier, L., Barré-Sinoussi, F. and Chermann, J. C. (1984). Inactivation of lymphadenopathy-associated virus by chemical disinfectants. *Lancet* **2**: 899–901.

106. Spire, B., Barré-Sinoussi, F., Dormont, D., Montagnier, L. and Chermann, J. C. (1985). Inactivation of lymphadenopathy-associated virus by heat, gamma rays, and ultraviolet light. *Lancet* **1**: 188–189.

107. Statland, B. E. and Winkel, P. (1977). Effects of preanalytical factors on the intra-individual variation of analytes in the blood of healthy subjects: consideration of preparation of subject and time of venipuncture. *C.R.C. Critical Reviews in Clinical Laboratory Science* **8**: 105–144.

108. Statland, B. E. and Winkel, P. (1977). The relationship of the day-to-day variation of serum iron concentration values to the iron binding capacity values in a group of healthy young women. *American Journal of Clinical Pathology* **67**: 84–90.

109. Statland, B. E., Bokelund, H. and Winkel, P. (1974). Factors contributing to intra-individual variation

of serum constituents. IV. Effects of posture and tourniquet application on variation of serum constituents in healthy subjects. *Clinical Chemistry* **20:** 1513–1519.

110.   Statland, B. E., Winkel, P. and Bokelund, H. (1976). Variations of serum iron concentration in young healthy men: within-day and day-to-day changes. *Clinical Biochemistry* **9:** 26–29.

111.   Statland, B. E., Winkel, P. and Killingsworth, L. M. (1976). Factors contributing to intra-individual variation of serum constituents. VI. Physiologic day-to-day variation of concentration values of ten specific proteins in the sera of healthy subjects. *Clinical Chemistry* **22:** 1635–1638.

112.   Statland, B. E., Winkel, P., Harris, S. C., Burdsall, M. J. and Saunders, A. M. (1978). Evaluation of biological sources of variation of leukocyte counts and other hematological quantities using very precise automated analyzers. *American Journal of Clinical Pathology* **69:** 48–54.

113.   Steige, H. and Jones, J. D. (1971). Evaluation of pneumatic tube system for delivery of blood specimens. *Clinical Chemistry* **17:** 1160–1164.

114.   Stengle, J. M. and Schade, A. L. (1957). Diurnal-nocturnal variations of certain blood constituents in normal human subjects. *British Journal of Haematology* **3:** 117–124.

115.   Stuart, J., Barrett, B. A. and Prangnell, D. R. (1974). Capillary blood collection in haematology. *Journal of Clinical Pathology* **27:** 869–874.

116.   Sturgis, C. C. and Bethell, F. H. (1943). Quantitative and qualitative variations in normal leukocytes. *Physiological Reviews* **23:** 279–303.

117.   Taswell, F. H., Smith, A. M., Sweatt, M. A. and Pfaff, K. J. (1974). Quality control in the blood bank – a new approach. *American Journal of Clinical Pathology* **62:** 491–495.

118.   Thomson, J. M. (1984). Specimen collection for blood coagulation testing. In Koepke, J. A. (ed.) *Laboratory Hematology*, Vol. 2, pp. 833–863. New York: Churchill Livingstone.

119.   Tombridge, T. L. (1978). Effect of posture on hematology results. *American Journal of Clinical Pathology* **49:** 491–493.

120.   Treacy, M. and Marsh, W. L. (1987). Enhancement of the sensitivity of the antiglobulin test. *American Clinical Products Review* **6:** 24–27.

121.   van den Besselaar, A. M. H. P. and Loeliger, E. A. (1982). The effect of contact activation on the prothrombin time with special reference to insufficiently siliconised vacutainers and venoject devices. In Triplett, D. A. (ed.) *Standardization of Coagulation Assays*, p. 95. Skokie, Ill: College of American Pathologists.

122.   Vanzetti, G. and Valente, D. (1965). A sensitive method for the determination of hemoglobin in plasma. *Clinica Chimica Acta* **11:** 442–446.

123.   Wald, N. and Howard, S. (1975). Letter: variations in carboxyhaemoglobin levels in smokers. *British Medical Journal* **1:** 393.

124.   Weaver, D. K. and Miller, D. (1978). Evaluation of a computer-directed pneumatic tube system for pneumatic transport of blood specimens. *American Journal of Clinical Pathology* **70:** 400–405.

125.   Winkel, P. and Statland, B. E. (1981). The acute effect of smoking on the concentrations of blood leukocyte types in healthy young women. *American Journal of Clinical Pathology* **75:** 781–785.

126.   Winkel, P., Statland, B. E., Saunders, R. M., Osborn, H. and Kupperman, H. (1981). Within-day physiologic variation of leukocyte types in healthy subjects as assayed by two automated leukocyte differential analyzers. *American Journal of Clinical Pathology* **75:** 693–700.

3

The Use of Reference Values

R L Verwilghen

Introduction

Interpretation of any observation can only be done by comparing it with other (previous) observations. While this is evident for measured results of laboratory tests in a patient, it might seem less relevant for clinical observations. However, we 'know' if somebody is tall or short, obese or underweight, plethoric or pale, because earlier experience has given us enough information (about shape, weight and colour of fellow-man) to reach approximate conclusions by comparing the physical state of our own patient with what we consider to be a normal population. In haematology, analytic test results are compared with values measured previously, either in the same individual or in an appropriate population, to allow us to state if the result is 'normal' or 'abnormal', and if abnormal, whether increased or decreased; the previous data provide a yardstick to assess if the patient is in good health or not, the effect of the treatment and whether aggressive treatment, rather than the underlying condition has resulted in abnormal biochemistry, making further drugs hazardous.

Traditionally, comparison has been with 'normal values'. Major problems are encountered, however, mainly due to lack of a clear definition of what is 'normal'. The existence of a theoretical 'normal man' was postulated a long time ago by physiologists on the basis of a height of 1.70 m, weight of 70 kg, age under 70 years. But this is not a helpful model for use in determination of 'normal' laboratory values. Normal values are often assumed indiscriminately in a laboratory from those used in other laboratories, usually with little or no knowledge about their origin, about the population from which they were derived or about the technique used for the measurement. Part of the confusion is due to the fact that there are many definitions of the word 'normal' (1). Normal can be used as a statistical term (a normal or Gaussian distribution) but it can also represent widely divergent conditions ranging from 'average' to 'habitual' and 'conventional' to 'optimal', 'ideal' or 'giving longest survival'.

It is thus clear that there is a need for adequate values for comparison and that previous 'normal values' are often useless for this purpose. What we need are values measured in a well-defined and adequately described population. We need to know the techniques used for the measurement, their accuracy and their precision; then, when similar techniques are used in a patient from this same population, we will obtain useful information for diagnosis and for treatment. Gräsbeck *et al.* (2) proposed the term 'reference values' for such population results.

The International Federation of Clinical Chemistry (IFCC) and the International Committee for Standardization in Haematology (ICSH) have made recommendations on the use of reference values (3–5). As a prerequisite for this it was first necessary to define clearly the concept of *reference individuals* who form a *reference population*. If the population is small the measurement can be done on each of these individuals, but nearly always this is not feasible and only a small group will be available for the determination. Care should be taken to ensure that the selection from the group provides a representative sample. An *individual reference value* is obtained from each member of this *reference sample group*. From the totality of values, a *reference interval* is determined. Unless otherwise specified this reference interval will contain the 95% central values, with the lowest and highest 2.5% values falling outside the *reference limits* (4) (Fig. 3.1).

Reference population

Composition of the reference population

By definition, the reference population is composed of all reference individuals. However, this can vary from only one reference individual (the patient himself at an earlier date) to very large reference populations (e.g. all inhabitants of a country or a continent). With large reference populations, representative sampling becomes a major difficulty. Many criteria (e.g. age, sex, race, health condition) can be used to define a reference population further.

Groups of patients suffering from a defined disease can form useful reference populations for individual patients with that disease. These types of haematological reference values are useful during remission of acute leukaemia, after bone marrow transplantation, during pregnancy, etc.

'Healthy' reference populations

The most frequently used reference values are expected to come from a healthy (normal) population. When measurements are known to differ between sexes or with ageing, adapted subgroups of reference individuals are required. There are problems in defining the relevant populations. Thus, major biases are often seen during the recruitment of healthy populations for measurement of reference values: medical students, laboratory technicians and blood donors are over-represented and thus they are not representative of a random population. A second problem is the definition of 'health'. There are no clear criteria to eliminate 'ill' people from reference populations. When only 'healthy' people are used (e.g. 'normal' weight, blood pressure, no known disease, no drug intake) many individuals will be excluded and it becomes difficult, if not impossible, to determine reference values for geriatric populations: no 'healthy' subjects remain if the screening is too rigid.

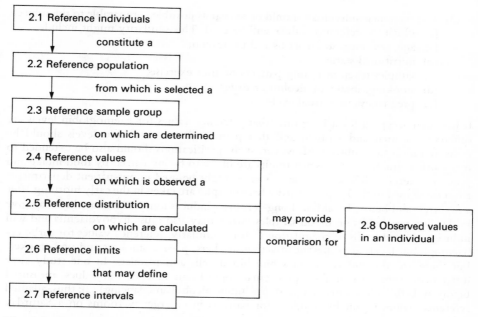

Fig. 3.1   Concept of reference values; relationship of recommended terms.

It is useful to note the frequent difference between a 'mean' value measured in a healthy population and the 'optimal' value from the group of longest survivors. For many parameters, longest survival is seen in individuals who differ significantly from the mean value (lower bodyweight, lower cholesterol level, etc.).

Description of the reference population

A careful description of the procedure used for the recruitment of the reference population is needed to make the reference values useful. Proof is required that the 'patient' is part of this population and that observations are compared with the appropriate values.

(1) This description must include the purpose for which the reference values will be used. It is clear that the same reference values cannot be used for physiological studies in sportsmen, for early detection of occupational disease in workers exposed to toxic substances, in health check-up and/or in life insurance screening, in general hospital practice, in differential diagnosis between defined diseases or in monitoring of therapy given for a known disease.

(2) The criteria on which individuals were included in or excluded from the reference population must be clearly stated. If the population is to be subdivided (e.g. according to age or sex) this information too should be known for each reference individual.

(3) The reference individuals should be as near as possible comparable to the subjects for which the reference values will be used. This similarity might include:
   (a) age, sex, race, social status and profession;
   (b) nutritional status;
   (c) samples taken in resting patients or after exercise;
   (d) smoking, intake of alcohol or drugs;
   (e) pregnancy, menstrual cycle.

It has been accepted for a long time that reference values for haemoglobin levels are different for men and women and that plasma glucose and lipid levels should be measured in fasting subjects. However, such specifications should also be extended to many other situations, e.g. when results are likely to be influenced by food intake and previous exercise, different reference values might be used in out-patient departments from those used in the hospital ward where samples are taken in the early morning after a nightrest and before breakfast. Long-term rest induces hypovolaemia which can give misleading test results on blood samples. Stress may also cause hypovolaemia and will induce increased levels of coagulation factors. Similarly, reference values for carboxy-haemoglobin levels are different in active smokers, passive smokers and non-smokers but there are also differences in white blood cells and platelets. In one study clear differences were seen in a set of haematological and biochemical values, measured before and after a Scandinavian party (including alcohol and dancing) (2); thus, adapted reference values might be required for patients in emergency rooms on a Saturday night.

Sites of blood sampling are important:

(a) Venous blood may differ between samples taken with the arm extended or flexed.
(b) Capillary blood will vary in its content of components depending on whether it has been obtained by deep puncture (which is really arterial blood) or light puncture in which there might be an accumulation of neutrophils and mono-cytes.

Individual or group-based reference values

When a given value shows marked variations between individuals (high inter-individual variations) but remains fairly constant in the same person (low intra-individual variations) during the day (low diurnal variations) and also over the years, individual reference values provide more useful information than population values. An example of this is body weight, but the concept also applies to some biochemical values which show large inter-individual variation (for example immunoglobin concentration). Many haematological values (haemoglobin level, white cell count) also show wide variations from one person to another but remain stable in the individual person. Thus, a decrease of 20 g/l in haemoglobin concentration (e.g. from 160 to 140 g/l) can be an important sign of disease *for that individual* although the lower value is still well inside the 'normal' limits for the population as a whole. Group-based reference values are useful for parameters with a wider intra-individual variation (e.g. body temperature, plasma iron and glucose level) or when no previous result is known in a 'new' patient.

Measurement of the reference value

In principle, the set of measurements used to produce the reference value should be obtained by a method as similar as possible to that used to obtain patient values. For this reason, values are often only useful in the laboratory in which the values were established. Use of reference values obtained in a different laboratory on a similar population is often not acceptable; not only do the techniques have to be the same but the whole procedure and the levels of precision and accuracy of the measurement must be no less than those in the original survey.

Inter-laboratory comparability can be achieved by standardization of methods. This allows one to use the reference values obtained at other centres, if they have been established with similar methods.

Statistical procedure

For practical use, a statistical analysis of the results obtained in each reference individual is needed (3). In many instances the purpose will be to establish reference limits defining a reference interval containing the 95% central values.

If results follow a normal or Gaussian distribution, computation of mean and standard deviation are easy and the reference interval will be defined by the mean ±2 standard deviations (parametric method). However, often biological data have a log-normal rather than a normal distribution. In such cases the logarithms of the observed values have a Gaussian distribution, so that the raw data can be treated by mathematical procedures to derive a normal distribution which can then be used to compute mean and standard deviation.

When possible, a parametric method should be used, since it is easy to perform and reliable results can be obtained from relatively small numbers of data. Only 30–40 measurements are needed with a parametric approach, while a significantly higher number is necessary for a non-parametric method.

In essence, the non-parametric method is simple: all observed values are ordered according to increasing value and the 2.5% lowest and 2.5% highest measurements are discarded, thus giving the limits of the 95% central observations. Reliable computer programs are available to perform such statistical analysis easily (6). For a more exhaustive discussion see Ref. 3.

Presentation of data

Often we will only need the reference limits, given as a low and a high value between which the central 95% are situated or as a mean and its standard deviation.

A frequency distribution curve (Fig. 3.2a) or a cumulative number fraction distribution curve (Fig. 3.2b) can be used. This last representation shows directly where

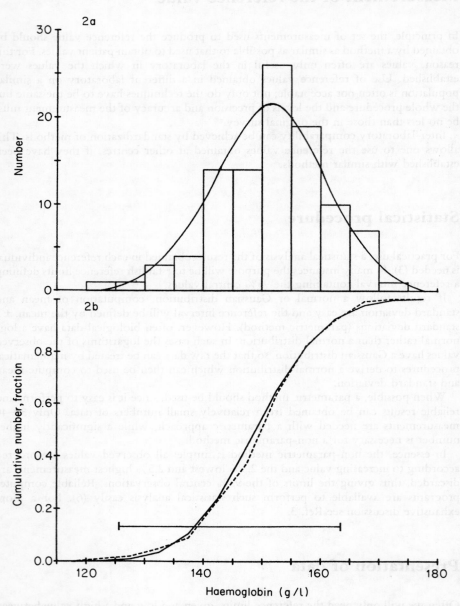

Fig. 3.2 Reference values, haemoglobin concentration. Reference population: 100 adult men, age 18–73 years. (a) Frequency distribution of observed values: histogram and Gaussian probability plot. (b) Cumulative number fraction of observed values. —— parametric (Gaussian) distribution; ---- non-parametric (observed) distribution; ⊢⊣ 95% reference interval.

the individual patient's value is situated in relation to the whole population, i.e. what proportion has higher or lower values than the individual.

Examples of determination of reference values

Example 1: Haemoglobin concentration in a healthy male Belgian population

The reference population consisted of 100 adult (age 18–73 years) males investigated as potential donors of blood or bone marrow. All were family members of patients treated for different haematological malignancies. They had undergone a routine clinical check-up in which no significant abnormalities were detected. A blood sample was taken into EDTA and the haemoglobin level was measured with a Coulter S-Plus IV counter. The distribution of measured values is shown in Fig. 3.2.

Analysis by the REFVAL computer program (6) showed that the distribution could be considered as normal reference limits (95% central values) and their confidence intervals as shown in Table 3.1. The number of measurements was too small to define confidence limits using a non-parametric method for this particular program.

Example 2: Reference values for patients in remission from acute leukaemia

The reference population consisted of 89 adult (15–77 years) male patients in remission from acute leukaemia.

Three months (± 1 week) after the first normal bone marrow smear subsequent to aggressive chemotherapy, measurements were obtained on EDTA blood samples with a Coulter S-Plus IV.

Figure 3.3 shows the reference values for haemoglobin levels, red cell count, packed cell volume (PCV) and mean cell volume (MCV). The distribution is not Gaussian and only a non-parametric approach is possible. These patients have markedly decreased values for red cell parameters while macrocytosis is prominent. Further subdivision of

Table 3.1 Reference limits and confidence intervals for Example 1

	Fraction	Reference limit	0.90 Confidence interval
Parametric determi-			
nation:	0.025	131.2	127.4–134.7
	0.975	168.3	166.0–170.6
Non-parametric de-			
termination:	0.025	129.7	
	0.975	168.5	

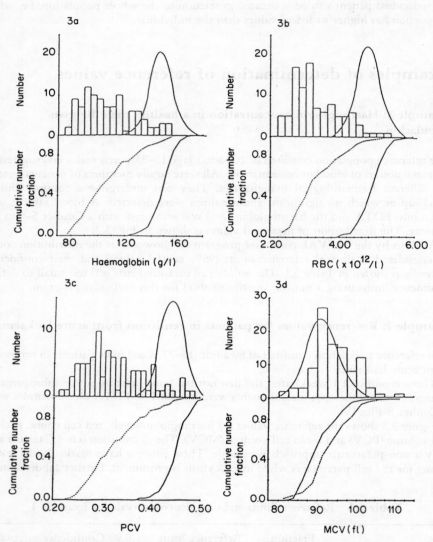

Fig. 3.3 Frequency distribution and cumulative number fraction of measurements in a population of 89 male patients (age 15–77 years) in remission from acute leukaemia since 3 months: Haemoglobin concentration (a), red cell count (b), packed cell value (PVC) (c), mean cell volume (MCV) (d). ---- Patients population; —— healthy adult males (population used for Fig. 3.2).

the reference population according to leukaemia type (lymphoblastic/non-lymphoblastic) showed no significant differences for red cell parameters between both subgroups.

These examples illustrate the need for reference values adapted to the patients treated in specialized units.

References

1. Alström, T. (1981). Evolution and nomenclature of the reference value concept. In Gräsbeck, R. and Alström, T. (eds) *Reference Values in Laboratory Medicine*, pp. 3–13. Chichester: Wiley.
2. Gräsbeck, R., Tikkanen, I., Yki-Jarvinen, H., Ojala, K. and Weber, T. (1981). Common types of quantities in laboratory personnel under standardized conditions, in the afternoon (1430 h) and following an evening party. In Gräsbeck, R. and Alström, T. (eds) *Reference Values in Laboratory Medicine*, pp. 369–375. Chichester: Wiley.
3. IFCC/ICSH (1983/84). The theory of reference values. Part 5: Statistical treatment of collected reference values. Determination of reference limits. *Journal of Clinical Chemistry and Biochemistry* **21**: 749–760, 1983; *Clinica Chimica Acta* 97F–114F, 1984; *Clinical Chemistry Newsletter (Milan)* **4**: 2–10, 1984.
4. IFCC/ICSH (1987). Approved recommendation (1986) on the theory of reference values. Part 1: The concept of reference values. *Journal of Clinical Chemistry and Clinical Biochemistry* **25**: 337–342.
5. IFCC/ICSH (1987). The theory of reference values. Part 6: Presentation of observed values related to reference values. *Journal of Clinical Chemistry and Biochemistry* **25**: 657–662.
6. Solberg, H. E. (1983). REFVAL. Technical Report, February 1983, Department of Clinical Chemistry, Rikshospitalet, N-0027 Oslo 1, Norway. The report, including FORTRAN source program listings, is available upon request to the author. Other versions of the program, suitable for personal computers (PC/MS-DOS), are also available.

4

Statistics Used in Quality Control and Quality Assessment

J M England

Introduction

Quality assurance programmes are intended to minimize imprecision and inaccuracy in laboratory data so ensuring that results are comparable from method to method and from laboratory to laboratory.

Imprecision is determined by repeatedly testing the same specimen. Laboratory workers therefore need to be familiar with the normal distribution and how it can be applied to the study of analytical variation. Imprecision within a particular laboratory is monitored by an internal quality control (IQC) programme (Chapter 5). Between-laboratory imprecision is assessed by external quality assessment (EQA) schemes (Chapter 7).

Inaccuracy can only be investigated by comparing results by a particular method with those obtained by a reference method. Such data always require careful statistical analysis and an understanding of the basis of significance tests such as the t- and F-tests. These will be explained and examples of the calculations will be provided using imaginary data.

Comparability between different methods or between different laboratories can be assessed both graphically and by regression techniques. It is important both for instrument and kit evaluation (Chapters 8 and 9) and for Youden plots which have important applications in IQC and EQA schemes.

The normal distribution

The normal distribution was apparently first described by De Moivre in 1753 but is often called the Gaussian or Laplacean distribution. In theory, it forms a typical 'bell-shaped' curve if a measurement, x, is plotted against the frequency, y, with which a particular measurement is observed (Fig. 4.1). One of the most important points to note

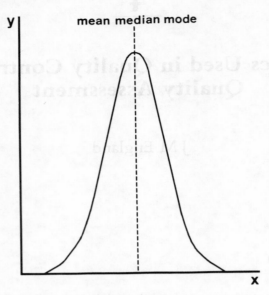

Fig. 4.1 The symmetrical 'bell-shaped' normal distribution.

about the distribution is that it is symmetrical, so that the mean, median and mode are identical.

Measures of central tendency

The mean, median and mode can be used to indicate the centre of the bell-shaped curve. Hence they are termed measures of central tendency.

The **mean** is the most important measure which can be calculated. It is usually obtained as the arithmetic mean by summing all of the *x* values (the symbol Σ means the sum of) and dividing the total by the number of *x* values. The number is usually given the abbreviation *n*.

$$\text{Mean} = \frac{\Sigma x}{n}$$

The **median** is the mid-point value, i.e. there are as many observations above the median as there are below. Thus if five observations are put in ascending order then the third would be the median (Fig. 4.2). More generally, if *n* is an odd number then the $(n+1)/2$th observation is the median. When *n* is an even number then the median is taken mid-way between the $(n/2)$th and the $((n/2+1))$th observation, e.g. for six observations the median is mid-way between the third and fourth (Fig. 4.3).

The median is less susceptible to extreme or out-lying values than is the mean. In Fig. 4.4a, for example, there is a reasonably concordant set of five values whereas in Fig. 4.4b

Median = 144
↓

Order	1	2	3	4	5
Observation	129	134	144	147	149

Fig. 4.2 The median of a set of observations (odd number), placed in ascending order.

$$\text{Median} = \frac{144 + 147}{2} = 145.5$$

↓

Order	1	2	3	4	5	6
Observation	129	134	144	147	149	152

Fig. 4.3 The median of a set of observations (even number), placed in ascending order.

(a)

Median = 144
↓

Order	1	2	3	4	5
Observation	129	134	144	147	149

Mean = 140.6

(b)

Median = 144
↓

Order	1	2	3	4	5
Observation	129	134	144	147	195

Mean = 149.8

Fig. 4.4 Observations placed in ascending order. Change in the highest number between (a) and (b) has no effect on the median whilst causing marked shift in the mean.

an outlier has been substituted for the highest observation. It can be seen that this substitution has no effect on the median but it has caused a marked change in the mean. This robustness of the median is of particular value when samples are small; a number of EQA schemes prefer the median to the mean for this reason.

This advantage of the median over the mean in no way means that it is superior to the mean. The mean is always the best measure if the data are distributed normally. The median is of advantage when outliers are present, since the data may not be distributed normally.

The **mode** is simply the commonest value and is represented by the value of x corresponding to the peak of the bell-shaped curve. Obviously with a theoretical curve there is no problem in locating the peak but with real data the peak may be uneven, with several possible candidates for the mode. Various formulae can be used to deal with this problem but, as the mode has no practical use in haematology, it will not be considered further.

Measures of dispersion

As well as central tendency there must be some measure of dispersion. In Fig. 4.5a, for example, both curves have the same dispersion but different means, whereas in Fig. 4.5b they have the same mean but different dispersion.

Deviation

Dispersion or deviation is taken as difference from the mean:

$$\text{Deviation} = x - \bar{x}$$

where $\bar{x}$ is the mean of the sample. The problem with using the deviation is that it has an average value of zero for all samples. To solve this one could square the deviations:

$$\text{Squared deviation} = (x - \bar{x})^2$$

so that all the deviations with a negative sign now become positive and the average is always a real value. The problem then is how to get the mean deviation.

Mean squared deviation: variance

Unfortunately, the mean squared deviation cannot be calculated by using the formula:

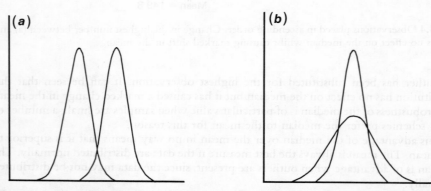

Fig. 4.5 Normal distributions. Central tendency and dispersion are indicated by the mean (μ) and standard deviation (σ), respectively. (a) Same σ, different μ. (b) Same μ, different σ.

$$\frac{\Sigma(x - \bar{x})^2}{n} \text{ Incorrect formula}$$

because the individual deviations should really be calculated by subtracting the mean of the population from which the sample was drawn rather than by subtracting the mean of the sample itself. Obviously the deviations will always be less about the sample mean than they are about the true mean so that the above formula will underestimate the mean squared deviation. The correct formula is:

$$\frac{\Sigma(x - \bar{x})^2}{n - 1} \text{ Correct formula}$$

and when $n - 1$ is used the mean squared deviation is the **variance** of the sample.

Analysis of variance

The importance of variance, statistically speaking, is that it can be analysed into components in such a way as to provide an endless scope for statistical significance testing. Suppose, for example, one measured haemoglobin levels on subjects from a number of different hospitals and calculated the overall variance. One could then ask the question, 'What is responsible for all of this variance?', and break down the results according to the sex of the person, their age group and the hospital at which they were tested, so giving three variables: sex, age and hospital. If any of these three variables is important, then variance should be less in the relevant subgroups than in the group overall. Thus an analysis of variance can determine whether sex, age or hospital significantly affect the haemoglobin measurement. Obviously a hospital effect could arise from differences in catchment population, measurement method or a combination of both.

The analysis of variance is a very powerful technique which is much more flexible than t-testing. Indeed paired and unpaired t-testing can be thought of as special cases of the analysis of variance. More details are given later in this chapter (p. 54–57).

Degrees of freedom

The term n-1, which has been introduced into the calculation of variance, is the degrees of freedom. This rather complicated concept is important to understand because it forms an essential part of the basis for statistical significance testing.

If one has a sample of n observations then, conceptually speaking, all n could vary. However, once one calculates $\bar{x}$, one of the degrees of freedom is used up, e.g. if there were five observations and the mean was calculated then only four of the observations could vary since the fifth may be calculated by subtracting the total for the four from $5 \times \bar{x}$.

When various dispersion measurements are calculated there may be different degrees of freedom. In regression analysis, for example, one can calculate the variance of the vertical distance of the points about the regression line (Fig. 4.6); under these circumstances there are $n - 2$ degrees of freedom and the formula is:

$$\text{Variance} = \frac{\Sigma(y - y')^2}{n - 2}$$

where y is the observation and y' is the value corresponding to the intersection of the regression line and a vertical line through y. Two degrees of freedom have been used up in calculating the mean value of y, $\bar{y}$, and the slope of the regression line, e.g. if there are five points and $\bar{y}$ and the slope are calculated then only three of the observations are free to vary (see p. 60–65 for further details of regression analysis).

Standard deviation (SD)

This is calculated as the square root of the variance:

$$\text{SD} = \sqrt{\text{Variance}} = s$$

The SD is sometimes called the root mean square deviation which explains how it is calculated. It is usually expressed as s. An advantage of the SD over the variance is that the former is expressed in the same units as the measurements themselves. However,

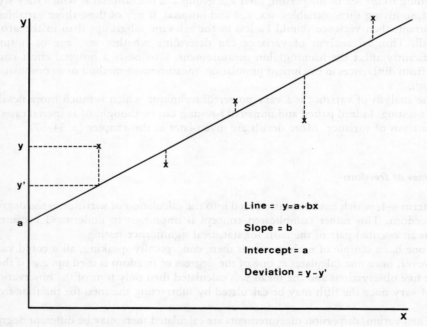

Line = y = a + bx

Slope = b

Intercept = a

Deviation = y – y'

Fig. 4.6 Deviation $y - y'$ for points about the regression line $y = a + bx$.

from a purely statistical point of view the variance is to be preferred because of its importance for the analysis of variance.

Coefficient of variation (CV)

The CV is calculated by expressing the SD as a percentage of the mean:

$$CV = \frac{s}{\bar{x}} \times 100\%$$

It is always useful to calculate the CV because high values ($\geqslant 12\%$) indicate serious deviations of the data from a normal distribution. This is important to recognize because many statistical techniques, including all those described in this chapter, are based on the assumption that the data are normally distributed. Methods for checking on the normality of the distribution are available and there are various possible ways of dealing with the problem of non-normality (2).

Another advantage of the CV, as compared to the SD, is that the former is dimensionless, e.g. for haemoglobin one divides an SD in g/l by a mean in g/l and the resulting quantity has no dimension. This is quite useful when studying analytical imprecision, biological variation, etc., since data for different measurements can be compared.

Standard error of the mean (SEM)

This term is confusing because it is used to describe the SD of the mean, i.e. if one takes a sample of n measurements and calculates the SD or s then:

$$SEM = \frac{SD}{\sqrt{n}} \text{ or } \frac{s}{\sqrt{n}}$$

It is, literally, the SD one might expect to get between the means of a large number of samples, each of which contained n measurements.

As a concept the SEM is useful in significance testing since, as part of the calculations, one may need the standard error of the mean or the standard error of the difference between two means etc.

However as a pure measure of central tendency to use when describing results there is little to be said for the SEM. Some experimenters like the fact that the SEM is less than the SD and might give other workers a better impression. This approach should be discouraged.

Theory of the normal distribution

Before embarking on the theory of the normal distribution it is important to clarify the relevant terminology. Normal distribution theory describes how an infinite population behaves whose mean is μ and whose SD is σ. Note that these symbols are different from those for the mean, $\bar{x}$ and SD, s, of a finite sample drawn from the infinite theoretical population.

The theory of the normal distribution predicts that measurements, x, will be observed with frequency, y, according to the formula:

$$y = \frac{N\ i}{\sigma\sqrt{(2\pi)}} \exp -\frac{(x-\mu)^2}{2\sigma^2}$$

where N is the total number of measurements, i is the measurement interval which is usually unity and π is approximately 3.1416. An example of such a curve is given in Fig. 4.7a.

There are a number of ways in which the theory can be simplified. The first is to set $N\ i = 1$ so that:

$$y = \frac{1}{\sigma\sqrt{(2\pi)}} \exp -\frac{(x-\mu)^2}{2\sigma^2}$$

This new relationship has then been generalized (Fig. 4.7b) so that it will show no dependence on sample size. However, for the construction of mathematical tables even this relationship is too complex so it has to be further assumed that $\mu = 0$ and that $\sigma = 1$, so giving:

$$y = \frac{1}{\sqrt{(2\pi)}} \exp -\frac{x^2}{2}$$

This relationship, shown in Fig. 4.7c, is termed a standardized normal distribution. To summarize, the differences from 4.7a are that: y does not depend on sample size; and x is expressed in SD units either above or below the mean.

Application to analytical variation

The normal distribution has a long history of application to the study of experimental

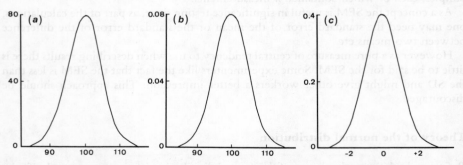

Fig. 4.7 Normal distributions. (a) $N = 1000$, $i = 1$, $\mu = 100$ and $\sigma = 5$. (b) $Ni = 1$, $\mu = 100$ and $\sigma = 5$. (c) $Ni = 1$, $\mu = 0$ and $\sigma = 1$.

error, first being used by Gauss in astronomy. It can be shown that the normal distribution will apply if one assumes that a measurement is liable to be affected by an infinite number of errors, each of which cause a minute under- or over-estimation. It has to be further assumed that there is an equal probability of the error causing an under- or over-estimation. These are, of course, quite reasonable assumptions, so it is not surprising that the normal distribution has such wide application both in terms of within-hospital precision testing (IQC, Chapter 5) or between-hospital precision testing (EQA, Chapter 7). In both of these situations decisions are based on the number of outliers beyond specified limits.

Figure 4.8 illustrates the areas under the normal distribution. It can be seen that 95.44% of all observations should fall within $\mu \pm 2\sigma$ with 2.28% below $\mu - 2\sigma$ and 2.28% above $\mu + 2\sigma$. Within the tails of the distribution observations become increasingly rare, as shown in Fig. 4.9 which enlarges the right-hand tail from Fig. 4.8 (the left-hand tail is symmetrical).

These facts can be used to define 'action limits' for Shewhart charts or to define 'poor performance' in EQA surveys. Suppose, in either instance, one takes five IQC or EQA results and considers the probability that 0, 1, 2, 3, 4 or 5 might be outside various limits. To do the calculation one applies the binomial distribution:

$$\text{Probability of } n \text{ results outside action limits} = P^n (1-P)^{N-n} \frac{N!}{(N-n)! \; n!}$$

where P is the probability of one result outside the action limits and N is the total number of results (five in the present example). The symbol ! after a letter means factorial, i.e. 4! would be $4 \times 3 \times 2 \times 1$.

As an example the calculation will be given for three results out of the five beyond

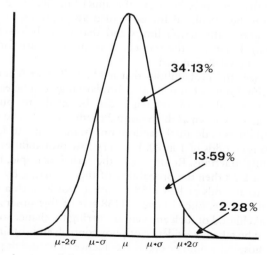

Fig. 4.8 Areas under the normal distribution.

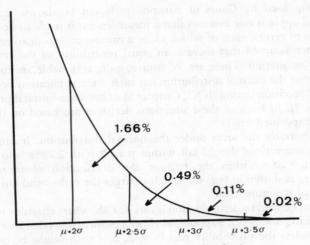

Fig. 4.9 Areas under the right-hand tail of the normal distribution.

the $\mu \pm 2\sigma$ limits (Fig. 4.10). The probability of being in one tail is 0.0228, so the probability of being in either tail is $P = 2 \times 0.0228 = 0.0456$, so giving:

$$\text{Probability of 3 results out of 5 beyond } \mu \pm 2\sigma \text{ limits} =$$
$$(0.0456)^3 \times (0.9544)^{5-3} \times \frac{5!}{(5-3)!\,3!} = 0.00086$$

It should be noted that there is a two–tailed assumption in this test, i.e. of the results outside the action limits some may be above the upper limit and some below the lower limit. Probabilities can be calculated for one-tailed assumptions, i.e. that one is only interested in results above the action limits and that those below the limits can be ignored (or *vice versa*). However, the one-tailed assumptions are totally unrealistic in haematology and can be safely ignored.

Table 4.1 summarizes the probabilities that $n = 0$, 1, 2, 3 or 5 results out of $N = 5$ might be outside action limits set at $\mu \pm 2.0\sigma$. Similar tables can be easily drawn up for any other values of n and N or reference can be made to published tables of $N!/((N-n)!\,n!)$, which is known as the binomial coefficient (4). The data are presented in Table 4.1 as probabilities in decimal fractions on a scale from 0 to 1.0 and as odds, i.e. a probability of 0.05 is an odds of 1 in 20. For very low probabilities odds are easier to appreciate than decimal fractions. Returning to the earlier example, if three out of five results were outside $\mu \pm 2\sigma$ then the probability of this occurring by chance is 0.00086, which is equivalent to an odds of 1 in 1158. In other words, such a result would only occur by chance, on average, once in every 1158 sets of five observations. This gives some idea of the unlikelihood of such an event occurring by chance so that: (a) such data in an IQC run would be taken as evidence of poor control; and (b) such data in a run of EQA results from a hospital would be taken as evidence of persistent poor performance.

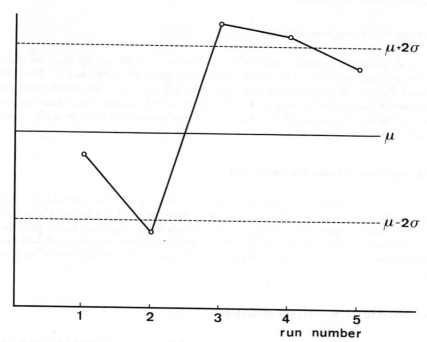

Fig. 4.10 IQC results in five runs with three observations outside $\mu \pm 2\sigma$ limits.

Table 4.1 Probability and odds of getting n results out of $N=5$ outside action limits set at $\mu \pm 2\sigma$, i.e. $P=0.0456$

n	Probability	Odds
0	0.79187	1 in 1.3
1	0.18917	1 in 5.3
2	0.01807	1 in 55
3	0.000864	1 in 1,158
4	0.0000206	1 in 48,466
5	0.000000197	1 in 5,071,960

Example of calculation: Using binomial coefficient from tables for $n=2$, $N=5$ gives $\log_{10} (5!/3!\,2!) = 1$ so that $5!/3!\,2! =$ antilog $(1) = 10$.
Then the probability is given by: $(0.0456)^2 \times (0.9544)^{5-2} \times 10 = 0.01807$.

Application to biological variation

Biological variation between subjects in a reference sample group may be used to calculate a reference range. It is conventional to calculate the range as $\bar{x} \pm 1.96s$ which, provided the sample is sufficiently large ($n > 30$), will provide a reasonable estimate of the reference range which encloses 95.0% of the sample group. Note that the range should not really be calculated as $\bar{x} \pm 2.0s$ since this encloses 95.44% of subjects rather than the conventional 95.00%.

Validating a normal distribution of data

The calculation of a reference range is based on the assumption that the underlying data are normally distributed and this assumption should be validated before the reference range can be relied upon. One of the easiest methods for doing this is to use probability paper (2) and this approach can also be used to determine how non–normal data should be transformed, e.g. by taking its logarithm, to make the assumption of normality valid.

The Student's *t* distribution

So far the discussion has centred around the probability that an individual result will fall outside certain limits, e.g. $\mu \pm 2\sigma$, if the overall population is normally distributed. The approach is helpful for IQC or EQA but it is not of much value for other studies in which, for example, measurements made by a new method may be compared with reference results (Table 4.2). Because two results are obtained on each specimen the data are said to be 'paired' so that differences between each pair can be calculated as can the mean difference, $\bar{d}$ and the SD of the difference, s_d. The question can then be asked: If there is really no difference between the results by the two methods i.e. $\bar{d} = 0$ then how often, by chance, might one expect to find a mean difference as large as $\bar{d} = 5.4$ or greater?

Note firstly that the question is posed against a background of 'If there really is no difference' – this hypothesis being called the **'null hypothesis'.** Secondly the probability of the result occurring by chance is to be calculated on the assumption that the null hypothesis is true. If the calculated probability is very low then it will be reasonable to conclude that the null hypothesis is untrue, i.e. there is a difference between the results by the two methods ($\bar{d} \neq 0$). This is the basis of statistical significance testing but the methodology could not be implemented until there was a better understanding of the behaviour of samples drawn from a normal distribution.

Theory of Student's *t*-test

It was not until 1908 that W. S. Gosset, a brewer working for Guinness, published the solution to this problem under the pseudonym 'Student'. In his paper he described the behaviour of samples drawn from a normal distribution and showed that, for example:

$$\frac{\text{Quantity being assessed from sample}}{\text{Standard error of quantity being assessed}}$$

would have a special distribution called Student's *t* distribution. Student's *t* distribution, like the normal distribution, is bell-shaped and symmetrical but there are differences in that the tails are larger for Student's *t* distribution (Fig. 4.11). Student's *t* distribution is a series of curves for particular degrees of freedom (d.f.); differences from the normal

Table 4.2 Haemoglobin measurements on an automated counter compared with those by the ICSH reference method

Specimen 1	Haemoglobin measurements (g/l)		
	Automated	ICSH	d
1	170	183	+13
2	147	153	+6
3	149	154	+5
4	144	146	+2
5	134	134	0
6	155	165	+10
7	131	130	−1
8	182	197	+15
9	165	177	+12
10	102	94	−8

For simplicity ten ($n = 10$) results are presented, but in practice at least 30 comparisons would be made. The differences, d, are calculated retaining the ' + ' or ' − ' sign.

The mean difference is: $\bar{d} = \dfrac{\Sigma d}{n} = \dfrac{54}{10} = 5.400$

The SD of the differences is:

$$s_d = \sqrt{\left(\frac{\Sigma(d - \bar{d})^2}{(n-1)}\right)} = 7.276$$

Student's *t* for the paired test is:

$$t = \frac{\bar{d}}{s_d/\sqrt{n}} = 2.347$$

with $n - 1 = 9$ d.f. and $P = 0.01 - 0.05$.

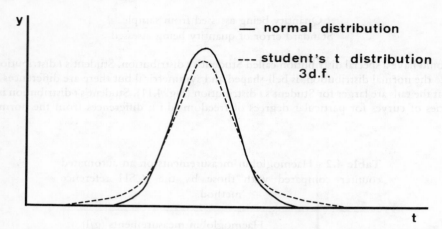

Fig. 4.11 A comparison of Student's *t* distribution (three d.f.) with the normal distribution.

distribution are especially apparent with low numbers of degrees of freedom, and they are lost when d.f. > 30.

In the example already considered it is possible to substitute:

$$t = \frac{\text{Quality being assessed}}{\text{Standard error}} = \frac{\bar{d} - 0}{s_d/\sqrt{n}} = \frac{\bar{d}}{s_d/\sqrt{n}}$$

where *n* is the number of pairs and the standard error of *d* is calculated as for any other mean by $s_d/\sqrt{n}$. The quantity being assessed is $\bar{d} - 0 = \bar{d}$ since we are testing the null hypothesis that $\bar{d}$ is zero. The value of *t* is then assessed by reference to the areas under Student's *t* distribution for $(n-1)$ d.f. Convenient tables are available (4, also see p. 286).

Student's *t*-test

There are as many possible *t*-tests as there are quantities which might be assessed; only the simplest ones will be described in this section though others will be considered in the discussion of regression (p. 72).

Comparison of a mean with a constant

If a number of observations are made with a mean of $\bar{x}$ then it is possible to test whether $\bar{x} = k$, where *k* is a constant. The value of *k* could, of course, be zero so the test would assess whether $\bar{x} = 0$. Using the familiar formula:

$$t = \frac{\bar{x} - k}{\text{Standard error}} = \frac{\bar{x} - k}{s/\sqrt{n}}$$

where there are n observations and their SD is s. The value of t is referred to tables for $n-1$ degrees of freedom. For example, if a run of 32 haemoglobin analyses on patients gave $\bar{x}=147$ g/l and $s=9$ g/l when the historical mean is $k=139$ g/l then:

$$t=\frac{147-139}{9/\sqrt{32}}=5.03$$

with $n-1=32-1=31$ d.f. and $P<0.001$.

The test is based on the assumption that the x values are normally distributed.

The paired t-test, already described on p. 56 and in Table 4.2 is, of course, merely an example of comparing $\bar{x}$ with a constant. In this case the individual x values are not the basic observations but the differences between the paired observations so that for $\bar{x}$ read $\bar{d}$ and for s read s_d. In this case k is zero so the equation becomes the same as the one in Table 4.2. The test is based on the assumption that the d values are normally distributed; provided this is true the distribution of the raw data from which the differences are calculated is immaterial.

Comparison of two means

Instead, for example, of comparing two methods on the same samples (Table 4.2), a worker may decide to assess whether the routine results from his analyser are the same in the morning or the afternoon. This would be a crude IQC method based on patient data but, like more sophisticated approaches (p. 80), it would detect changes in the underlying patient population as well as instrument drift.

The morning and afternoon data sets would be completely independent with no specimens being run twice, i.e. there is no pairing and the t-test required is termed an unpaired t-test. In this case t is calculated with the formula:

$$t=\frac{\bar{x}_1-\bar{x}_2}{\left[\left((n_1-1)s_1^2+(n_2-1)s_2^2\right)\frac{n_1+n_2}{(n_1+n_2-2)n_1n_2}\right]^{\frac{1}{2}}}$$

The value of t is referred to tables for n_1+n_2-2 degrees of freedom. For example if 32 haemoglobin analyses in the morning gave $\bar{x}_1=147$ and $s_1=9$ with 32 analyses in the afternoon giving $\bar{x}_2=135$ and $s_2=6$ (all in g/l) then:

$$t=\frac{147-135}{\left[\left((32-1)9^2+(32-1)6^2\right)\frac{32+32}{(32+32-2)\times32\times32}\right]^{\frac{1}{2}}}=6.28$$

with $32+32-2=62$ d.f. and $P<0.001$.

It should be noted that this formula for the unpaired Student's t-test is based on the assumption that the data are normally distributed and that both groups have the same variance.

Fisher's *F* distribution

Whilst the work by W. S. Gosset ('Student') enabled scientists to perform statistical significance tests, the methodology could only be applied to simple experimental designs. If one takes a more complex situation, such as within- and between-batch testing, it becomes very difficult to use Student's *t*-test in a meaningful way. An example of this is provided in Table 4.3 with four specimens being tested in triplicate in two batches. The objective of the exercise is to estimate both within- and between-batch precision and to see whether the latter is significantly greater than the former, i.e. are there differences between batches 1 and 2 which are greater than those which might have arisen by chance? Obviously an unpaired Student's *t*-test could be used for specimen 1 by comparing $\bar{x}_1$ with $\bar{x}_2$, where $\bar{x}_1$ is calculated from the triplicates in batch 1 and $\bar{x}_2$ from the triplicates in batch 2. However, such a test would only have $n_1 + n_2 - 2 = 4$ degrees of freedom and any inter-batch difference would have to be relatively enormous before it became statistically significant. The same considerations would apply to similar unpaired Student's *t*-tests performed on specimens 2, 3 and 4, and one could end up with a total of four *t* values none of which were statistically significant despite there being a manifest difference between the batches. Such a problem can only be resolved by amalgamating all the significance tests into one. This problem is best approached by an **analysis of variance** to see whether there is a significant overall inter-batch effect. The actual statistical significance test used is Fisher's *F*-test which is based on the distribution he described.

Theory of Fisher's *F*-test

In 1924 Fisher published his *F* distribution and explained how it described the behaviour of the ratio of the variances of two samples drawn from a normal distribution. For assessing whether there is a significant between-batch effect in the within- and between-batch study (Table 4.3) it is necessary to calculate:

Table 4.3   Within- and between-batch precision testing

	Red cell counts (10^{12} per litre)	
	Batch 1	Batch 2
Specimen 1	4.64, 4.66, 4.72	4.85, 4.91, 4.87
Specimen 2	4.17, 4.17, 4.17	4.28, 4.25, 4.28
Specimen 3	5.17, 5.20, 5.18	5.31, 5.35, 5.24
Specimen 4	5.43, 5.39, 5.44	5.51, 5.47, 5.51

Data are presented for red cell counts on specimens tested in triplicate in two batches. In practice a larger study would be performed.

$$F = \frac{\text{Variance between batches}}{\text{Variance due to analytical error}}$$

The detailed calculations are given in Appendix 4.A at the end of this chapter.

With significance tests based on Student's t distribution the value of t has to be assessed in the light of the relevant d.f. In contrast, with F both the numerator and the denominator have their own d.f. so that tables of F are more complicated than tables of Student's t and graphs of the F distribution have to be related to the two separate d.f. values (Fig. 4.12).

F-tests: analysis of variance

In order to explain the range of common use of F-tests the within- and between-batch study can be used as an example (Table 4.3). Each specimen is presented as a row and each batch as a column, i.e. there are four rows and two columns making a total of $4 \times 2 = 8$ cells, within each of which there are three replicate observations.

Three F-tests can be performed in this situation:

(a)   To assess between-batch variation:

$$F = \frac{\text{Variance between batches}}{\text{Variance due to analytical error}}$$

In the example chosen this is the most important F-test.

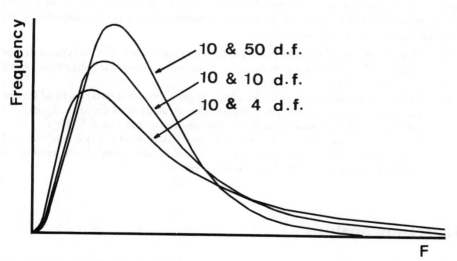

Fig. 4.12 Fisher's F distribution for various d.f., e.g. the curve for 10 and 50 d.f. is for the d.f. of the numerator and denominator respectively. (Adapted from Lentner, 1986, with permission.)

(b)   To assess between-specimen variation:

$$F = \frac{\text{Variance between specimens}}{\text{Variance due to analytical error}}$$

In the example chosen this is the least important F-test.

(c)   To assess interaction:

$$F = \frac{\text{Variance due to interaction}}{\text{Variance due to analytical error}}$$

An interaction effect is an exceptional result in a particular cell or cells, i.e. a result which does not comply with the predicted behaviour for the row(s) and the column(s) corresponding to the particular cell(s). Thus if the red cell counts in batch 2 were 0.10×10^{12} per litre above those in batch 1 (batch effect) and specimen 2 had a count 0.5×10^{12} per litre above that of specimen 1 (specimen effect) then the result for specimen 2 in batch 2 should be 0.6×10^{12} per litre in excess of that for specimen 1 in batch 1; any difference greater or less than this would indicate a possible interaction effect influencing either or both results. Such an interaction could arise from biased analysis on a particular specimen in a particular batch or it could come from a specimen which showed excessive inter-batch instability. In either case the interaction is important and would be recognized by the F value in (c) being statistically significant.

Because there is more than one column the data are said to have a two-way classification and their analysis is a two-way analysis of variance (Appendix 4.A, p. 68). If there had been only one row with several columns or *vice versa* a one-way analysis of variance would have been sufficient (Appendix 4.B, p. 70) though this is, of course, merely an abbreviated example of the two-way analysis. There are various other ways in which the analysis can be simplified:

(a)   A two-way classification with only one observation per cell. This type of design is not to be encouraged because it does not permit the identification of interaction effects.

(b)   A two-way classification with one observation per cell but two rows and several columns. This is the paired t-test expressed as an analysis of variance. Student's t and F are related inasmuch as, when the numerator has one d.f., $F = t^2$.

(c)   A one-way classification with more than one observation per cell, one row and two columns. This is the unpaired t-test and, again, t and F are related, as explained above, since the numerator has one d.f.

Regression analysis

Student's t-test and the F-test both have important applications in regression analysis. In this technique a regression line is drawn to describe the relationship between an independent variable, x, and a dependent variable, y. Classically it is assumed that x is measured without error and that only y is subject to error. The regression line which is fitted (Fig. 4.6) has the formula:

$$y = a + bx$$

where a is the intercept and b is the slope.

Theory of regression analysis

There is very little theory associated with this type of analysis (Appendix 4.C, p. 71). Essentially the regression line is a least-squares fit, i.e. it minimizes the squares of the distances of the points from the regression line so that the lowest possible value is obtained for:

$$\Sigma(y - y')^2$$

The actual line passes through the point corresponding to the mean values x and y and through the intercept a. Fitting the line uses up two d.f. so if there are n points then the variance of the points about the line has $n-2$ d.f.

Significance testing

Is the intercept a = 0?

In most dilution studies and in comparison studies with reference methods the fitted regression line should pass through the origin of the graph, i.e. $a = 0$. To test whether this is so use can be made of Student's t-test.

$$t = \frac{\text{Quantity being assessed from sample}}{\text{Standard error of quantity being assessed}}$$

The relevant calculations are given in Appendix 4.C, p. 72.

Is slope b = 1?

In most dilution studies the slope of the regression line is immaterial since the x axis is not graduated in any fixed manner. When evaluating an automated blood cell counter, for example, various mixtures are made of concentrated cells and cell-free autologous plasma. The mixtures, which vary from 0 to 100% cells, must be made accurately but the x axis itself is graduated arbitrarily in per cent and there is no requirement to graduate it metrologically.

However, when comparing a new method with a reference method it is important to assess whether the slope $b = 1$. Again use is made of Student's t-test (Appendix 4.C, p. 73).

Is slope b = 0?

In some dilution studies, e.g. of cell–plasma mixtures, measurements such as the red cell indices would not be expected to vary with dilution and the regression line should be horizontal. The intercept will not be zero and it is pointless to test if $a=0$ and $b=1$. Instead a test should be made to see if $b=0$ (Appendix 4.C, p. 72).

Is the relationship linear?

Strictly speaking, it is pointless to perform Student's t-tests to assess values of a and b unless the underlying relationship between x and y is linear. Whilst the term 'linear' has no precise meaning, in this chapter its use will be restricted to mean conformity to a straight line. There are several ways in which such conformity can be judged, but first it is necessary to discuss how points scatter about a regression line. This was illustrated earlier in Fig. 4.6 when considering the variance of the points about the regression line; the concept is expanded in Fig. 4.13. The vertical distances between the points and the regression line represent a combination of analytical error and any deviation from the simple linear regression. In Fig. 4.13a the points scatter fairly evenly about the regression line and it is obvious that the relationship is linear with the variance about the line arising only from analytical error. On the other hand, in Fig. 4.13b it can be seen that the lowest points are below the regression line, the middle points above and the highest points below. The scatter is not evenly about the line and clearly the relationship really is curvilinear with the points scattering evenly about an underlying curve (Fig. 4.13c). It would be perfectly feasible to assess linearity by using an F-test to compare the variance of the points about the line with the variance of the points about an underlying curve. Indeed this approach was adopted for assessing linearity by the British Committee for Standardization in Haematology (BCSH) (5). However, it suffers from two possible draw-backs:

(a) Measurements of y should be made for as many x values as possible and ten x values were suggested. However, it can be quite tedious, in dilution studies for instance, to prepare the required number of dilutions. (The large number of points suggested stems from the fact that, whilst fitting a line uses up two d.f., fitting a curve uses up at least three d.f. leaving seven or less d.f. for the variance of the points about the curve.)

(b) A decision has to be made as to the type of curve to be fitted. BCSH adopted the parabola and whilst this approach was used successfully in instrument evaluation (1) the choice inevitably is arbitrary and one is open to the criticism that 'you missed the non-linearity because you fitted the wrong curve'.

ICSH therefore decided to adopt a simpler method for assessing linearity which would be independent of choice of curve and less critically dependent on the number of x levels tested, though ten again were suggested (3). Their approach was based upon replication of y measurements at individual x levels. An example of this is in Fig. 4.14a where it can be seen that the replicated observations scatter evenly about the line and it is reasonable to infer that the data are linear. This could be confirmed by first performing a one-way analysis of variance (Appendix 4.B, p. 70) to estimate the

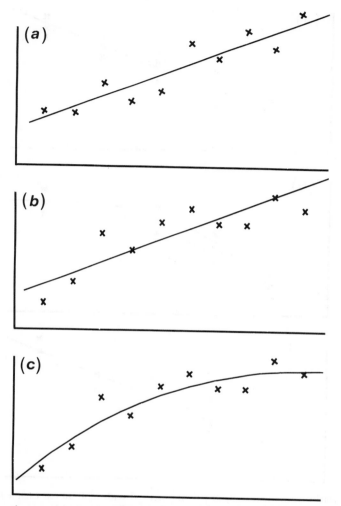

Fig. 4.13 Linearity assessment using the BCSH method with single determinations at each x level. (a) Data conforming to a straight line. (b) Data not conforming to a straight line with the points corresponding to the lower x levels tending to be below the line, the middle points above and the higher points below. (c) Same data as in b but with fitted curve.

variance due to analytical error, i.e. the variance between the replicates estimated from the triplicates at each of the five x levels. The within-group variance is then compared with the variance of the points about the regression line:

$$F = \frac{\text{Variance about regression line}}{\text{Variance due to analytical error}}$$

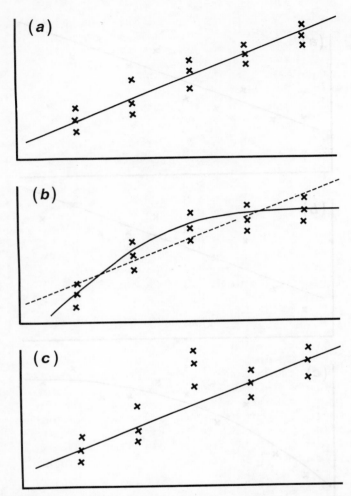

Fig. 4.14 Linearity assessment using the ICSH method with replicates at each *x* level. (a) Data conforming to a straight line. (b) Data not conforming to a straight line (---) with the points corresponding to the lower *x* levels tending to be below the line, the middle points above and the higher points below. A curve (——) fits better. (c) Data not conforming to a straight line because the points corresponding to the central *x* level are discordant.

The calculations are given in Appendix 4.C, p. 71. If the data are linear then the value will not be statistically significant.

Given that, in the context of this book, linearity is assessed in dilution studies (p. 183) or in comparing a new method with a reference method (p. 187), it is easy to justify the ICSH approach using replication since most of the work is involved in preparing the dilutions or performing the reference measurements (the *x* levels). The replication of the y values for each x level is not especially time-consuming so that experimenters could, say, study only five x levels rather than ten but replicate each y measurement three times. Provided that the five x levels chosen span the total range to be assessed, and that there are no non-linearities 'hidden' by the coarser graduation of the x axis, then it is perfectly satisfactory to test five x levels in triplicate instead of ten x levels singly. Nevertheless, the ICSH approach, like the BCSH approach has two disadvantages though these are obviously different:

(a) If the sample for one or more of the x levels is faulty because the dilution is not properly prepared or the reference measurement is wrong (Fig. 4.14c) then the analysis will show a statistically significant deviation from linearity by the F-test even though the results do not show the presence of a curve. In this respect the BCSH analysis is better since it is unlikely that parabola would fit such data better than a line. Hence the BCSH analysis leads to the meaningful conclusion that there is no evidence of a parabola being better than a line, whereas the ICSH analysis leads to the vague conclusion that there is some unspecified deviation from linearity.

(b) Another disadvantage of the ICSH approach is that where an obvious curve is present (Fig. 4.14b) the nature of the curve is not assessed. At least with the BCSH approach a parabola is fitted and its conformity to the data can be evaluated.

It is, of course, perfectly possible to combine the BCSH and ICSH approaches so obtaining the advantages of both. This can be done firstly by estimating whether there is significant variance of the fitted parabola about the fitted line; such an F-test will detect the sort of curvilinearity usually associated with haematological work without being 'confused' by the situation exemplified in Fig. 4.14c, where one of the x levels is in error. Secondly it is possible to estimate whether the variance about the fitted parabola is greater than the variance due to analytical error; if such an F-test shows statistical significance, then there is either curvilinearity not conforming to a parabola or there is error in measuring one or more of the x levels. Obviously the mathematics are much more complex than with either the BCSH or ICSH approaches individually. Nevertheless the method has been used successfully for assessing linearity (1).

Correlation analysis and the correlation coefficient, r

Correlation analysis is quite distinct from the type of regression analysis described above in which the x levels are deemed to be fixed and error-free (either accurately made dilutions or results by reference methods) and only the y values are subject to variation such that $y - y'$ is distributed normally (Figs 4.6 and 4.15a). In contrast, a correlation study is based on the random selection of 'subjects' on whom two measurements x and y are made, where both x and y are subject to variation in accordance with the normal distribution (Fig. 4.15b). It can be seen that such data tend to form an ellipse; this is also termed a bivariate normal distribution.

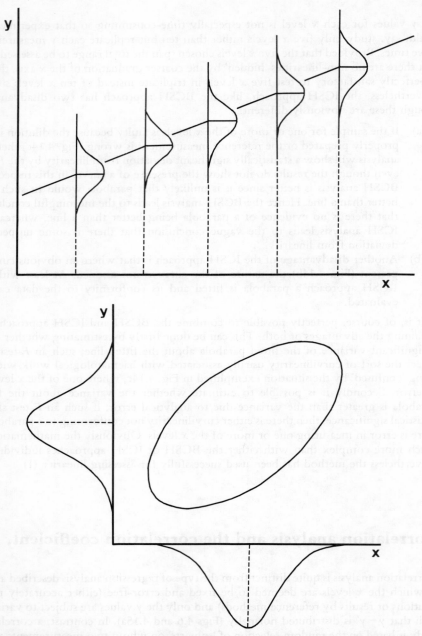

Fig. 4.15 Comparison of regression and correlation. (a) Regression with *y* normally distributed at each of five predetermined *x* levels. (b) Correlation with *x* and *y* both normally distributed when the values are projected onto the respective axes. Together the *x* and *y* points form an ellipse corresponding to their bivariate normal distribution.

Correlation analysis is often misapplied to linearity studies and to comparison of results with reference data. Such applications are invalid because:

(a) In dilution studies the dilutions are fixed in advance at equal intervals so x is not normally distributed.

(b) In comparison studies with reference methods samples should be selected to give as wide a range of x as possible, thus violating the assumption that x is random and normally distributed (correlation studies would be valid if random sampling took place and x and y were found to be normally distributed).

References

1. England, J. M., Chetty, M., Chadwick, R. and Woodhead, G. B. (1982). An assessment of the Ortho ELT-8. *Clinical and Laboratory Haematology* **4:** 187–199.
2. Healy, M. J. R. (1968). The disciplining of medical data. *British Medical Bulletin* **24:** 210–214.
3. ICSH (1984). Protocol for evaluation of automated blood cell counters. *Clinical and Laboratory Haematology* **6:** 69–84.
4. Lentner, C. (1986). *Geigy Scientific Tables* (8th edn), Vol. 2. Basle: Ciba-Geigy Ltd.
5. Shinton, N. K., England, J. M. and Kennedy, D. A. (1982). Guidelines for the evaluation of instruments used in haematology laboratories. *Journal of Clinical Pathology* **35:** 1095–1102.

Appendix 4.A: Two-way analysis of variance

The data on within- and between-batch precision testing (Table 4.3) may be analysed as follows:

	Batch B_1 Result	Sub-total	Batch B_2 Result	Sub-total	Totals
Specimen A_1	4.64 4.66 4.72	14.02	4.85 4.91 4.87	14.63	28.65
Specimen A_2	4.17 4.17 4.17	12.51	4.28 4.25 4.28	12.81	25.32
Specimen A_3	5.17 5.20 5.18	15.55	5.31 5.35 5.24	15.90	31.45
Specimen A_4	5.43 5.39 5.44	16.26	5.51 5.47 5.51	16.49	32.75
Totals		58.34		59.83	118.17 Grand total

The calculations yield:
(a) Correction term

$$C = \frac{118.17^2}{4 \times 3 \times 2} = 581.84$$

(b) Between-As sum of squares

$$SSA = \frac{28.65^2 + 25.32^2 + 31.45^2 + 32.75^2}{3 \times 2} - 581.84$$
$$= 5.425$$

(c) Between-Bs sum of squares

$$SSB = \frac{58.34^2 + 59.83^2}{4 \times 3} - 581.84 = 0.093$$

(d) Between-means sum of squares

$$SSM = \frac{14.02^2 + 14.63^2 + \ldots + 16.26^2 + 16.49^2}{3} - 581.84$$
$$= 5.532$$

(e) Interaction sum of squares

$$SSI = 5.532 - 5.425 - 0.093 = 0.014$$

(f) Total sum of squares

$$SST = (4.64^2 + 4.66^2 + \ldots + 5.51^2) - 581.84$$
$$= 5.547$$

(g) Error sum of squares

$$SSE = 5.547 - 5.532 = 0.015$$

where 2 is the number of batches, 4 is the number of specimens, 3 is the number of replicates and the other entries are individual values, sub-totals, totals, and the grand total as shown above.

(h) Analysis of variance table

Source of variation	Degrees of freedom	Sum of squares	Mean square (MSQ)
Between-As	3	5.425	1.808
Between-Bs	1	0.093	0.093
Interaction	3	0.014	4.579×10^{-3}
Error	16	0.015	9.417×10^{-4}
Total	23	5.547	

where the between-As d.f. is one less than the number of specimens, the between-Bs d.f. is one less than the number of batches, the interaction d.f. is the product of the between-As d.f. and the between-Bs d.f. and the error d.f. is the number of specimens multiplied by the number of batches multiplied by one less than the number of replicates.

(i) $F_A = \dfrac{\text{Variance between specimens}}{\text{Variance due to analytical error}} = 1920.5$

$F_B = \dfrac{\text{Variance between batches}}{\text{Variance due to analytical error}} = 98.24$

$F_I = \dfrac{\text{Variance due to interaction}}{\text{Variance due to analytical error}} = 4.86$

(j) Between-replicate CV for single readings within the same batch:

$$= \frac{\sqrt{\text{Error mean square}}}{118.17/4 \times 3 \times 2} \times 100\% = 0.623\%$$

(k) Between replicate CV for single readings in different batches:

$$= \frac{\sqrt{\left(\dfrac{\text{Between Bs MSQ} + (((4 \times 3) - 1) \times \text{error MSQ})}{4 \times 3} \right)} \times 100\%}{118.17/4 \times 3 \times 2}$$

$$= 1.880\%$$

where in (j) and (k) 2 is the number of batches, 4 is the number of specimens and 3 is the number of replicates.

It is possible to calculate between-batch CV differently to take account of any significant interaction effects. The formula is more complicated and either statistical advice should be sought or the experimental work repeated.

The values of F_A, F_B and F_I are referred to tables (4) with d.f. values appropriate to the relevant numerators and denominators.

Appendix 4.B: One-way analysis of variance

For estimating overall reproducibility a one-way analysis of variance is employed. In the example below four random replicate counts were obtained on three samples and the totals and grand total calculated. For simplicity data are analysed from a much smaller study than would be performed in practice.

	Observations			Total
Sample 1	5.6	5.7	5.4	16.7
Sample 2	3.0	2.9	2.9	8.8
Sample 3	7.4	7.3	7.2	21.9
Sample 4	6.1	5.9	6.3	18.3
			Grand total	65.7

(a) Correction term

$$C = \frac{65.7^2}{4 \times 3} = 359.708$$

(b) Between-samples sum of squares

$$SSB = \frac{16.7^2 + 8.8^2 + 21.9^2 + 18.3^2}{3} - 359.708$$

$$= 30.569$$

(c) Total sum of squares

$$SST = (5.6^2 + 5.7^2 + \ldots + 6.3^2) - 359.708 = 30.722$$

(d) Error sum of squares

$$SSE = 30.722 - 30.569 = 0.153$$

where 4 is the number of samples and 3 is the number of replicates

(e) Analysis of variance table

Source of variation	Degrees of freedom	Sum of squares (SSQ)	Mean square
Between-samples	3	30.569	10.190
Error	8	0.153	0.019
Total	11	30.722	

where between-samples d.f. is one less than the number of samples and the error d.f. is the number of samples multiplied by one less than the number of replicates.

(f) *F* statistic

$$F = \frac{10.190}{0.019} = 531.64$$

(g) Between replicate $CV = \frac{\sqrt{\text{Error MSQ}}}{65.7/4 \times 3} \times 100\%$
$$= 2.529\%$$

where 4 is the number of samples and 3 is the number of replicates.

(h) The value of *F* is referred to tables (4) with d.f. values appropriate to the numerator and denominator.

Appendix 4.C: Regression, *t* tests and analysis of variance

Effect of dilution

The effect of dilution is tested by making replicate measurements on a series of dilutions of packed cells and plasma. In the example below a concentration of 10% represents 10 parts cells to 90 parts plasma by volume. For simplicity three replicate values are analysed though it would be usual to make more replicate analyses.

Concentration (%)	Hb (g/dl)		
10	2.1	1.8	1.9
20	4.6	4.6	4.8
30	7.6	7.6	7.5
40	10.2	10.2	10.2
50	12.8	12.6	12.7
60	15.5	15.6	15.5
70	18.2	17.8	18.0
80	20.3	20.4	20.5
90	22.9	22.9	23.0
100	25.3	25.6	25.5

The zero point is not included in the analysis if the instrument is unable to record a negative value. From the concentration values (x), taken for simplicity to range from 1 to 10, the Hb values (y) and the total number of observations (N) calculate:

$$N = 30 \qquad \Sigma x = 165 \qquad \Sigma x^2 = 1155$$
$$\Sigma y = 418.2 \qquad \Sigma y^2 = 7512.36 \qquad \Sigma xy = 2945.2$$

The linear fit, $y = a + bx$, can then be derived:

Term $1 = \Sigma xy - \Sigma x \Sigma y/N) = 645.1$
Term $2 = \Sigma x^2 - (\Sigma x \Sigma x/N) = 247.5$
Term $3 = \Sigma y^2 - (\Sigma y \Sigma y/N) = 1682.652$
$b = $ Term $1/$Term $2 = 2.6065$
$a = (\Sigma y/N) - (b\Sigma x/N) = -0.39556$

To assess whether the relationship is linear it is necessary to compare the variance for deviation from the regression with the between-replicate variance which is estimated as in Appendix 4.B by treating each dilution as a sample so giving:
Between-replicate

Sum of squares (SSQ) $= 0.26$
Degrees of freedom (d.f.) $= u(n-1) = 20$
Variance $= $ SSQ/d.f. $= 0.013$

where u is the number of dilutions and n is the number of replicates.
Then calculate:
Deviation of the mean at each dilution from regression line

SSQ $= $ term $3 - $ between-replicate SSQ $- ((\text{term } 1)^2/\text{term } 2) = 0.96166$
$d.f. = u - 2 = 8$
Variance $= $ SSQ/d.f. $= 0.1202$
Variance ratio $= F = 0.1202/0.013 = 9.246$ with 8 and 20 d.f.

Since this value of F means $P < 0.01$ one can conclude that the relationship is not linear and the analysis is then terminated. If the value of F had meant that $P > 0.05$ there would have been no evidence of departure from linearity and one should than test whether:

$a = 0$ if the magnitude of the variable should be proportional to dilution and have a zero intercept,

e.g. Hb, or

$b = 0$ if the magnitude of the variable should be independent of dilution having a zero slope, e.g. MCV.

To test whether a or b is zero a Student's t-test can be used as follows:

$$t = \frac{a}{s}\sqrt{\left(\frac{\text{term } 2}{\Sigma x^2/N}\right)}$$

$$t = \frac{b}{s}\sqrt{\text{term } 2}$$

where s is the square root of the variance about the regression line. The value of t has $(N-2)$ degrees of freedom and s is calculated from:

$$s = \sqrt{[(\text{term } 3 - (b \times \text{term } 1))/(N-2)]}$$

To test whether $b=1$, substitute $b-1$ for b in the above Student's t-test (From ICSH, 1984, with permission.)

5

Internal Quality Control

5.1 Quantitative Assays

I Cavill

Introduction

The aim of any clinical laboratory providing a service to patients is to ensure that the right results are produced for the right patient at the (clinically) right time (5). In the early days of haematology this was brought about by the personal and individual attention to each sample and request of the consultant and a small band of laboratory staff. In the last three decades, however, the explosive increase in workload demanded of the laboratory has meant that the laboratory must increasingly resort to mass production techniques. The problem for the laboratory is to increase its capacity to deal with this workload without sacrificing the quality of its service. By using automated equipment to deal with as high a proportion of the workload as possible the haematologist will have more time to devote to those problems which demand personal attention. At the same time, however, this hands the responsibility for the technical production of results over to a machine. In order for the haematologist to be able to have confidence in such an impersonal system the machine's performance must be continually monitored. Thus quality control becomes a vital part of the strategy by which the laboratory copes with the increasing and increasingly varied demand placed upon it.

This chapter will deal with the means by which the production of quantitative analysis of results from samples presented to the laboratory may be monitored in the laboratory in real laboratory time. It must be emphasized that the aim of this internal quality control is not just to detect faults. Rather, it is to put the stamp of approval on what, with modern technology, is likely to be a very reliable result–producing service. By making the assessment of the quality of the data an objective process it removes the need for the laboratory staff to be forever hovering anxiously over the outgoing results. A proper and effective system of internal quality control thus allows the full benefits of automation to be achieved. It must, however, be recognized that the validity of any result is only as good as the quality of the sample. If the sample is in any way unsatisfactory, no amount of quality control can possibly rectify this. Similarly, and more importantly, if the sample is wrongly labelled a perfectly valid result may be attributed to the wrong patient. The potentially disastrous consequences of this are most evident in the blood bank but apply equally to all other investigations. Thus the total quality of the service starts at the bedside and ends with the clinician's interpretation of the results (see p. 2), and cannot be restricted to international quality controls alone.

Standardization

Haematological analysis is based largely on quantitation of cells, cellular constituents and cell characteristics. This presents a particular problem for standardization as there are very few standards available to the haematologist, and the laboratory must rely heavily on comparison with peer groups for this purpose. Inter-laboratory quality control, as practised through external quality assessment schemes, provides a means by which widely distributed laboratories may achieve an appropriate degree of sameness (see Chapter 8). There is no guarantee that either the mean, median or mode of any selection of laboratories will correspond with the *true* answer for any test parameter and it must be recognized that it is quite likely that in some circumstances laboratories may 'standardize' on the same incorrect value. However, the starting point for internal quality control is participation in an appropriate external quality assessment scheme.

Methodologies

Once the laboratory's compass has been set by the use of such standards as are available, and by the external schemes, the aim is to maintain a steady course on that setting. The first and most important element in achieving this is to ensure that methods do not deviate from the established procedure. It is difficult to over-emphasize the importance of having written standard operating procedures. There is no activity within the laboratory which is too trivial for such treatment. Bitter experience has shown that without strict adherence to a well-founded operating procedure a succession of marginal, unrecorded modifications made on the spur of a particular moment can, in a matter of months, transform a sound methodology into something quite different.

It has been very sensibly suggested (7) that the safest way of achieving this sort of control is to produce a detailed and itemized standard operating procedure which, if amended, should be clearly identified as such. Any amendments should be specific, dated and signed. The value of this in tracking down any cause of deviation in the quality of results is invaluable. In addition, it is prudent to keep a log book of all manipulations, changes of reagents and machine failures. This can then be related to the maintenance programme, which should itself be specified in advance. Adherence to a standard operating and maintenance procedure will avoid the problem of unintentional, or even intentional, modification of methods. It is not sufficient simply to refer to a published method because its local application will undoubtedly require minor modifications each of which will be important and variation of which may nullify the whole.

Quality control

A systematic approach to the problem of controlling the quality of any variable was born out of industrial development and automation (1). The concepts and techniques developed 40 or more years ago in industry can be applied with equal success to the numerical output of laboratories. In essence, all quality control schemes are predicated on the notion that some quantifiable aspect of the particular process will remain stable in the absence of any change in that process. This concept is referred to as the **process mean** and is usually directly equated with the characteristics of the particular product. This stability will not, however, be absolute and whether the product is nylon fibre or a blood count there will be random variation about some underlying process mean. However, in a stable process the data will be random variation about some underlying process mean. However, in a stable process the data will show no more variability over a prolonged time span than would be expected if the measurements were made repeatedly at one time.

In the haematological context the application of this concept is not quite as straightforward as in a factory. The individual products of the process, the patients' results, will themselves vary, not because there is any moment-to-moment variation in the underlying process mean but because patients are different from one another! In addition to this patient variation, the results will also contain an element which is attributable to variation in the underlying analytical process. The problem for the laboratory is thus to separate this analytical process variability from the inherent variability in the patient samples. The solution to this particular problem can take one of two forms. The first depends upon the identification of some aspect of patients' results which will remain stable whatever the nature of those results. The second depends upon including further samples which will be independent of any patient-to-patient variation in the analytical process. The target mean for these control samples will then be equated with the process mean, and variation in the control samples will allow the process mean to be monitored. This fundamental divide in the approaches to quality control in the haematology laboratory is independent of any method for analysing either the patient data or control data. While different analytical techniques have become associated with these processes it would be wrong to associate them directly with either the analysis of patient or control samples. Indeed, it may be appropriate to apply any of the statistical techniques to either patient data or control data.

It is important to realize that where control preparations are used these must not be confused with calibrating materials (see Chapters 5.4 and 9). There is no sense in trying to search for the true value of any parameter in a control material. Indeed, because the controls must remain stable with time they must be treated in such a way as to preserve the blood cells. This will itself make the control sample quite unlike the fresh sample and would render it unsuitable for standardization by any of the old manual methods for blood cell counting. When such preserved materials are assayed they may well give different answers in different machines even though the fresh blood samples analysed on each machine may give identical results. Further, for a number of haematological parameters there may be no such thing as the true answer. The mean cell volume, for example, is simply a measurement of the relative size of the red cell balloon in particular circumstances and after a particular time of exposure to a lysing agent. None of the measurements made in automated cell counters, nor indeed any estimate based on more manual, *in vitro* measurements, will necessarily reflect the size of the red cell *in vivo*.

Automated blood cell counters

The major demand of a haematology laboratory is for good reliable blood cell counts. Modern automated counters, whether based on cell impedance or laser light scattering, are becoming increasingly stable and reliable. This technological sophistication should not, however, blind the laboratory to the need to maintain a continuous programme of performance-monitoring. This is necessary not only to detect those occasions when machine performance changes, but also to certify that any result issued from the laboratory has been positively verified as having come from a machine which can be shown to have been in control. This will not mean, however, that a result produced on one patient on one day will be exactly the same as that on the same patient on another day. All the blood count parameters are subject to a degree of normal *in vivo* variation and this biological variation will affect both normal and pathological samples. The magnitude of this variation will determine the degree to which the laboratory must aim to control variation in the blood counting apparatus itself. In general it will be profitable for the laboratory to aim to control machine variation so that it is less than biological variation. Of course, if the parameter is to be of any value in detecting pathology, the sum of both biological and machine variation must be less than that seen between normal and pathological samples.

Control materials

The desirable attributes of any control medium are easy to define. It should behave in the same way as fresh patient material, it should be stable over a reasonably long time (weeks rather than days), and it should be readily available. While laboratories may well also wish that it should be inexpensive this is not a necessary attribute! The aim must be to have functionally adequate control material and laboratories should regard this as a necessary and valued reagent, not a desirable cost-free adjunct. After all, there is no economic sense in installing an expensive and sophisticated automated analyser and then producing unreliable results. The direct cost, not to mention the consequential costs that litigation may bring, of uncontrolled results would far exceed that of any control material. It may be worth looking on the provision of control material as insurance against such consequences.

Control media for automated blood counters divide into two categories, patient samples or stabilized cellular materials. For other haematological assays the appropriate materials may also be patient–derived material. When extra samples or larger volumes are taken from patients for this purpose this can only be done if the ethics of the donation are properly covered. In addition, where sera are stored for use at a later date it will be necessary to ensure that they do not present any infective problems to those who may use them without any knowledge of the specific source.

Patient samples

Despite the individual variation between patients' results it has been shown that the mean value for the red cell parameters, MCV, MCH and MCHC, remain remarkably similar across the globe (2). This led to the development of the notion that subsets drawn from within the local population should also produce mean estimates which would be normally distributed about the mean of the whole population. The subset means should thus approximate to the population mean and the mean calculated from successive samples of the population should remain stable. It was estimated that in practice a batch size of 20 would be appropriate. This appeared to be generally true for the red cell indices, MCV, MCH and MCHC. Bull *et al.* (4), in the pioneering study in this field, found that the stability of the subpopulations was enhanced when a running geometric mean was calculated rather than a simple arithmetic mean. However, the validity of this approach is dependent upon the 20 patients selected for each batch being a representative subset of the whole population. This may require active randomization of the samples. It certainly requires strict adherence to the rule that no more than one-third of any 20 patients' samples should come from a chemotherapy clinic, a group of iron–deficient patients or a unit where abnormal red cell indices are particularly common. Where this cannot be strictly adhered to there will be variations in the mean for each batch of 20 patient samples which will reflect changes in the sample rather than changes in the underlying process mean. As it is only the latter that is of interest to the laboratory as far as quality control is concerned, it is clear that failure to randomize and select correctly the patient samples to be analysed by the Bull algorithm will invalidate the use of patient results as a control medium.

Control samples

Preserved whole–blood material which mimics the behaviour of fresh blood samples is available from the manufacturers of the major automated cell counters. These will usually allow haemoglobin concentration, the red cell parameters, the white cell count and platelet count to be monitored. The degree to which these materials simulate fresh blood is sometimes limited and 'embalmed' blood may introduce variables into the system which do not reflect machine performance with fresh whole–blood samples (8).

While these materials might clearly be labelled for use as a control they are often expensive and this is a natural disincentive to their frequent use in the routine procedure. As a result many laboratories have either individually or collectively prepared their own material. Originally these materials were designed for the now relatively simple Coulter S counter (14, 15). This formulation has subsequently been modified to take account of the different characteristics of more modern counters and in particular to allow the platelet count to be monitored (13) although the material is not suitable for use in the Technicon family of instruments.

Where one laboratory takes on the task of preparing large volumes of control material the problem of maintaining homogeneity and sterility must be dealt with. It is essential that when distributing a medium such as blood the efficacy of the mixing process is tested by taking sample aliquots at a rate of about 1 in 50 and measuring the blood cell counts ten times in each sample. The variation between the sample means should not exceed that of the variation within the samples themselves. This may be assessed by a simple *F*-test. Although these materials are usually prepared in a sterile manner and suspended in a bacteriostatic medium the ubiquitous *Pseudomonas* is an ever-present problem. There are, indeed, strains of *Pseudomonas* which clearly flourish in glutaraldehyde at 0–4°C. These will produce gradual changes in the MCV and will render the material useless as a control. In our own laboratory we culture samples taken from the control batch and ensure its sterility before it is issued to laboratories.

Analytical techniques

Where the control medium is based on random patient samples then the control of the blood count data must be exercised indirectly through the red cell indices. These parameters may be analysed using a statistical averaging technique and of these the algorithm derived by Bull *et al.* (4) is the best known. The data from 15–20 patients, not more than one-third of whom should come from any particular source and whose red cell indices appear to lie within 'normal limits', should form the basis for each batch in the algorithm. This Bull algorithm has the property of minimizing the effect of variation within the sample and as the running mean progresses this tends to increase the stability of the parameter. In the scheme proposed by Bull and Korpman (3) this running mean is simply compared with a target for the population. This target may be an estimate of the true population mean for normal subjects either from a particular laboratory or from previously-determined worldwide data (2).

The algorithm which they derived was:

$$\bar{X}_{B,i} = \bar{X}_{B,i-1} + \mathrm{sgn}\left(\sum_{j=1}^{N} \mathrm{sgn}\ (X_{ji} - \bar{X}_{B,i-1}) \sqrt{(|X_{ji} - \bar{X}_{B,i-1}|)} \right) \times$$

$$\frac{\left(\sum_{j=1}^{N} \mathrm{sgn}(X_{ji} - \bar{X}_{B,i-1}) \sqrt{(|X_{ji} - \bar{X}_{B,i-1}|)} \right)^2}{N}$$

Although this expression may appear complex it is basically and functionally quite simple. The nomenclature is based on considering 20 samples within a succession of batches. The samples are numbered 1–20 but in the generalized expression are called j. Similarly the batches are numbered in sequence and the batch number is designated as i in the expression. It is easiest to approach the expression backwards, starting with the term contained within the right-hand brackets. This is simply the difference between the patient result for the jth sample in the ith batch and the geometric mean for the previous batch. The vertical lines around this term indicate that this difference is taken without regard to its sign. Only by treating this as positive is it then possible to take the square root of that difference. This has the immediate effect of trimming the data by minimizing the disruptive effect of any single deviant value. The sign of the difference is then simply given back to the square root of the difference by the term sgn $(X_{ji} - \bar{X}_{B,i-1})$. Although it may seem a long way around this is just an arithmetic device to get the square root of the difference between the current result and the previous mean. These differences can then be added together. The sign of this sum then reflects the distribution of results which are greater or less than the previous mean. This sum is then squared and divided by the number of samples in the batch. The result is a value which is a measure of the average deviation of the patients' results from the previous mean. This value is, of course, always positive. Whether it is to be either added or subtracted from that previous mean is determined by the term contained within the left-hand pair of brackets. This can be seen to be similar to that in the right-hand pair except that the square roots of the individual deviations are summed without being squared or averaged. It is basically the sum of the square roots of the deviations in which the sign, $+$ or $-$, is retained but the rest is discarded. Finally the average deviation with its sign is added to the previously established geometric mean, $\bar{X}_B$, for the batch before the current ith batch, i.e. batch $i-1$, to produce the new mean $\bar{X}_{B,i}$. The square root element of the calculation trims the data while building up a running mean from an initial population mean and the subsequent deviations have an additional smoothing or stabilizing effect. All in all, the effect of any individual result is minimized in an attempt to extract the underlying current estimate of the population mean.

This approach aims to keep the variation in the running mean to within ±3% of the population mean value. Deviations greater than 3% produce characteristic patterns which by logic and previous experience may allow the machine operator to infer which principle parameter has changed and the nature of that change (3). This, of course, is a relatively simple approach and it may well be that the running mean produced by the algorithm could be equally effectively assessed using other statistical trend analysis techniques. A modification of this method of analysis, based on detecting consistent changes of 2%, has been applied to $\bar{X}_B$ data to enhance its sensitivity to smaller changes and has been included in an appropriate multirule scheme (12).

Changes in machine performance may be of two basic types. The first is a sudden jump in some attribute. If this change persists it will be detected by that change manifesting itself in the results for any control samples that are included in the routine procedure. However, if it is not a persistent change and if the counter quickly reverts to the previous state it may remain undetected. The chance of detecting such a change is then directly related to the frequency with which controls are included in the routine procedure. Where a change is persistent it is susceptible to detection by a number of methods of trend analysis. The detection of stepwise changes is clearly made easier the larger and more prominent they are. Small changes demand a more sophisticated approach which, at its extreme, is equivalent to that for the detection of the second type of change: that is, a steadily incremental change which begins at a minimally detectable level and progresses to the frank and easily detectable level comparable to a large stepwise change.

It is in the interest of the laboratory to be able to detect either small persistent or incremental changes before they become clinically significant. In that way the laboratory can avoid the consequences of a simplistic approach to quality control where change is only detected once it has become significant. With such a procedure it will be necessary to halt the procedure until the fault is detected and corrected. It may also be necessary to recall, amend or delete results that have been issued. In the strategy which we have adopted this is not necessary and the aim is to detect any nascent change early enough so that the analytical process may continue uninterrupted. Laboratory control procedures can then be seen as a means of validating and assisting the production and issue of results rather than as a simple negative fault-finding exercise.

A detailed comparison of a wide range of control rules and procedures has been undertaken largely in relation to chemical pathology but apply equally to haematology (17). The optimum approach to different laboratory demands recognizes the advantages of a 'multirule' scheme (9). However, it is clear that one technique above all others is more powerful and more effective at detecting either persistent small changes or incremental changes. That is the CUSUM analysis of control data (see below).

The earliest rule devised for quality control was that of Shewhart (16). This seminal work is frequently attributed to 'Levey Jennings' as a result of the application of the Shewhart method to clinical laboratories (11). Using this method the data are plotted graphically against time. When the process is in control then the result will be seen to oscillate about the mean value for the control sample. Moreover, the majority of the results will lie within ±1 SD of that mean and less than 5% will exceed the mean ±2 SD. Shewhart proposed drawing warning lines and action lines on this chart. Each warning line is generally located at a level which only 1 in 40 of the results may exceed when there is no change in the underlying mean. If the data are normally distributed about the control mean this will be equal to ±2 SD. That is, for every 40 control samples one may be expected to lie above that line and one may be expected below that line. If the frequency with which control results lie outside the warning lines is greater than 1 in 40 this may be taken as a warning to the operator that the process is becoming more variable than heretofore. Action lines in this scheme commonly correspond to the points outside which only 1 in 1000 control results would be found by chance alone. If these limits are breached more frequently then it is a clear indication that either the mean may have changed or the process has become more variable. If two or more results in succession are outside the same limit then it is clear that the process mean has changed.

The Shewhart approach has the virtue of great simplicity. It is, however, relatively inefficient in that decisions are based on only the most recent data values. The magnitude of the change that can be detected may be large and this may also limit the use of this method in detecting small pre-symptomatic changes but at least gross faults will not be missed. This approach has been most comprehensively evaluated by the power function analysis of Westgard and Groth (17) and, from a specifically haematological point of view, by Hackney *et al.* (9). These studies emphasize the relatively high probability of false rejection at low levels of systematic or random error and the high error level needed to achieve a probability of detection greater than 0.5. This remains true even when more elaborate rules are applied such as would indicate a violation if two out of the last three control observations were beyond either the same or the opposite 2 SD limits.

In all these analyses it is important to realize that the SD of the control data must be established in the laboratory concerned. The use of the control limits supplied by the manufacturer of the material is inappropriate. These limits usually refer to the range of mean results that may be expected if a large number of laboratories assay the material. This range of values will be considerably greater than those which should be found in an individual laboratory where the variation is about only one of those mean values. In establishing the laboratory mean and standard deviation it is important to derive the estimate from analyses carried out over a number of days. Thus the variation should reflect that which might be expected not only within the day but between days. Where this between-day variation is significant the analyses should be spread over 5 and preferably 10 days.

CUSUM analyses

Where the detection of small but sustained changes in a target level are important then the cumulative sum (CUSUM) analysis has major advantages (1). As an arithmetic procedure it is perhaps even simpler than the Shewhart analysis and it is certainly less complex than any other algorithm. It consists simply of adding the successive differences between the control value and its target. These differences are summed taking regard of the sign so that results that fall persistently above the target value will produce larger and larger cumulative sums. Conversely, results which consistently fall below the target value will produce an increasingly negative cumulative sum. Where the deviation is randomly distributed about the target mean then positive and negative deviations will cancel out and the cumulative sum will oscillate around zero.

In functional terms this arithmetic process is a way of enhancing the informative signal and suppressing background noise. By subtracting the mean from the data the variation about the mean is allowed to stand out in its own right. By enhancing the impact of this variation the CUSUM technique can be used as a sensitive indicator of pre-symptomatic change. It is, however, no more than a tool or instrument for seeing change more easily – the arithmetic equivalent of the microscope – and not an end in itself. It should be tailored to the requirements of each laboratory and to the size of the change that is to be detected for each assay procedure according to the methodological limitations and clinical requirements of each parameter. In general the detection sensitivity should be based upon the standard deviation for the method, but in some circumstances modern automated counters are so consistent that this would be inappropriately small. In this case it is better to base the definition of the level of variation that will be accepted on the clinical significance of different magnitudes of change. The aim should be to detect a consistent change which is well within any clinically significant variation.

The original approach to CUSUM analysis was graphical but, in a busy laboratory and with automated counters producing a large number of parameters, plotting either control data or cumulative sums on graph paper is just not possible. Numerical analysis is not only necessary from this point of view but also because it allows the laboratory to set objective rules for the implementation of the scheme. If a scheme is well founded it will indicate either that the laboratory may safely continue to produce results or that there is a need to return to the calibrating material. This objectivity removes the need for laboratory staff to agonize over the control data.

The decision interval analysis of CUSUM data is operationally simple and eminently amenable to computer analysis. The first step in this process is to define the sensitivity of the application (15). This means that the machine variation of all the results issued by the laboratory will be less than this figure. This is usually equal to 2 SD for the particular method. However, because successive samples coming in to the laboratory from the same patient will be affected by biological as well as machine variation the maximum difference between successive samples on the same unchanging patient may be much greater, and more practical values may be selected.

The decision interval scheme defines a narrow band about the mean which is limited by the upper and lower reference values (URV and LRV). As long as control results lie within these reference values no action is taken. These values are defined as half the minimum significant change (C) which the laboratory wishes to detect. Thus, if the mean value of the control material $= m$, then $URV = m + (C/2)$ and $LRV = m - (C/2)$. When either of these reference values is reached, a CUSUM is calculated about whichever value was transgressed. This CUSUM is continued either until it returns to zero or until it exceeds the previously determined decision interval (DI). The decision interval is $1.3 \times$ the minimum significant change to be detected. At this level of sensitivity the scheme will detect that change within three control samples of it taking place. It will only falsely indicate a change once in every 500 samples. Single large changes will produce a CUSUM greater than the decision interval in one step and thereby indicate immediate loss of control. Abrupt changes may also be monitored by following the sign of the CUSUM. When this goes from $+$ to $-$ or *vice versa* it is prudent to increase the rate at which the control samples are analysed. If three control samples are then analysed consecutively, either the change will be confirmed or the cause for concern will be eliminated. Although this method is ideally suited for automation, either on a laboratory computer or as an integral part of the blood count analyser, it may nevertheless be used manually (15).

Reproducibility

All the systems considered thus far monitor the underlying process mean. This is related to, but separate from, any consideration of the reproducibility of the counters. Indeed if the apparatus is not stable then any attempt to monitor the mean will be confounded. In practice all modern automated counters are highly reproducible and it is for this reason that this important aspect can be relegated to a relatively minor consideration. Nevertheless, there will be occasions when the laboratory may suspect that blood counters are malfunctioning in such a way as to impair their reproducibility. These occasions may be indicated by increased oscillation in the control results and this can be checked by calculating the variance over the last 20 controls and comparing it with the variance calculated initially. In addition, some laboratories may gain extra confidence by repeating the analysis of some samples. The differences between these duplicate analyses should be analysed and again the variance of this may be calculated and compared with the variance calculated from the initial control value.

Another approach that has been adopted is to look at successive results from the same patient. This is sometimes described as delta (Δ or δ) checking. It is particularly inappropriate as a quality control procedure in hospitals where patients are being actively treated or where some clinical intervention may result in a change in the patient's blood count. Establishing a sophisticated automated data-processing system in the laboratory to recognize a consecutive result from the same patient and to calculate the differences between the two is pointless if, for example, one sample was pre- and the other post-operative. Indeed, it could well be argued that if a high proportion of patients' results do not differ on successive occasions then there must be real doubt as to the clinical need for these repeated blood counts.

Of course it is obviously sensible to ensure that the results produced by the automated apparatus are consistent with the patient's condition, but the clinician should not be too ready to ascribe any inconsistency to machine malfunctions. An unusual result may well be correct for a particular sample but if that sample had been mislabelled and was from another patient it would indicate the need for quality control closer to the bedside. In addition, an inexplicable result produced from a correctly taken and identified sample and produced on a counter which was demonstrably in control should not be dismissed. An inconvenient result may well be right and perhaps it should form the basis for developing a new understanding of the situation.

Batched assays

Thus far, discussion has centred on automated blood counting and its control. All other activities of the laboratory are equally worth controlling. However, not all of these have reached the same systematic level and qualitative investigations must be handled individually. The measurement of serum vitamin B_{12}, folate and ferritin epitomizes the problems of controlling quantitative assays which are carried out in batches. It is difficult in such assays to treat the results as one continuum and a modification of the procedure used for automated counters is required. The first step is to ensure, particularly where radioactive isotopes are used, that the individual measurements are sufficiently precise. This means that in order to achieve a reproducibility of $\pm 3\%$ it is necessary to collect at least 1000 counts for each sample, including the background count. Wherever possible, machines should be set to collect the same total number of counts from each sample rather than setting a fixed counting time regardless of activity. If samples are counted for a fixed time but with different total counts, it will be necessary to weight the results to take account of the different accuracy of each estimate. It is particularly important that there is a statistically significant difference between the background activity and the activity of the lowest standard.

The strategy that we have adopted is to insert control samples regularly throughout each batch (10). These control data are then assessed for each batch to ensure a maximum variation of less than 10%. This is a measure and an indication of the reproducibility of the assay across the batch as a whole. If there is any heterogeneity indicated in the controls or any progressive change across the run then the batch as a whole must be discarded. If the batch is acceptable, the mean of the controls for that batch is calculated. This mean is then assessed by the same CUSUM technique as used for the routine blood count. The variation which is tolerated in the mean is defined by the standard deviation of the reproducibility of the assay method. This is established when the assays are introduced but is remeasured every time any significant alteration in the procedure is introduced. Although a coefficient of variation of 5% is the aim, this may not always be achievable and in the ferritin assay 10% is the norm.

Conclusion

It is important that every laboratory operates a system of quality control and this should be particularly active for automated blood counters. The choice of control materials and the means by which these are analysed can only be decided in the light of local circumstances. Where patient samples are used and the data is analysed by the Bull algorithm the strict rules for the inclusion and randomization of data must be observed. Indeed, every laboratory proposing to use this approach must first establish the local validity of the approach. In many hospital service laboratories, where there is a high proportion of abnormal counts and insufficient time to select samples and to randomize the order of analysis, this approach will not be applicable (6). The European Committee for Clinical Laboratory Standards has identified the use of control material analysed by the CUSUM technique as a standard approach to internal quality control (6). The development and supply of stabilized control material which is suitable for modern automated cell counts may still present problems. In these cases laboratories should continue to press manufacturers to ensure that control material is readily available. This is just as important as the ability to produce yet another fascinating parameter and should be considered as an integral part of any automation package.

Finally, it is not sufficient for a laboratory to operate an effective system of quality control and then to rest on its laurels. The system must be clearly documented, diligently operated and, above all, its existence made known to the users of the laboratory. It is, after all, they who must have confidence in the data which they use.

References

1. Bissell, A. F. (1982). Statistical foreword. In Cavill, I. (ed.) *Quality Control: Methods in Haematology*, Vol. 4, pp. 1–12. Edinburgh and New York: Churchill Livingstone.
2. Bull, B. S. and Hay, K. L. (1985). Are red blood indices international? *Archives of Pathology and Laboratory Medicine* 109: 604–606.
3. Bull, B. S. and Korpman, R. A. (1982). Intralaboratory quality control using patients' data. In Cavill, I. (ed.) *Quality Control: Methods in Haematology*, Vol. 4, pp. 121–150. Edinburgh and New York: Churchill Livingstone.
4. Bull, B. S., Elashoff, R. M., Heilbron, D. C. and Couperus, J. (1974). A study of various estimators for the derivation of quality control procedures from patient erythrocyte indices. *American Journal of Clinical Pathology* 61: 473–481.
5. Cavill, I., Ricketts, C. and Jacobs, A. (1975). *Computers in Haematology*, p. 9. London and Boston: Butterworths.
6. ECCLS (1987). Standard for Quality Assurance. Part 4: Internal Quality Control in Haematology. ECCLS Document Vol. 4 No. 2. Berlin and Koln: Beuth Verlag.
7. Fowler, J. S. L. (1982). Quality control of batch assays. In Cavill, I. (ed.) *Quality Control in Haematology*, Vol. 4, pp. 87–101. Edinburgh and New York: Churchill Livingstone.
8. Gibson, J. M. (1985). Quality control of automated cellular analyses – the fallibility of embalmed blood. *Blood Cells* 11: 301–307.
9. Hackney, J. R., Cembrowski, G. and Carey, J. (1988). Quality control in the haematology laboratory. In Cembrowski, G. (ed.) *The Essential Guide to Quality Control*. ASCP Press.
10. Jones, B. M. (In press). Quality control of ferritin assays. In *Quality Control II. Methods in Haematology*, Vol. 18.
11. Levey, S. and Jennings, E. R. (1950). The use of control charts in clinical laboratories. *American Journal of Clinical Pathology* 20: 1059–1066.
12. Levy, W. C., Hay, K. L. and Bull, B. S. (1986). Preserved blood versus patient data for quality control – Bulls algorithm revisited. *American Journal of Clinical Pathology* 85: 719–721.
13. Morgan, L. O. and Hunt, J. (1984). A whole blood control for Coulter electronic particle counters. *Medical Laboratory Sciences* 41: 209–218.
14. Morgan, L. O., Jones, W. G., Fisher, J. and Cavill, I. (1978). A whole blood control for the Coulter Model S. *Journal of Clinical Pathology* 31: 50–53.
15. Ricketts, C. (1982). Intralaboratory quality control using control samples. In Cavill, I. (ed.) *Quality Control: Methods in Haematology*, Vol. 4, pp. 151–172. Edinburgh and New York: Churchill Livingstone.
16. Shewhart, W. A. (1931). *Economic Control of Quality of Manufactured Products*. New York: van Nostrand.
17. Westgard, J. O. and Groth, T. (1979). Power functions for statistical control rules. *Clinical Chemistry* 25: 863–869.

5.2 Blood Films and Differential Counting

K C Carstairs

There is no laboratory test so informative on a vast range of clinical conditions as the examination of a blood film. This is especially true if film, equipment and observer are of high quality and clinician has been astute enough to reveal the clinical problem. The test is not cheap but the two main items of equipment, microscope and morphologist, can both work for decades if not too much abused.

Reporting a blood film is dependent on human judgement. Although there are computerized pattern recognition devices no manufacturer claims a complete film analysis. Every human component is different and changes from hour to hour: boredom, fatigue, distractions, fear of error, desire to please, all affect the output. Probably many know morphologists who rush headlong to the dramatic diagnosis and others who cannot make a firm statement. It is impracticable to have every film examined by a panel of experts, so how is one to exert quality control over such complexity? The answer is simple: it cannot be done. What can be achieved is a set of circumstances which will increase the likelihood of success. It is attention to detail which ensures high quality of blood film reporting and white cell differential counting, the latter frequently being the more time-consuming and less informative portion.

Sample

Blood may be capillary, venous or arterial. If capillary, blood must be free flowing before collection: 'milking' must be avoided. Contamination with skin cleanser should be prevented. No matter how skilled the operator, platelet aggregation and clotting soon occur and it is essential to make the film expeditiously. Alternatively, blood may be collected drop by drop in commercially available 200–500 µl containers with EDTA (e.g. Becton–Dickinson 'Microtainers').

For routine venepuncture samples the universally preferred anticoagulant is a sodium or potassium salt of EDTA. The tripotassium salt is popular because of its high solubility, but for the morphologist it matters little which is used; what is important is that sufficient but not excessive anticoagulant is effectively present. The amount of anticoagulant needed will vary with the salt used. Approximately 0.75–1.2 mg of

EDTA per ml is recommended (23). If blood is to be taken through an in-dwelling catheter large quantities of blood may have to be aspirated and discarded to ensure that there is no contamination by heparin or infusion fluid.

Films should be made within 6 h, preferably within 4, to avoid changes which will interfere with morphological interpretation.

Prolonged exposure to EDTA increases the risk of platelet aggregation and satellism. Both granulocytes and monocytes show increasing cytoplasmic vacuolation; polymorph nuclei may condense and become rounded, so the cells resemble erythroblasts. Platelets may swell and lose their granules. Erythrocytes may crenate to such an extent that the true morphology is entirely obscured.

Blood film

There are two classical methods for making blood films: the 'wedge' and the 'coverslip'. The second is now used in few laboratories possibly because of the difficulty of the technique, fragility of the cover glass, and problems with processing and storage. In the wedge technique a small drop of blood is placed centrally at one end of a glass slide which should be flat, of uniform thickness and completely clean. A spreader, making an angle of between 20 and 30° with the slide, is placed in front of the drop and brought back into contact with the blood which is allowed to flow evenly along the entire base of the spreader. Immediately, the spreader is moved rapidly and evenly along the slide, thereby making the film. It is important that the spreader be narrower than the slide, clean and have an absolutely smooth edge in contact with the slide. A slide with polished edges and bevelled corners makes a good spreader. If thought to be too wide, the corners can be nipped off with pliers, the new edges being smoothed with emery paper. If all has gone well, the entire drop will have been used, the film will be rectangular with little 'feathering' at the thin end and will taper uniformly in thickness from origin to tail.

The wedge film has serious drawbacks even when well made: granulocytes and monocytes are concentrated at the sides and ends of the film; there is cell damage, especially in chronic lymphocytic leukaemia; and most of the film is either too thick or too thin for good morphology. The uneven cell distribution is exaggerated when there is a delay in spreading the drop, when all the drop is not used or spreading is started before blood has flowed along the entire width of the spreader (see excellent review by Stiene-Martin, 26). Only practice will teach the correct angle and speed.

It is always difficult to make a good film when the haemoglobin concentration is high and frequently extremely difficult when it is very low. Removal of sufficient plasma to raise the haemoglobin content to normal will produce excellent red cell morphology. The slide should be prominently labelled as being made from plasma-depleted blood.

Some workers rarely make good films and clinical pathologists have constructed mechanical spreaders to lessen skill required. Geometric Data Corporation's Hemaprep was a mechanical film-maker for use with pattern-recognition machines. These films were intentionally thin and allowances had to be made for the extra target cells and spherocytes that were sometimes induced. The best method of preparing blood films uses a well designed centrifugal device resulting in a 'spun' film giving a monolayer of evenly distributed leucocytes, erythrocytes and platelets, with almost perfect morphology for all series in the entire coverslipped area. Rarely, very 'toxic' granulocytes are distorted. The beautifully preserved lymphocyte morphology in chronic lymphocytic leukaemia contrasting with the cell havoc that the wedge film causes, is but one example of the high quality of this type of preparation. One has to get used to the additional nuclear detail visible to avoid over diagnosis of lymphoproliferative disorders. Much larger numbers of intact white cells free of distortion can be examined, especially useful when there is severe leucopenia, or a very small percentage of abnormal cells. Erythrocytes are perfectly arranged for microscopy throughout, and rouleaux formation is uniform, in sharp contrast to the extreme variability present in the wedge. It is much easier to make estimates of platelet and leucocyte numbers.

Such machines were developed to facilitate the operation of the pattern recognition devices (10). Prototypes produced their own set of artefacts but these were eliminated (2, 9). Unfortunately, very few such devices are now being made.

Koepke (14) provides a table listing the advantages and disadvantages of the three main ways of making blood films and refers to published papers by Rogers (20) and Shafer (25) based on prototype equipments but these publications do not give any detailed comparisons of the three methods. The influences of various factors on the films are illustrated in Fig. 5.2.1.

Labelling

A firm link between blood film and sample is best made by a legible inscription on the slide either on a frosted area or with a reagent-proof label. It is dangerous to rely on a name and date written on the film itself because damage to the film may remove all identification. Each slide should be identified as it is made. As a minimum the slide should have patient's family name and initials, date, clinical area, laboratory accession number (this in itself provides a great deal of security) and an identification of the person making the film. All of these data can be written in an area 2.5 × 2 cm at one end of the slide. A hard lead provides less debris in the staining dish than does a soft one.

Fixation

As soon as the blood film is made it should be air-dried rapidly and fixed in methanol for 5–10 min. If methanol contains much more than 3% water much artefact will be produced (5). This may be very difficult to ensure for methanol is hygroscopic. Relief may be obtained by putting in 'tea-bags' containing Sephadex. Frequent changes of fixative, filling the fixing jar to the brim and keeping it covered by a well-fitting lid may all be required. The fixation step can be omitted when an alcohol-based stain such as Leishman's is used, but it is still essential to avoid aqueous contamination.

Staining

For a short but comprehensive review of the problems besetting users of 'Roma-

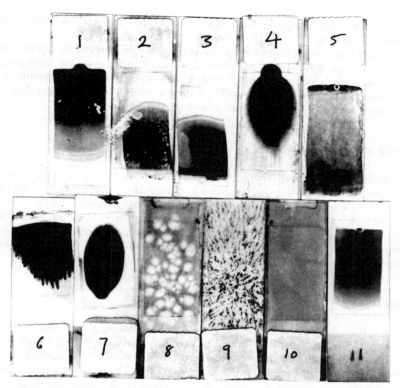

Fig. 5.2.1 A collection of blood films. (1) Made by a semi-automated spreader. (2) Film made on a dirty slide. (3) Uneven staining. (4) Too much blood and spread too soon. (5) Poor quality 'wedge' with tail almost as thick as origin. (6) Cryoglobulinaemia. (7) Poor quality film (cf. number 4) and patient had multiple myeloma. (8) Spun film, from a hyperlipaemic sample. (9) Spun film, with cold agglutinins. (10) Spun film, normal sample. (11) Reasonable quality wedge preparation.

nowsky' stains see Wittekind and Löhr (28). Marshall *et al.* (16) compared different types of commercial Romanowsky stains and also differing batches of the same stain. Grading results from 'excellent' to 'useless' they found almost as much variation between batches as between types of stain.

A stain for routine use should clearly show nuclear structure, nucleoli, demonstrate all the different types of cytoplasmic granules and permit the ready separation of mature and immature erythroid cytoplasm. Some stains are incapable of demonstrating the granules of basophils and eosinophils and should never be used. A simple staining technique is preferred over one that is complex, even if the end results are marginally more attractive. Subtleties of colouring are of little practical use. Most cell types can be easily distinguished when rendered in monochrome providing that internal structures are stained. Marshall *et al.* (17) give, as well as useful general tips, a formula for a reasonably easily prepared stable stock solution which provides all the better qualities of a Romanowsky stain. This is the basis of the ICSH reference method for standardized Romanowsky staining (11).

When small numbers of slides have to be processed excellent results can be obtained by manual staining. With large numbers some form of automation becomes preferable and the choice lies between machines which stain individual slides sequentially, e.g. Ames HemaTek, USA or batch stainers, e.g. Shandon–Elliot, UK; Sakura, Japan. The batch stainers provide a greater degree of versatility.

Coverslip and mountant

The coverslip and mountant form the front element of all but the simplest low–power lenses and as such must meet specifications as indicated by the figure 0.17 on the lens barrel showing the optimum thickness of the two in millimetres. The tolerance is 0.02 mm. Thick coverslips seriously degrade optical performance. The better the lens the more important is the coverslip. It is obvious that painting a plastic coating over the film or using a layer of immersion oil may degrade performance. Mountant should be free flowing and quick drying. It is better to use too little than too much.

The microscope

The prime function of a microscope is the demonstration, or resolution, of detail; magnification exists to facilitate this and to save eye-strain. Resolving power is a term used to define the ability of showing detail and is determined by the smallest distance between two points that can exist if the two objects are to be seen as separate. Resolving power implies nothing about the quality of the images. High resolution and poor image quality can co-exist. The numerical aperture (NA) of a lens system defines the maximum resolving power of the lens. The maximum practicable NA for visible light is 1.4, permitting a resolution of better than $0.2\,\mu m$. NA and resolution are linearly related. It is rare for the useful magnification of a microscope to exceed 1000 times the NA of the objective. With cheap optics this value is much less.

The effective NA of a lens is much affected by the condenser, which has its own NA value, controlled by the aperture diaphragm. Because the condenser's function is to focus light onto the subject there is only one correct position for it for any given slide thickness (Fig. 5.2.2). Errors in condenser setting destroy the optical properties of the objective. The condenser must be oiled to the slide to achieve NA values greater than 1.0. Fortunately, this is rarely required because most condensers are not sealed against oil! Decreasing the NA with the aperture diaphragm will cause a loss of resolution but will often enhance the image by increasing contrast and depth of field, analogous to setting a smaller *f*-stop in a camera lens. If the NA is much greater than that of the objective an undesirable veiling glare may be produced. A similar effect may occur if the field diaphragm is open too wide.

The practice of moving the condenser to control illumination shows ignorance of the function of both microscope and rheostat. Condenser performance determines the performance of the entire microscope and much care and thought should go into its purchase and use.

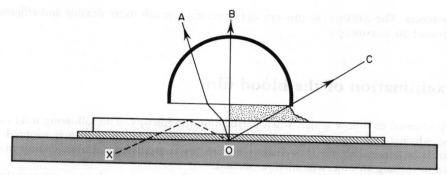

Fig. 5.2.2 Sketch to show idealized pathways of light through slide, mountant and cover-glass. O→A: Pathway for a dry lens. Angle AOB indicates a low numerical aperture and therefore low resolution. O→C: pathway for an oil-immersion lens. Angle BOC is large and therefore numerical aperture is large. O→X: light ray reflected from glass–air interface, which limits numerical aperture of a 'dry' system. Note that angle BOC can only be of maximum size if condenser is also oiled to underside of slide and has an equivalent numerical aperture.

Modern oculars can have a magnification of 12.5 × without any narrowing of the field of view and there is no longer anything to be gained from using lower-power eye-pieces unless it is to mask deficiencies in objectives or to economize.

Flat-field low power lenses with very high NA values and excellent image quality are available. For example, a plan-apochromat 40 × dry lens adjustable for different cover-glass thicknesses is available with an NA of 0.95. This value is as high as the effective working aperture of a 100 ×, NA 1.3 oil-immersion objective used with a dry condenser and partially closed aperture diaphragm. Similarly there is a flat field 25 × oil-immersion lens with NA of 0.8, a value at least twice that of an equivalent dry lens. With this lens it is easy to see basophilic stippling or trophozoites in red cells. The total magnification is 312.5, well within the maximum useful magnification of 800 × (0.8 × 1000). One can use this type of lens to perform safely and rapidly most haematological morphology. Superb lenses command high prices and it is difficult to persuade administrators to invest in such expensive equipment. Also, many morphologists cannot adapt and do not trust what they see at the low power. A compromise is to purchase a high NA 10 × or 16 × flat-field dry lens and a 40 × with NA of at least 0.6, preferably 0.95. A cheap 100 × can be bought because it will only be used to examine an individual cell, and central performance of almost any such lens will be adequate. Of course it will be essential to use good quality coverslips, small amounts of mountant and correctly adjusted condenser.

The reader should be advised that the advice to buy expensive lower power lenses and cheaper high power is not orthodox. In the manual *Hematology: Principles and Procedures* (3) it is stated that the 10 × should be used to assess the white cell count and to find anything large or unusual. Thereafter all microscopy is to be performed with the 100 × oil-immersion lens. Dacie and Lewis (5) recommend the inspection of a mounted film with the 16 mm (10 ×) lens followed by a 4 mm (dry 40 ×) or 3.5 mm (40 or 45 × oil?). Fine detail is to be examined using the 2 mm (100 ×) lens in conjunction with 6 ×

eye-pieces. The advances in modern optics permit a much more flexible and efficient approach to microscopy.

Examination of the blood film

It is essential to follow a plan when performing microscopy. The following indicates one which I and my colleagues have found efficient. Whichever plan is adopted it should be adhered to: the excitement generated by recognizing one abnormality may lead to missing an otherwise obvious second.

The film should first be examined macroscopically to confirm identity, assess quality and find diagnostic clues. Obvious defects such as clots, bad staining, dirty slides and poor technique will alert the observer to potential problems. Deep coloration may indicate hypergammaglobulinaemia, and a granular appearance may indicate red cell agglutination. Severe hyperlipidaemia gives a peculiar mottled appearance.

Next, using a low power lens gather as much information as the quality of the lens system permits. At a minimum the following should be part of a checklist: background; red cell pattern; approximate leucocyte count; approximate differential; platelets; and anything unusual. This brief list is expanded in Tables 5.2.1 and 5.2.2. If necessary the next higher power lens is used to confirm or refute impressions and extend the search for abnormalities.

The morphologist must be concentrating and working all the time, extending the search for specific abnormalities as clues are detected and looking for confirmation of earlier findings and always, always completing the local morphological protocol. Specific abnormalities may be hinted at or indicated by machine-generated data or

Table 5.2.1 Checklist of points to note in low power scan of blood film

General quality of slide, stain, and cell distributions		
Background	Colour	Hypoproteinaemia, hyperproteinaemia heparin, cryoglobulin, hyperlipidaemia, parasites
Erythrocytes	Arrangement	Agglutinates, rouleaux
	Uniformity	Anisochromia, some poikilocytes, erythroblasts
Leucocytes	Number	Number
	Quality	Rough differential
	Arrangement	Agglutinates Rosettes
Others		Possible malignant cells, histiocytes

Table 5.2.2   Checklist of points to note in higher power scan of blood film

Background	Confirmation of low power findings	
Erythrocytes	Size	Uniformity, degree of anisocytosis, separate populations
	Colour	Hypochromia, hyperchromia
	Shape	Poikilocytes, e.g. targets, spherocytes
	Inclusions	Nuclei, Howell–Jolly bodies, haemoglobin precipitates, coarse stippling, Pappenheimer bodies, parasites, bacteria
Leucocytes	Polymorphs	Hypergranulation, hypogranulation, vacuolation, bacteria, nuclear hypersegmentation or hyposegmentation, basophils, eosinophils
	Lymphocytes	Reactive, suppresser, malignant
	Monocytes	Maturity, phagocytosis
	Others	Blasts, hairy cells, unknown

clinical information. A good practice, after determining an abnormality with the high power lens, is to review it with one of lower power, so that recognition may be earlier next time.

The differential count

In 1938 Goldner and Mann emphasized that even if one could deal with a perfect sample a differential count would still be subject to the error of random sampling or the statistical error. They calculated the likely range for truth (19 times out of 20) for each value in 200 and 500 cell differentials, thus considerably anticipating the more widely quoted work of Rümke (22). Although the mathematical approaches differ, the two sets of tables are almost identical. For a value of 10 obtained for a cell class the likely range (19 times out of 20) is from 5.8 to 14.2 in a 200 count and from 7.4 to 12.6 with a 500 count. With a 100 cell differential the range is larger, 5 to 16! *By definition, in 1 of every 20 times, the result will fall outside the range.*

Much work has gone into circumventing the inherent problems of cell distribution in the wedge film (Fig. 5.2.3). Scott MacGregor *et al.* (24) made an extensive and detailed study and determined that best results were obtained by performing a battlement count along a narrow strip each side of the film. The NCCLS proposed standard (19) for leucocyte differentials recommends a broad battlement track running transversely across that area of the film best for red cell morphology. Dacie and Lewis (5) suggest counting within a strip extending the entire length of the film avoiding the edges completely. Many use a 'battlement' pathway down one side of the film.

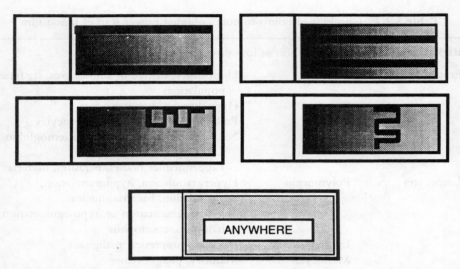

Fig. 5.2.3 The black bands indicate suggested pathways for performing white cell differentials. Top row: left, a narrow strip along each edge (24); right, two strips running parallel from end to end within the blood film (5). Middle row: left, commonly used 'battlement' path; right, transverse battlement (19). Bottom: spun film, anywhere in the entire area may be used.

Whichever technique is followed it is obvious from the above that with a 100 cell differential there will be frequent errors and many small populations of abnormal cells missed. In a spun film of blood with normal counts there will be 40–60 leucocytes per low power field. With good optics each is recognizable and so several hundred cells can be scanned before starting a formal differential.

Arkin *et al.* (1) compared scanning, i.e. a qualitative report with no formal differential, to the formal 100 cell differential. Although no details are provided on the microscopes and the 'scanners' were allowed only 1.5 min microscopy per slide to generate a complete morphology report (no mention is made of time allowed those performing the test routinely), they detected small populations of blasts in 31 of 36 opportunities, while the standard approach succeeded in only 24 of 36. The morphologist will be reassured that each differential will be much closer to 'truth' than would be expected by the mindless counting of the first 100 cells seen and that the chance of missing numerous abnormalities have been much reduced. Although 'technologists do not scan in most laboratories' (6), this must be taken as admission of poor technique, not as proper methodology.

It is axiomatic that the more cells seen the greater the opportunity to detect small populations of cells. Rock *et al.* (21) showed that by increasing the number of leucocytes counted on a pattern-recognition machine from 100 to 400, the number of slides found to have abnormal cells increased from 59 to 141 in a batch of 260. In contrast, Lewis (15) described a practical experiment in microscopy which suggested that little was gained by counting more than 300 cells.

The function of blood film microscopy is to find information useful to patient management and the formal differential is often unnecessarily detailed and wasteful of precious resources. 'Differential normal' is a report that tells the requesting clinician all that is needed, to wit that the leucocytes are normal in number, distribution and morphology. Similarly, 'Mostly neutrophils with a mild left shift and severe toxic changes' is a report not improved by adding numbers.

Machine differentials

There are five types of machine differentials: (1) three-part, and the more recently developed five-part, differentials from cell counters based on the impedance principle, as exemplified by Coulter Electronics' S-Plus series or TOA-Sysmex E series; (2) opticals with Ortho's ELT series; (3) pattern–recognition devices, e.g. from Abbott, Geometric Data, Hitachi and Omron; (4) combined optical and enzymatic analysis of Technicon's H1 equipment; and (5) the QBC centrifugation system of Becton Dickinson and Company which is intended for decentralized office use rather than for the laboratory. Most manufacturers have stopped making pattern–recognition devices and they will not be discussed further; nor will such specialized techniques as flow cytometry and surface markers.

There are, as yet, no control or calibration materials available for the differential portion of any of the above white cell differential systems and it is imperative to understand the mode of operation of one's machine and know its limitations and quirks of performance. It takes a lot of practice to get the most from the histograms. Excellent illustrated manuals are available from Coulter Electronics (7) for the S-Plus series and from American Scientific Products for the TOA E series (27).

Criteria for normality and patient population will both affect the estimation of the false negative rate for the three-part differential. In a community (non-teaching) hospital Kalish and Becker (12) showed a false negative rate of 9% while Miers *et al.* (18) give rates of 15.7–10.1% according to rules applied. Cox *et al.* (4) found five patients with acute lymphoblastic leukaemia (ALL) who had normal white cell histograms. Presumably there were similar instances with acute myeloblastic leukaemia (AML) for in the same paper they state 'no cases ... with myeloblasts that did not have an abnormality in the histogram or cell number'. ALL blasts also gave problems with the Technicon H1: all four false negatives found in 45 leukaemias were ALL (13).

The safest policy is to perform microscopy on all new patients. If any of the automated cell counters are to be used to decide what further investigation is required then any flag or abnormality should be taken as an indication to go to the microscope. The false positive rate should be accepted.

The manufacturers' recommendations for the timing of testing should be followed. Samples less than 30 min old or more than 4, 8 or 12 h old (according to machine) may not give accurate differentials.

The morphologist

How to quality control the key factor in the entire process? A good morphologist can successfully compensate for numerous deficiencies in film, staining, microscope, patient identification and clinical information. Moreover, he or she may discover something new. Morphology reports may affect patient investigation and treatment by providing information not available from any machine.

The morphologist must be thoroughly grounded in the ranges of normality and have a wide knowledge – even if some is theoretical – of pathological and artefactual changes. The morphologist must be disciplined to see what is to be seen, not what is expected or desirable, and assess correctly the possible significance of the findings. It is probable that all good morphologists enjoy their work, have an ability to recognize and dissect patterns and have enough self-assurance to commit themselves to a short and informative report (as a rule the longer the report, the less information).

Common sense, adaptability, inquisitiveness and willingness to seek other opinions are all useful attributes but which may be hard to acquire. It is possible to improve mediocre morphologists, medical or technological, by intensive exposure to pathological samples and by providing support and encouragement, but there are some that can barely cope with normals and cannot be relied upon to detect abnormals. It is better and safer to have them transferred to other duties.

It is good practice to follow up all new abnormals to ensure the validity of both findings and conclusions. Information so gathered, whether from the clinical area or from other laboratory areas should be brought back to the morphologist. Allegedly normal blood films can be retrieved on a regular basis and reviewed. Striking a balance between under- and over-reporting is extremely difficult at all skill levels. Over-reporting is the commonest problem, particularly with red cell morphology; every film shows variation in red cell size and shape to some extent and moderate increases in these variations are non-diagnostic: describing them wastes everybody's time. Most films should be reported as 'normal' or 'non-specific changes'. Then, when something useful is described the report will probably be read. The use of an extensive and easily accessible slide file is of great value in assessing the quality of reporting. Any slide may suddenly become quality control material and the original morphologist asked to justify the report. Annual collation and review of major diagnoses may also help to show unusual patterns of reporting. In-house teaching sessions and group discussions are both useful. Participation in external quality assurance programmes which use blood films are of benefit to laboratories both large and small. The larger may unexpectedly broaden their experience and the smaller gain expertise and a valuable collection of abnormals.

References

1. Arkin, C. F., Medeiros, L. J., Pevzner, L. Z., Guertin, B. P., Kobos, P. J., Phelps, J. W. and Smith, S. J. (1987). The white blood cell differential. Evaluation of rapid impression scanning versus the routine manual count. *American Journal of Clinical Pathology* **87**: 628–632.
2. Bacus, J. W. (1974). Erythrocyte morphology and centrifugal 'spinner' blood film preparations. *Journal of Histochemistry and Cytochemistry* **22**: 506–516.
3. Brown, B. A. (1984). *Hematology: Principles and Procedures* (4th edn), pp. 1–28. Philadelphia: Lea & Febiger.

4. Cox, C. J., Haberman, T. M., Payne, B. A., Klee, G. G. and Pierre, R. V. (1985). Evaluation of the Coulter Counter mode S-Plus IV. *American Journal of Clinical Pathology* **84**: 297–306.
5. Dacie, J. V. and Lewis, S. M. (1984). *Practical Haematology* (6th edn), pp. 62–83. Edinburgh: Churchill Livingstone.
6. Dutcher, T. F. (1985). Discussion in *Blood Cells* **11**: 58.
7. Gibson, J. M. (1984). *Coulter Casebook*. UK: Coulter Electronics Ltd.
8. Goldner, F. M. and Mann, W. N. (1938). The statistical error of the differential white count. *Guy's Hospital Reports* **88**: 54–65.
9. Green, J. E., Weintraub, H. A., Donnelly, B. S. and Mordecai, B. G. (1979). Sample preparation variation and its effects on automated blood cell differential analysis. *Analytical and Quantitative Cytology Journal* **1**: 187–201.
10. Ingram, M. and Minter, F. M. (1969). Semiautomatic preparation of coverglass blood smears using a centrifugal device. *American Journal of Clinical Pathology* **51**: 214–221.
11. ICSH (1984). Reference method for staining of blood and bone marrow films by azure B and eosin Y (Romanowsky stain). *British Journal of Haematology* **57**: 707–710.
12. Kalish, J. R. and Becker, K. (1986). Evaluation of the Coulter S-Plus V three-part differential in a community hospital including criteria for its use. *American Journal of Clinical Pathology* **86**: 751–755.
13. Kawarabayashi, K., Tsuda, I., Tatsumi, N. and Okuda, K. (1987). Leukemic blasts detected by H-1® blood cell counter. *American Journal of Clinical Pathology* **88**: 624–627.
14. Koepke, J. A. (1982). Differential white cell counting and the NCCLS method. In van Assendelft, O. W. and England, J. M. (eds) *Advances in Hematological Methods: the Blood Count*, pp. 99–106. Florida: CRC Press.
15. Lewis, S. M. (1985). Discussion in *Blood Cells* **11**: 182–183.
16. Marshall, P. N., Bentley, S. A. and Lewis, S. M. (1975). An evaluation of some commercial Romanowsky stains. *Journal of Clinical Pathology* **28**: 680–685.
17. Marshall, P. N., Bentley, S. A. and Lewis, S. M. (1975). A standardized Romanowsky stain prepared from purified dyes. *Journal of Clinical Pathology* **28**: 920–923.
18. Miers, M. K., Fogo, A. B., Federspiel, C. F., McAllister, N. W., Phillips, P. A. and Cousar, J. B. (1987). Evaluation of the Coulter S-Plus IV three-part differential as a screening tool in a tertiary care hospital. *American Journal of Clinical Pathology* **87**: 745–751.
19. NCCLS (proposed standard) (1981). Koepke, J. A., Bauer, S., Green, J., Marshall, P., Stiene-Martin, E. A., Pierre, R. V., Saunders, A. M., Schmidt, R. M. and Triplett, D. A. Proposed Standard for Leukocyte Differential Counting. NCCLS Vol. 1, 425–460.
20. Rogers, C. H. (1973). Blood sample preparation for automated differential systems. *American Journal of Medical Technology* **39**: 435–442.
21. Rock, W. A., Miale, J. B. and Johnson, W. D. (1984). Detection of abnormal cells in white cell differentials: comparison of the Hematrak® automated system with manual method. *American Journal of Clinical Pathology* **81**: 233–236.
22. Rümke, C. L. (1960). Variability of results in differential cell counts on blood smears. *Triangle* **4**: 154–158.
23. Sacker, L. S. (1975). *Specimen collection*. In Lewis, S. M. and Coster, J. F. (eds) *Quality Control in Haematology*, pp. 211–229. London: Academic Press.
24. Scott MacGregor, R. G., Richards, W. and Loh, G. L. (1940). The differential leucocyte count. *Journal of Pathology* **51**: 337–368.
25. Shafer, J. A. (1978). Quality assurance for differential white cell counts performed manually. In Koepke, J. A. (ed.) *Differential Leukocyte Counting*, pp. 197–204. College of American Pathologists Conference, Aspen, 1977.
26. Stiene-Martin, E. A. (1982). Causes for poor leukocyte distribution in manual spreader-slide blood films. *American Journal of Medical Technology* **46**: 624–632.
27. Walters, J. G. and Garrity, P. F. (1987). *Case Studies in the New Morphology*. McGaw Park, Illinois: American Scientific Products.
28. Wittekind, D. and Löhr, W. (1975). Purification, standardization and quality control of Romanowsky dyes. In Lewis, S. M. and Coster, J. F. (eds) *Quality Control in Haematology*, pp. 143–152. London: Academic Press.

5.3 Quality Assurance in the Transfusion Service

J A Koepke

Introduction

Probably because of the direct relationship of crossmatch tests with the safety of blood transfusion, quality control and quality assurance programmes were implemented into blood bank laboratories earlier than was done in most other clinical laboratories. The setting of standards for blood banking in the United States has been centred at the governmental regulatory and professional organizational level rather than at the individual institutional level. Thus, a fairly complete set of standards has been extant for many years and it is infrequently called into question. Innovative quality assurance schemes are rarely implemented (12) with the notable exception of the widespread implementation of the abbreviated crossmatch procedures which have gained acceptance (5). The formation of the American Association of Blood Banks in 1947 was associated with the early development of standards of laboratory practice for transfusion medicine. Consecutive editions of *Standards for Blood Banks and Transfusion Services*, now in its 12th edition (1) and the *Technical Manual*, most recently in its 9th edition (14), along with *Federal Regulations* (7) developed by the former Bureau of Biologics, have served to put into place a more or less standard approach to blood banking quality assurance in North America as well as elsewhere in developed countries.

The American Red Cross (3) with its network of 58 regional blood donor services as well as the Council of Community Blood Centers have effectively standardized the donor eligibility requirements as well as the processing of donor blood and components.

Although the requirements for processing blood and compatability testing are extensive, there remain several gaps in this system of controls. These primarily concern the quality control of newer blood component preparations such as platelets, and cryoprecipitate.

Haematologists, with their special expertise in cell counting and coagulation testing, coupled with their direct responsibilities for patient care, are in a rather unique position to assess both the *in vitro* and the *in vivo* acceptability of blood products, especially Factor VIII (2) and platelet preparations.

In the sections which follow, the present state of the art of blood banking quality control will be outlined rather than extensively reviewed, since comprehensive discussions have been published elsewhere. In addition, however, a programme for the on-going assessment of the acceptable quality of blood products is presented, since this is an area in which haematologists can make a significant contribution to patient care.

Basic quality assurance practices

As noted above, several sources for quality assurance programmes are available. This chapter will focus its discussions on the transfusion service within the hospital. The AABB Standards includes a fairly succinct requirement for quality assurance which reads as follows:

> A8.000 All blood banks and transfusion services shall use a programme of quality control that is sufficiently comprehensive to ensure that reagents, equipment and methods function as expected, and that there is compliance with the Standards. Each blood bank and transfusion service shall participate in a proficiency testing programme. (1)

Note that the standard merely requires such a programme but does not prescribe a standard method. The choice of methodology is left to the medical director and his staff. Ample publications are available for study, the most comprehensive being the AABB *Technical Manual* (14). A recent publication of the Council of Europe (6) outlines the apparent consensus for quality assurance practices for Europe. Whilst these two publications agree in principle on most essentials, several discrepancies exist. For example, the European standards require duplicate but entirely separate ABO and Rh typing as a method for error prevention.

The monograph by Myhre (9) provided a practical guide to quality control in blood banks. Unfortunately a 2nd edition did not follow in due time. A more recent conference updates much of quality control especially in regard to component acceptability, and while not a listing of standards, this book provides some new perspectives to quality assurance in clinical transfusion medicine (11).

Donor screening for infectious diseases

Although screening blood donors for syphilis has been a time-honoured practice, it has proven to be almost useless in the prevention of that disease. Nevertheless, in many places the practice continues. More recently, the screening for hepatitis B has become standard practice and this testing has proved to be quite successful in the prevention of that infectious complication of transfusion.

More problematic have been the recently instituted screening programmes for the prevention of cytomegalovirus (CMV) infections by using immunologic screening tests on donor units. Finally, a new development has been the use of so-called surrogate tests for the identification of donor units which, on a statistical basis, have been shown to be associated with a higher transmission of non-A non-B hepatitis. But the implementation of these tests has been associated with a higher rejection rate ($\sim$3–5%) of donor units.

Despite the long experience with testing of blood for the prevention of infectious disease, the blood banking community has been hard pressed in mounting a programme for the prevention of acquired immune deficiency syndrome (AIDS) secondary to blood transfusion. Presently, however, screening of donor units for the possible presence of human immunodeficiency virus (HIV) appears to be fairly effective (either directly or by the Hawthorn effect) in significantly reducing transfusion-related AIDS, although only the passage of time will allow us to draw a firm conclusion on this point. Blood donor centres are primarily responsible for the accurate performance of these tests and as far as one can ascertain these systems are quite successful in the prevention of infection secondary to blood transfusion.

The reporting of post-transfusion hepatitis to the donor service has long been a responsibility assigned to the transfusing facility. However, since the onset of symptoms of hepatitis almost always occurs long after the patient has been discharged from the hospital, such reporting as there is, is incomplete and often undocumented.

However, the individual transfusion services have now acquired additional responsibilities in the study of the epidemiology of AIDS. The process of reporting is even more problematic for obvious reasons, including the apparently long incubation period for AIDS. This incubation period, at times, seems to be considerably shorter with transfusion-acquired AIDS. In the United States an epidemiology programme called 'Lookback' has been undertaken by all blood banks. In this programme, a donor giving a positive test result for AIDS antibody is checked for any previous donation. If he had donated, that donor unit with any of its components is traced to its recipient(s). When the recipient is identified, the medical director of the transfusion service discusses the case with the patient's physician and together they try to determine if the recipient may have any clinical or laboratory evidence of AIDS or its precursor states. While presently primarily an epidemiologic study, if and when effective therapy for AIDS is found, these individuals would be candidates for such treatment.

The medical director of the transfusion service reviews any transfusion-acquired AIDS in an effort to prevent transfusion-acquired infection and close liaison with the donor service is necessary when working through these difficult problems.

Shared quality assurance

In the increasingly complex world of transfusion medicine the provision of blood products has in many places been divided between the donor facility and the transfusion service. In the past these two entities may have been co-existent within the hospital but more recently they have been geographically and administratively separated. In the United States blood drawing has moved out of the hospital toward the American Red Cross Blood Services and/or the community blood banks. Although there has been a recent trend to incorporate donor rooms into hospitals again as a way to collect blood from autologous and directed blood donors, more conveniently and efficiently this has not yet had a significant impact on the division noted above.

Since whole-blood units provide the source for the various components used in transfusion medicine, the blood collection facility is responsible for the testing of the original source of the blood as well as for the production of the several components (Tables 5.3.1 and 5.3.2). The test results on the original unit are thus directly valid for the components prepared from that unit.

Components produced by apheresis techniques are likewise tested for the several factors noted in Table 5.3.2.

However, the transfusion service is required by regulation to repeat certain tests on previously tested units. These confirmatory tests are noted in the right-hand column of Table 5.3.2. These studies have become standard practice for transfusion services and are carried out on all units received from outside sources. Any discrepancies between the original and confirmatory testing must be resolved before transfusion. Usually the unit is returned to the original donor facility.

Quality control of blood components

With the evolution of blood component therapy, criteria for acceptability of such products were promulgated first by the developers of the manufacturing method. These were subsequently incorporated into the *Code of Federal Regulations* of the Food and Drug Administration (7) in the United States. The criteria of the Council of Europe (6) are similar and are also included in Table 5.3.3. At present the criteria for quality of product are *in vitro* measurements; *in vivo* testing is not yet required.

Significant problems can exist in the quality assurance of blood components which are not covered by standards. As an example, cryoprecipitate formerly was used for the treatment of Factor VIII deficiency. However, with the development of purified Factor VIII concentrates (which are also essentially non–infectious) clinicians are increasingly using cryoprecipitate for its fibrinogen content rather than to replace Factor VIII; for

Table 5.3.1 Blood components

Red cells products	Plasma products	Other cellular products
Leucocyte-poor red cells (filtered, washed)	Cryoprecipitate	Apheresis platelets
Plasma-poor red cells (washed)	Cryo-poor plasma	Buffy coat leucocytes
Frozen deglycerolysed red cells		Apheresis granulocytes
Packed red cells	Fresh frozen plasma	Platelet concentrate

Table 5.3.2 Quality assurance of donor units

Factor to be checked	Quality specification	Frequency of control	Control executed by	Confirmation by central transfusion service
ABO and Rh	Grouping	All units	Donor facility	Required
HBsAg	Negative by approved screening test[a]	All units	Donor facility	Not required
Unexpected antibodies	Negative[a]	All units	Donor facility	Not required
HIV	Negative by ELISA test[a]	All units	Donor facility	Not required
Syphilis (when required)	Negative screening test[a]	All units	Donor facility	Not required
Volume, excluding anticoagulant	450 ml ± 45 ml	Weighing of 1% of all units	Donor facility	Not required
Packed red cells	280 ± 60 ml		Donor facility or transfusion service	Not required
CPDA-1	PCV 0.70–0.80			
Adsol	PCV 0.50–0.60			

[a]Positive units not sent to transfusion service.

Table 5.3.3 Quality assurance of blood components

Product	In vitro volume (ml)	In vitro criteria	Proposed in vivo criteria
Fresh frozen plasma	225–250	>5.1 g/dl protein	None
Cryoprecipitate	10–20 or 8–15 (dry button)	>80 IU F VIII >150 mg Fibrinogen[a]	F VIII increment and/or fibrinogen increment
Platelet concentrates	40–55	Platelets >5.5×10^{10}[b] pH >6.0	Corrected count increment or % expected increment
Apheresis units	180–220	Platelets >3.0×10^{11}[b] pH >6.0 WBC <1.5×10^9	

[a] Proposed standard.
[b] 75% of units tested.

this property no standards exist. Published estimates of fibrinogen content range up to 250 mg/bag but extensive testing shows levels significantly lower than these amounts of fibrinogen (8).

Two actions are anticipated. Firstly, cryoprecipitate production methods should be optimized for fibrinogen rather than for Factor VIII. Secondly, standards for this new use of this product should be put in place, so that there may be more rational use of this product.

Another procedure which could improve the quality of platelet therapy would be the routine measurement of the platelet count increment expressed in either absolute terms (corrected count increment) or as a percentage of expected increment. It is proposed that pre- and post-transfusion (1–4 h) counts be routinely done and the platelet transfusion be evaluated for effectiveness as well as to discover the onset of a refractory state (10).

Internal quality control of laboratory testing

This aspect of quality control has been extensively used in developed as well as in developing countries. The details have been incorporated into systems of control which have been extensively documented (e.g. Ref. 13). The essentials of ABO and Rh testing are outlined in Tables 5.3.4 and 5.3.5. These control systems cover both the reagents and the methods used in the blood bank. American and European standards are similar except that duplicate ABO and Rh testing is recommended by the Council of Europe (6), whereas the AABB Standards (1) indicate that single testing is adequate.

The haematologist's role in changing transfusion practices

With the development of new blood components comes the need for quality assurance standards which should become part of the operation. However, should clinical needs change, the methods of manufacture and the assurance of quality may lag behind. A good example is the evolution of cryoprecipitate, noted above. In the early 1970s it was the first concentrated Factor VIII product. When first used, blood banks did not have the expertise to determine the actual Factor VIII content of these concentrates and haematologists interested in coagulation provided such assays. Subsequently these assays became widely available as well as standardized (2).

With the present concern about HIV infection, newer concentrates which do not transmit HIV have become the product of choice for the treatment of classic haemophilia. Cryoprecipitate has become popular for the replacement of fibrinogen, e.g. in the treatment of disseminated intravascular coagulation, when the prescribed dose of cryoprecipitate must take into account the measured fibrinogen content of such units.

Table 5.3.4 Internal quality control of ABO-antisera and Rh antisera

Parameter to be checked	Quality requirements	Frequency of control
Appearance	No haemolysis, precipitate, particles or gel-formation by visual inspection	Daily
Reactivity and specificity	No immune haemolysis, rouleaux formation or prozone phenomenon. Clear-cut reactions with RBC bearing the corresponding antigen(s): no false reactions	Daily
Potency	Undiluted serum should give a 3–4 plus reaction in saline tube test using a 3% RBC suspension at room temperature	Each new lot
Avidity	Macroscopic agglutination promptly appearing with a 50% RBC suspension in homologous serum, using the slide test	Each new lot

Table 5.3.5 Quality control of ABO- and Rh-typing

Parameter to be checked	Minimal requirements for testing	Control samples	Frequency of control
ABO-typing	Use of anti-A and anti-B AB-serum as a negative control if reversed typing cannot be performed	One blood sample of each of the following types: O, A_1, A_2, B and A_2B	Daily
ABO reverse typing	Use of reagent A and B cells		Daily
$Rh^0(D)$-typing (incl. D^u)	Typing in duplicate[a] using two different anti-D sera: use of the indirect antiglobulin test for D^u-confirmation in donors	One $Rh_0(D)$ pos, one $Rh_0(d)$ neg sample	Daily
Rh phenotyping	Typing in duplicate[a] using two different antisera for each Rh-factor	For complete Rh-phenotyping one sample of each of the following Rh-types: R_1r, R_2, $R'r$, $R''r$ and rr	Daily

[a]AABB standards do not require duplicate testing.

The use of monitoring functions for blood usage review

Comprehensive hospital-wide quality assurance programmes have become a requirement for hospital accreditation in the United States. Blood transfusion constitutes a significant aspect of patient care and therefore is one of the major areas that requires review by the medical staff of a hospital. Reviews of the appropriateness of blood transfusion (both red cells and components) are performed periodically. As part of this process it is required that all confirmed transfusion reactions are evaluated.

Blood usage reviews also include the development of policies and procedures for the administration of blood products, the review of the adequacy of the transfusion service as well as a review of ordering practices for blood products. To perform these functions, criteria for appropriate transfusion usage must be developed by the clinical staff (4).

References

1. AABB (1987). *Standards for Blood Banks and Transfusion Services* (12th edn), pp. 1–52. Arlington, VA: American Association of Blood Banks.
2. Allain, J-P (1984). Clinical efficacy and safety of Factor VIII concentrate. In Smit Sibinga, C. T. S., Das, P. C. and Taswell, H. F. (eds) *Quality Assurance in Blood Banking and its Clinical Impact*, pp. 187–193. Boston: Martinus Nijhoff.
3. American Red Cross (1987). Blood Services Directives, Sections 6.12, 6.13, 6.14, 6.17, 6.20, 6.21, 6.37, 6.46. Washington, D.C.: American Red Cross.
4. Anon. (1987). *Medical Staff Monitoring Functions – Blood Usage Review* (1st edn), pp. 1–36. Chicago, IL: Joint Commission on Accreditation of Hospitals.
5. Boral, L. I. and Henry, J. B. (1977). The type and screen: a safe alternative and supplement in selected surgical procedures. *Transfusion* 17: 163–168.
6. Council of Europe (1984). *Quality Control in Blood Transfusion Service*, pp. 28–35, 39–48. Strasbourg, France: Council of Europe.
7. FDA (1985). Code of Federal Regulations, Food and Drugs, No. 21, Parts 600–799 (1985), pp. 131, 137, 138, 150, 152. Washington, D.C.: Office of the Federal Register, General Services Administration.
8. Hoffman, M., Koepke, J. A. and Widmann, F. K. (1987). Fibrinogen content of low-volume cryoprecipitate. *Transfusion* 27: 56–358.
9. Myhre, B. A. (1974). *Quality Control in Blood Banking*, pp. 1–227, New York: John Wiley & Sons.
10. Schiffer, C. A. (1984). Platelet transfusion: Quality control. In Smit Sibinga, C. T. S, Das, P. C. and Taswell, H. F. (eds) *Quality Assurance in Blood Banking and Its Clinical Impact*, pp. 177–185. Boston: Martinus Nijhoff.
11. Smit Sibinga, C. T. S., Das, P. C. and Taswell, H. F. (eds) (1984). *Quality Assurance in Blood Banking and Its Clinical Impact*. Boston: Martinus Nijhoff.
12. Taswell, H. F., Smith, A. M., Sweatt, M. A. and Pfaff, K. J. (1974). Quality control in the blood bank – a new approach. *Transfusion* 62: 451–495.
13. Thurrell, T. (1987). Quality assurance in the transfusion service. In Stewart, C. E. and Koepke, J. A. (eds) *Basic Quality Assurance Practices for Clinical Laboratories*, pp. 179–185. Philadelphia: J. B. Lippincott.
14. Widmann, F. K. (ed.) (1985). *Technical Manual* (9th edn), pp. 369–381. Arlington, VA: American Association of Blood Banks.

5.4 Control Materials and Calibrators

S M Lewis

The International Committee for Standardization in Haematology has defined reference standards, calibrators and controls as follows:

A **reference standard** is a substance or device, one or more properties of which are sufficiently well established to be used for the calibration of an apparatus, the assessment of a measurement method or for assigning values to a material. Where possible, it must be based on or traceable to an exactly defined physical or chemical measurement.

A **calibrator** is a substance or device used to calibrate, graduate or adjust a measurement. It must be traceable to a reference standard.

A **control** is a substance, device or procedure for checking that the performance of an analytic instrument is constant.

Calibrators and controls both have a place in internal quality control; they have interrelated but different functions. A control must be stable and homogenous; the exact analytic value is not important although the approximate value should be known in order to select a preparation at the upper or lower limit of the normal reference range or at other clinically important levels. By contrast, a calibrator must have an assigned value as close to the true value as can be established. The essential difference is that a calibrator is used for accuracy and inter-laboratory harmonization, whilst a control is used for precision.

The materials used as calibrators and controls are, in general, interchangeable but establishing an assigned value is an expensive, time-consuming procedure which makes it sensible to use it sparingly, whereas a control should be used with each batch of tests. Some controls are provided with stated values but this information should be treated with caution unless their accuracy can be confirmed independently by reference methods in expert laboratories. Material used in an external quality assessment scheme will usually have value obtained as consensus mean or median value when results from all participants are analysed (see Chapter 7). However, it is not good practice to regard the material with that assigned value retrospectively as a calibrator, and to use it to re-adjust an instrument.

A control is used alongside patients' samples in a batch of tests. It is subjected to the same reactions and the end-point of reaction is read in the same way as in the adjacent samples. Thus, it must closely resemble test specimens in its behaviour. This is not always easy to achieve and for the blood count, especially, there is an inverse relationship between specimen-like behaviour and stability: blood in EDTA is unstable within a few hours of collection, mixing the blood with formaldehyde or glutaraldehyde will prolong its stability to years but this will seriously affect its physical properties (see later). Human blood preserved in acid citrate dextrose (ACD) or citrate phosphate dextrose (CPD) anticoagulant (p. 157) is stable at 20°C for several days and at 4°C for 3–4 weeks, while equine (horse or donkey) blood is stable even longer, up to 3 months for most red cell parameters. There are certain differences in the way in which ACD/CPD blood and EDTA blood react in various tests, including cell counting systems, but they behave sufficiently alike for ACD or CPD blood to be used as a control, with the advantage of having a reasonably long stability (9).

A reference standard need not behave in the same way as natural blood, but it is important to ensure that the instrument that is to be calibrated is not adversely affected by the material, e.g. by blocking the system's pathway or by giving an inconsistent reaction with its reagents or diluent. It may also be necessary to convert measurement obtained with the standard to the measurement which would have been obtained on the same instrument with a fresh blood with equivalent dimensions. It has been suggested that glutaraldehyde-fixed blood cells might make a suitable reference preparation (10, 12). When blood is fixed there will be an alteration in its density, flexibility, shape and rheological properties; this will affect its behaviour as it flows through a counting–sizing system to the sensing zone, as well as affecting the response of the system's sensor. Thus, before fixed cells can be used as a calibrator for a system these differences may have to be taken into account by applying correction factors (2, 14).

With an automated blood counting system which will not process a fixed cell preparation directly, it may be necessary to introduce an intermediate step in which the reference preparation is used to calibrate a single-channel counter which is then used to assign values to an intermedium of fresh blood which can be used directly to calibrate the automated system (Fig. 5.4.1). This system can then be used to assign values to other calibrators.

Other materials have also been suggested as surrogate blood cells for calibrating automated counters. These include spherical polystyrene latex particles which are now available in a series of defined sizes, each in a narrow range with a CV less than 1%. From their diameters (obtained by direct microscopic measurement) their volumes as spheres are calculated as $\frac{4}{3}\pi r^3$. They can then be used to calibrate pulse-sizes in a blood counting system, provided that a 'shape factor' can be established to take account of the difference between pulses generated by the latex which present at the sensing zone as inflexible spheres and those generated by fresh red blood cells which present at the sensing zone as ellipsoids (10, 14, 15). Monosized latex particles, with diameters of 2.2, 4.8 and 9.5 μm respectively, are available as certified reference materials from BCR (see below); they are being developed as blood cell sizing and counting standards in a collaborative study by ICSH and BCR.

Primary reference materials (reference standards) are available for a number of haematological tests. The main international authorities for this are World Health Organization (WHO), International Committee for Standardization in Haematology (ICSH) and Bureau of Reference of the European Communities (BCR). Several national standardizing bodies are also active in this work, notably the UK National Institute for Biological Standards and Control (NIBSC) and the Central Laboratory of the Netherlands Red Cross Blood Transfusion Service (CLB); these institutes are also responsible for maintaining certain WHO standards.

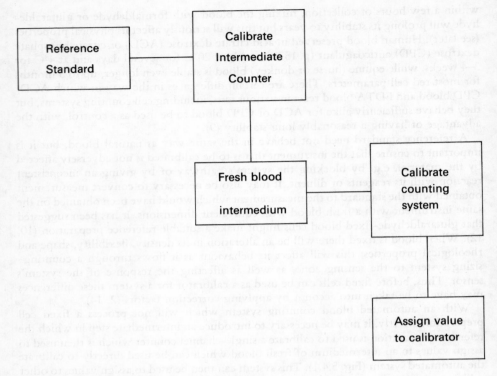

Fig. 5.4.1 Use of Calibrator in Blood counting.

The standards which are available are as follows:

Haemoglobin (WHO, ICSH)
Erythropoietin (WHO, NIBSC)
Ferritin (WHO, ICSH, NIBSC)
Vitamin B₁₂ (NIBSC)
Thromboplastin (WHO, ICSH, BCR, CLB)
    Rabbit
    Bovine
    Human
Blood typing sera (WHO, CLB)
    Anti-A human
    Anti-B human
    Anti-AB human
    Anti Rh₀ (anti-D)
    Anti-rh′ (anti-C)

Immunoglobulins (WHO, NIBSC)
  Human IgG
  Human IgA
  Human IgM
  Human IgE
Antinuclear factor (WHO, CLB)
Human serum complement components (WHO, CLB)
Antihuman globulin reagent (ICSH)
Abnormal haemoglobins (ICSH)
HbA$_2$ (ICSH)
Fetal haemoglobin (ICSH)
Blood coagulation factors (WHO, NIBSC)
  Antithrombin III
  Factor VIII:C
  Factor VIII related activity
  Factor IX
  Plasmin
  Thrombin
  Urokinase
Sized latex particles (surrogate blood cells) (see text above) (BCR)

Details of the various products and the conditions under which they are supplied may be obtained as follows:

(1) WHO—World Health Organization, Biological Standards Division, CH–1211 Geneva-27, Switzerland.
(2) ICSH—c/o Dr S M Lewis, Royal Postgraduate Medical School, Du Cane Road, London W12 0HS, UK.
(3) BCR—Community Bureau of Reference, Rue de la Loi 200, B–1049 Brussels, Belgium.
(4) NIBSC—National Institute for Biological Standards and Control, Blanche Lane, South Mimms, Potters Bar, Hertfordshire EN6 3QG, UK.
(5) CLB—Central Laboratory of the Netherlands Red Cross Blood Transfusion Service, Plesmanlaan 125, 1066 CX Amsterdam, The Netherlands.

Traceability

The science of measurement is known as metrology. There are certain measurements which have such well defined physical properties that any other material measured against these metrological standards will be equally well defined. The fundamental measurements in this context include length, mass and molar concentration. If a ruler is calibrated directly and precisely against the defined reference standard meter this will give a measure of its true length. If a second ruler is calibrated against the first ruler this will give a measure of *its* true length (within limits of precision), and similarly with a third, fourth and many more rulers, all of which will have been calibrated indirectly against the original meter. Thus, these successive measurements are **traceable** to the metrological standard of length. There are similar examples of standards based on weight and traceable to the gram. Included in this group are chemical standards which can be defined in terms of their molecular weight. Haemoglobin belongs to this category (6).

When a biological substance cannot be expressed directly in terms of either chemical and physical quantities, it may be defined in terms of international units. These are arbitrary units based on some type of reaction which relates to its biological activity. The unit concentration of any other preparation which reacts in the same way can be determined by comparing their reactions, thus making the second preparation traceable to the primary standard. Thromboplastin provides an example of this (8, 11).

As described above, metrological standards ensure accuracy (truth); on the other hand, biological standards are arbitrary, and thus cannot be claimed to be 'accurate' but at least they ensure consistency.

Primary international standards and reference materials are only available in restricted amounts. **Secondary standards** are established by direct comparison with a primary standard, usually by a national authority. They are more freely available and are intended for assigning values to **testing standards** or calibrators, which are commercial (or privately) manufactured products. Some calibrators are clearly seen to be traceable to the relevant primary standard; with other materials labelled as calibrators the link is tenuous and unfortunately sometimes non-existent.

Preparation of blood count calibrators

Calibrators and controls are now available commercially for a number of haematological tests, and details can be found in various manufacturers' catalogues. In Chapter 7 details are given for preparation of materials for external quality assessment. These are equally suitable for internal quality control. They may also be used as calibrators provided that values can be assigned to them reliably. In the following section preparation of blood count calibrators and methods for assigning values will be described.

Haemoglobin (haemiglobincyanide)

For calibrating a haemoglobinometer or a photometer for measuring haemoglobin the ICSH haemiglobincyanide reference preparation, or a solution derived from it, should be used (16). The standard is an aqueous solution of haemiglobincyanide with a concentration in the range 550–850 mg/l.

The method is as follows (4):

(1) Prepare a haemolysate as described on p. 159.
(2) Measure the Hb concentration in the lysate. Then convert the haemoglobin to haemiglobincyanide by adding sufficient cyanide–ferricyanide (modified Drabkin) reagent to the lysate to obtain a concentration of *ca* 700 mg/l. Allow to stand at room temperature for about 1 h.

(3) Filter through a micropore filter at 0.2 μm, and dispense 10 ml volumes aseptically into sterile containers, preferably ampoules of amber glass. Heat-seal the ampoules or if vials are used cap and seal them. The material will be satisfactory for several years if kept at 4°C, provided that it is sterile.

(4) Measure absorbance in a spectrophotometer against reagent blank at 540 nm and also at 504 nm and 750 nm. The ratio of A^{540}/A^{504} should be 1.59–1.63 and A^{750} should be < 0.002 per 1.000 cm lightpath length. The spectrophotometer should be checked by means of the ICSH haemiglobincyanide standard.

(5) Calculate Hb concentration $(mg/l) = \dfrac{(A^{540} \times 16114.5)}{(11.0 \times 1.000)}$, where $11.0 =$ coefficient extinction and $16114.5 =$ monomeric mol. wt of haemoglobin.

Haemoglobin (lysate)

This is intended for use when haemoglobin is one of the tests in an automated blood counting system with an automated diluter.

The method for preparation of a lysate is described on p. 157. To assign a value for haemoglobin concentration use the ICSH reference method (6) with a spectrophotometer, the calibration of which has been checked against the ICSH haemiglobincyanide standard or a secondary standard derived from it. Establish the coefficient of variation (CV) by ten replicate tests, sampling from several tubes taken at random from the batch. The CV should not exceed 2%.

When the instrument to be calibrated is an automated counting system in which haemoglobin is one of a set of interrelated parameters, whole-blood preparations should be used (see next section). The value of haemoglobin concentration is assigned to this material in the same way as for lysate.

Red cell parameters

The preparation of preserved blood is described on p. 157. For analysis take several vials at random, gently mix their contents on a roller mix for 10 min.

Establish the RBC by ten replicate measurements from each of the vials, using a standardized single-channel aperture-impedance electronic cell counter (7), and making the appropriate dilutions by pre-calibrated pipettes.

Inter-vial and intra-vial CV should be less than 2%.

Establish packed cell volume (PCV, haematocrit) on samples from the same vials by microhaematocrit, spun at more than $12,000 \times \boldsymbol{g}$ for at least 5 min and if necessary corrected for trapped plasma as described in the ICSH recommendations (5), modified for capillary tubes instead of Wintrobe tubes. CV should not exceed 2%.

White blood cells

Preparation of fixed blood cells as pseudo-leucocytes is described on p. 159. The concentrated preparation is unsuitable for use in fully automated cell counters but can be used when it is added to preserved blood or haemolysate or after diluting appropriately in glycerol–saline as described on p. 160.

For analysis take several vials, re-suspend by vigorous shaking by hand or by vortex mixing, following by mixing on a roller mix for 10 min. Then establish the cell count by ten replicate measurements from each of the vials, using a standardized single channel aperture-impedance electronic cell counter (7) and making the appropriate dilutions by pre-calibrated pipettes. The CV should not exceed 2%.

Platelets

Method for preparing platelets is described on p. 160. To assign values carry out haemocytometry by four replicate counts on each of three vials from the batch, using a standardized method (13). The CV should not exceed 3%. Intra-vial consistency can be checked by counting five to ten randomly selected vials by an electronic counter (13). The CV of these counts should also not exceed 3%.

Precision and Accuracy

The level of precision and accuracy with which the assigned values have been established depends largely on technical skill, and especially on diluting accuracy. Individual bias can be overcome, or at least identified, by having the measurements carried out by two technicians in each of two or three separate laboratories. This is the basis of a protocol devised by the British Committee for Standardization in Haematology for testing calibration and quality control material used with automatic blood counting apparatus (1, 3). The objectives of the protocol are to ensure that manufactured preparations conform to their claimed performance and to check their continuing performance in routine use. Essentially the procedure is as follows:

(a) On three fresh blood samples Hb, RBC, PCV and WBC are obtained by *direct measurement* using reference methods as described above. The red cell indices are calculated from these measurements.

(b) The same parameters are obtained on the fresh blood samples and also on the quality control material which is being evaluated by *indirect measurement* on an automated cell counter.

Then the value which should be assigned to the quality control material (by one laboratory) can be calculated by:

$$d_q = i_q \times \sqrt[3]{\left(\frac{d_1}{i_1} \times \frac{d_2}{i_2} \times \frac{d_3}{i_3} \right)}$$

where d_1, d_2, d_3 are the direct values on the fresh bloods 1, 2, 3, respectively; i_1, i_2, i_3 are the indirect values on the fresh bloods 1, 2, 3, respectively, and i_q is the indirect value of the control material (i.e. on the automated counter).

When results from three laboratories (a, b and c) are used, the assigned value (d_q) will be:

$$d_q = \sqrt[3]{\left(d_{q_a} \times d_{q_b} \times d_{q_c} \right)}$$

On subsequent days the stability of the material can be tested on the same automated cell counter(s) provided that performance of the counter itself is checked by an independent procedure such as constancy of mean MCV, MCH and MCHC (see p. 80).

References

1. Crosland-Taylor, P. J., Allen, R. W. B., England, J. M., Fielding, J. F., Lewis, S. M., Shinton, N. K. and White, J. M. (1979). Draft protocol for testing calibration and quality control material used with automatic blood counting apparatus. *Clinical and Laboratory Haematology* **1**: 61–64.
2. England, J. M. and van Assendelft, O. W. (1986). Automated blood counters and their evaluation. In Rowan, R. M. and England, J. M. (eds) *Automation and Quality Assurance in Haematology*, pp. 87–128. Oxford: Blackwell Scientific.
3. England, J. M., Chetty, M. C., Garvey, B., Lewis, S. M., Wardle, J., Cousins, S., Crosland-Taylor, P. J. and Syndercombe-Court, D. (1983). Testing of calibration and quality control material used with automatic blood counting apparatus: application of the protocol devised by the British Committee for Standardization in Haematology. *Clinical and Laboratory Haematology* **5**: 83–92.
4. Holtz, A. H. (1965). Some experience with a cyanhemiglobin solution. *Bibliotheca haematologica* **21**: 75–78.
5. ICSH (1980). Recommendations for reference method for determination by centrifugation of packed cell volume of blood. *Journal of Clinical Pathology* **33**: 1–2.
6. ICSH (1987). Recommendations for reference method for haemoglobinometry in human blood (ICSH Standard 1986) and specifications for international haemiglobincyanide reference preparation (3rd edn). *Clinical and Laboratory Haematology* **9**: 73–79.
7. ICSH (1988). The assignment of values to fresh blood used for calibrating automated blood cell counters. *Clinical and Laboratory Haematology* **10**: 203–212.
8. Kirkwood, T. B. L. and Lewis, S. M. (1983). Requirements for thromboplastins and plasma used to control oral anticoagulant therapy. *WHO Technical Report Series* **687**: 81–105.
9. Lewis, S. M. (1975). Standards and reference preparations. In Lewis, S. M. and Coster, J. F. (eds) *Quality Control in Haematology*, pp. 79–95. London: Academic Press.
10. Lewis, S. M. (1982). The philosophy of value assignment. In van Assendelft, O. W. and England, J. M. (eds) *Advances in Hematological Methods: the Blood Count*, pp. 232–237. Boca Raton, Florida: CRC Press.
11. Lewis, S. M. (1987). Thromboplastin and oral anticoagulant control. *British Journal of Haematology* **66**: 1–4.
12. Lewis, S. M. and Burgess, B. J. (1966). A stable standard suspension for red-cell counts. *Laboratory Practice* **15**: 305.
13. Lewis, S. M., Wardle, J., Cousins, S. and Skelly, J. V. (1979). Platelet counting in development of reference method and a reference preparation. *Clinical and Laboratory Haematology* **1**: 227–237.
14. Richardson Jones, A. (1982). Counting and sizing of blood cells using aperture-impedance systems. In van Assendelft, O. W. and England, J. M. (eds) *Advances in Hematological Methods: the Blood Count*, pp. 50–72. Boca Raton, Florida: CRC Press.
15. Thom, R., Marchandise, H. and Colinet, E. (1985). The certification of monosized latex spheres in aqueous suspensions with nominal diameters 2.0 μm, 4.8 μm and 96.6 μm. BCR Information EUR 9662. Brussels: Commission of European Communities.
16. van Assendelft, O. W., Holtz, A. H. and Lewis, S. M. (1984). Recommended method for the determination of the haemoglobin concentration of blood. WHO Document, LAB 84.10. Geneva: World Health Organization.

6

Standardization and Quality Control in Blood Coagulation Assays

A M H P van den Besselaar and R M Bertina

Introduction

The reliability of the result of coagulation tests is as much dependent upon the care and attention given to the collection and subsequent handling of the blood samples as to quality control of the tests themselves. Accordingly, part of this chapter is concerned with the pre-test variables in blood coagulation testing, especially for the prothrombin time, activated partial thromboplastin time, and Factor VIIIC assay. Equally important and intimately related is standardization of coagulation assays in order to ensure that measurements give the same results when carried out at different times, in different laboratories and by different methods.

A distinction should be made between standardization of global tests such as prothrombin time (PT) and activated partial thromboplastin time (APTT) and standardization of specific clotting factor assays. Standardization of a clotting factor assay involves the use of a material standard, i.e. a sample of potency agreed locally or internationally. Standardization of the PT for oral anticoagulant treatment has now been agreed internationally and involves the use of thromboplastin standards.

The quality of oral anticoagulant treatment is also dependent on skilful dosage regulation and adequate patient education. Part of this chapter will be concerned with therapeutic control, i.e. assessment of the proportion of time that the patients are within the therapeutic range.

Normal and, where possible, abnormal controls should be included in each run of PT and APTT testing. Lyophilized controls in both the normal and abnormal range are commercially available. The requirements for and use of plasma controls will be discussed.

Pre-analytical variables

The coagulation system consists of enzymes and proenzymes which are easily activated or denatured. The sample must be collected in such a manner that the integrity of the coagulation factors is preserved. There are general rules which must be followed to achieve this goal. However, depending on the specific assay to be performed, there may be modifications in pre-analytical conditions for optimum stability of the constituent to be assayed.

A comprehensive discussion of pre-test variables in blood coagulation testing has been given by Thomson (80, 81).

Venepuncture technique

Venous blood may be collected using needle and syringe, or evacuated-tube system. There are conflicting opinions in the literature concerning the suitability of evacuated tubes on account of deleterious effects on haemostatic components which have been observed by some investigators (80). In either circumstance, blood specimens must be collected or stored in containers made from non-reactive materials, such as polypropylene or siliconized glass.

The needle and syringe technique allows the phlebotomist to draw the blood sample gently, without forced pressure. However, if the blood is drawn too slowly or obtained with difficulty, the clotting mechanism may be activated.

Traditionally, the two-syringe technique has been used to collect blood for most coagulation tests. The first millilitres drawn in the first syringe may be contaminated with tissue thromboplastin, which would activate the clotting sequence, thereby invalidating test results. The blood collected in the second syringe is used for most coagulation tests. However, no significant differences were observed in PTs or APTTs of normal samples between the first and second tubes using an evacuated system (26). In samples obtained from heparinized patients, the APTT of the first tube plasma was about 20% shorter than the APTT of the second tube plasma (96).

The following procedures for venepuncture technique are recommended:

(1) Prolonged tourniquet application and stasis should be avoided. One minute seems to be a reasonable limit. Expert phlebotomists can accomplish the task in a much shorter time, and in a patient with good veins, some do not even require a tourniquet. If the tourniquet is applied, it is probably best to leave it on during the collection of samples (26).

(2) Tubes for coagulation tests should be filled after those for other tests. In case of a single tube drawn for PT monitoring of oral anticoagulant therapy, it is not necessary to draw a preliminary sample (26). The sample for the coagulation testing should not be part of a blood specimen of more than 25 ml when a 20-gauge needle is used, or 50 ml when a 19-gauge needle is used (64). For APTT and factor assays, the reasonable approach is to allow common sense and informed judgement to prevail in each case. If venepuncture is prompt and atraumatic, and blood withdrawal is quick, one tube should suffice. If adverse conditions occur, a preliminary tube should be collected and discarded.

(3) Samples for PT and APTT tests from paediatric, burn, or other special patients may require small or microvolume samples. Capillary blood tests are particularly appropriate for use in babies and young children. A well collected, free-flowing capillary sample is likely to give a more reliable assessment of the patient's

coagulation profile than a venous sample which has been collected with trauma and difficulty (80).

(4) If blood for monitoring of heparin therapy is collected through indwelling catheters it may be contaminated by exogenous heparin (51). Blood for laboratory monitoring of heparin treatment should be collected by venepuncture.

(5) If a syringe is used, it should be emptied by placing the tip against the side of the tube and allowing the blood to run down the side so as to prevent frothing or excessive turbulence.

(6) Prompt and adequate mixing with the citrate solution by gentle inversion must be done to ensure immediate binding of calcium.

Specimen processing

The following checks should be made before a sample is accepted for coagulation assays:

(1) **Identification of patient.** In every case the full name of the patient should be checked to ensure the name entered on the request form is correct. Properly collected samples should be labelled at the time of collection and in the patient's presence. Unidentified or mislabelled tubes should be rejected by the laboratory.

(2) **The correct volume of whole blood** must be drawn for tube size and amount of anticoagulant. For accurate results, this must be within 10% of the stated volume. Each tube is compared with a reference tube containing the minimum acceptable volume. Any tubes that do not contain the minimum volume should be discarded, and another sample collected. The important factor is the plasma:citrate ratio. All of the calcium to be bound by citrate is in the plasma. If the haematocrit is very high and the usual relative volumes of blood and citrate solution are mixed, a prolonged PT or APTT results from overcitration of the reduced proportion of plasma in the blood sample (49). Polycythaemic samples can be recognized by checking for apparently high packed cell volumes in the centrifuged tubes. If the actual PCV (haematocrit) has been determined, the correct proportions of blood and citrate solution may be read from Fig. 6.1. In such a case the blood should be collected by syringe, because in evacuated tubes the blood:citrate ratio is fixed.

(3) **Clots** must be checked for in all blood samples. Even small clots render a sample completely unacceptable for investigation. Any clots present can be visualized by slowly tilting the container prior to centrifugation. All clotted specimens should be rejected.

(4) **Haemolysis** may affect APTT results but not PT results (26). Following centrifugation, the plasma should be observed for haemolysis. Haemolysis may be due to traumatic venepuncture, rupture of red cells and platelets during collection, or a contaminated syringe system. Haemolysed plasma should be rejected for APTT tests (26).

(5) **Jaundiced plasma** always should be noted on test reports. This should also alert the technologist to use special care in handling these potentially infectious specimens.

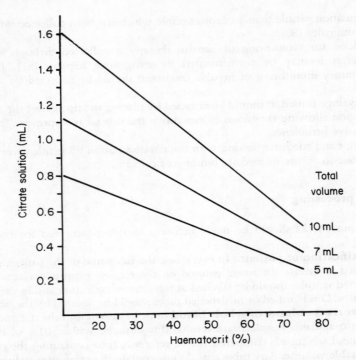

Fig. 6.1 Chart for determining the volume of citrate to be added to blood to make a total volume of 5, 7 or 10 ml. Determine the patient's haematocrit (PCV). Then select the line for the desired volume of citrated blood and read off the required volume of citrate solution corresponding to the patient's PCV. (From Ref. 37, with permission.)

Centrifugation

The speed and duration of centrifugation should be controlled and standardized, according to the requirements of the test. Platelets are the key variable affected by the speed or relative centrifugal field and time of centrifugation. They contain platelet factor 3 (a catalyst of the intrinsic coagulation pathway), platelet factor 4 (a heparin antagonist), and several of the blood coagulation factors.

In most routine plasma clotting tests (PT, APTT) excess phospholipids (platelet substitute) are contained in the reagent. For these tests, it may be sufficient to centrifuge at a minimum speed of $1000 \times g$ for 10 min (64).

When blood samples are to be assayed for control of heparin therapy, centrifugation at $600 \times g$ may result in shorter APTTs than centrifugation at $940 \times g$ or higher speeds (93). This might be due to release of platelet factor 4 in the low-spun samples.

A refrigerated centrifuge (4°C) is preferable for separation of plasma for Factor V and Factor VIII assays (80). Certain tests of platelet function require centrifugation at room temperature.

The containers should remain capped throughout to minimize pH changes and to prevent an aerosol effect or evaporation. For the one-stage assay of Factor VIII:C a higher minimum speed of centrifugation has been recommended, i.e. at $2500 \times g$ for 15 min at 15°C (16).

If the plasma cannot be assayed for Factor VIII:C within 2 h after blood collection, it is recommended that the plasma be centrifuged again under the above conditions. The sediment is then discarded carefully, and the sample frozen quickly at -70°C (16).

For the preparation of prothrombin time reference plasma two centrifugation steps are recommended, the first at a speed of $2000 \times g$ for 20 min at 15°C, the second at a speed of $20,000 \times g$ for 30 min at 15°C (17). The centrifuge brake should not be used. Following each step, the plasma should be drawn off carefully, without disturbing the buffy coat or sediment.

Anticoagulants and buffers for blood collection

Sodium citrate is the anticoagulant of choice for collecting blood specimens for coagulation testing. Sodium oxalate is not recommended. For PT testing, the International Committee for Standardization in Haematology (ICSH) and the International Committee on Thrombosis and Haemostasis (ICTH) have recommended 0.109 mol/l sodium citrate in a proportion of 9 volumes of blood to 1 volume of sodium citrate solution (37).

Despite this recommendation, other citrate concentrations are being used. In one study, 0.109 mol/l and 0.129 mol/l sodium citrate were compared (30). Within a normal range of haematocrits, the concentration of citrate used did not appear to be significant in the results of the PT or APTT in normals or in individuals receiving coumadin. However, the significance of the citrate concentration may be dependent on the type of reagent used. In a recent study we compared 0.109 mol/l with 0.136 mol/l sodium citrate, using three different thromboplastins. Significantly longer PTs were observed in anticoagulated patients in 0.136 mol/l, but not in normals (Table 6.1). This means that the PT-ratios of the patients in 0.136 mol/l are significantly higher than in 0.109 mol/l sodium citrate.

Non-buffered sodium citrate ($Na_3C_6H_5O_7$) solution has a pH > 8.0. If non-buffered sodium citrate is stored in siliconized glass tubes, the silicone layer may become unstable due to changes in the silica skeleton of the glass (90). This can be avoided by using buffered sodium citrate. Some manufacturers of evacuated tubes use a mixture of sodium citrate and citric acid at pH 5.8.

However, at pH 7.4 the buffering capacity of sodium citrate/citric acid is extremely low. Without additional buffering the pH of citrate plasma may rise to 8.5 due to loss of carbon dioxide. At high pH labile clotting factors, e.g. Factors V and VIII may deteriorate rapidly. Good results were obtained by buffering plasma with *N*-2-hydroxyethyl piperazine *N'*-2-ethane sulphonic acid (HEPES) in the preparation of lyophilized plasma samples for quality control (100).

It should be kept in mind that although HEPES prevents the deterioration of some clotting factors, it prolongs the clotting time in the PT test (80). The magnitude of the HEPES effect is shown for several thromboplastins in Table 6.2. In contrast, HEPES has been shown to shorten the APTT in patients receiving heparin by intravenous infusion (93).

Table 6.1   The effect of sodium citrate concentration on the prothrombin time

	Mean PT (s)			
	Normals (n = 10)		Patients (n = 13)	
	0.109 mol/l	0.136 mol/l	0.109 mol/l	0.136 mol/l
Thromboplastin–FS	14.1	14.1	37.0	38.6
Thrombotest	36.7	36.1	125.5	129.0
BCT/099	13.9	14.0	47.4	48.2

Blood was collected in tubes containing either 0.109 mol/l sodium citrate or 0.136 mol/l sodium citrate. The blood was centrifuged, plasma removed, and PTs determined. Results were obtained in 10 normal individuals and in 13 patients on oral anticoagulant treatment. Mean PTs are shown for three different thromboplastins: Thromboplastin–FS (American Dade), Thrombotest (Nycomed), and BCT/099 (human-brain reference material obtained from BCR). The differences in PT between the citrate concentrations are significant in the patients ($P < 0.05$), but not in the normals.

Specimen stability

Transport to the laboratory

The specimen should be transported to the laboratory as quickly as possible. It is important to maintain the containers in an upright position. Vigorous vibration, e.g.

Table 6.2   Effect of HEPES on prothrombin time

	Mean PT (s)			
	Normals (n = 4)		Patients (n = 10)	
	Citrate	Plus HEPES	Citrate	Plus HEPES
Thromboplastin–FS	15.0	15.1	30.9	31.6
Thrombotest	35.6	37.5	107.7	111.4
BCT/099	15.3	15.4	43.2	43.5

Blood was collected in tubes containing either 0.109 mol/l sodium citrate or 0.109 mol/l sodium citrate plus 0.27 mol/l HEPES (pH adjusted to 7.3 by NaOH). The blood was centrifuged, plasma removed, and PTs determined. Results were obtained in 4 normal individuals and in 10 patients on oral anticoagulant treatment.

caused by transportation on a trolley, must be avoided since haemolysis and damage to blood components could ensue.

There are conflicting opinions concerning the temperature at which the specimens should be maintained. NCCLS recommended that the blood specimen should be immediately placed in melting ice or equivalent (64). The rate of Factor VIII:C deterioration at 21°C is similar to that at 4°C (74), so that Factor VIII assay does not require the sample to be maintained at 4°C. More important than temperature is the delay between blood collection and Factor VIII assay, which should be less than 2 h (16). In view of the effect of cold-promoted activation of Factor VII, it would be preferable to maintain the blood samples at an ambient temperature of 15–20°C if a PT or Factor VII assay is required (80).

It is also important to keep the blood containers tightly capped to prevent loss of carbon dioxide and associated rise in pH. Koepke *et al.* (49) confirmed that no significant change in either PT or partial thromboplastin time occurred during storage of unopened citrated specimens at room temperature for as long as 6 h.

A decrease in APTT was observed in citrated blood specimens obtained from patients receiving heparin during storage at room temperature (93). However, an increase in APTT was observed when the specimens were stored at 4°C. When the blood was collected in a mixture of citrate, theophylline, adenosine and dipyridamole (CTAD), storage at room temperature resulted in much less shortening of the APTT (Fig. 6.2).

Release of platelet factor 4 during storage could be inhibited by CTAD mixture, which may explain why the effect of heparin on the APTT decays at a slower rate.

The effect of temperature on APTT stability may be dependent on the instrument used for the assessment. While the APTT of a normal plasma kept at 4°C did not change over a 6-h period with a turbidimetric procedure and the fibrometer (mechanical instrument), the same plasma incubated at 25°C gave longer APTTs with the turbidimetric method as the incubation progressed, but gave constant APTTs with the fibrometer (34).

Deep-frozen plasma

If fresh plasma cannot be tested within a limited time after venepuncture, it may be stored deep-frozen. It should be appreciated that some of the clotting factors even deteriorate in fresh-frozen plasma.

In general, the clotting factors in deep-frozen plasma will be more stable when the temperature of storage is lower. It is suggested that deterioration of clotting factors is minimized by rapid processing and double centrifugation to eliminate most cells (16). The manner in which the plasma is deep frozen is important, and even slight variations in technical procedure may affect the duration of stability. Storage in small aliquots in liquid nitrogen ($-196°C$) is the optimum if facilities are available. This is particularly desirable if the plasma is to be used repeatedly for assays extended over a period of time, e.g. as a reference material (94).

Comparison of Table 6.3 with Table 6.2 shows the effect of plasma freezing and thawing on the PT. Although the effect is relatively small, a prolongation of the clotting time could be observed with some thromboplastins. This effect does not seem to be of clinical significance.

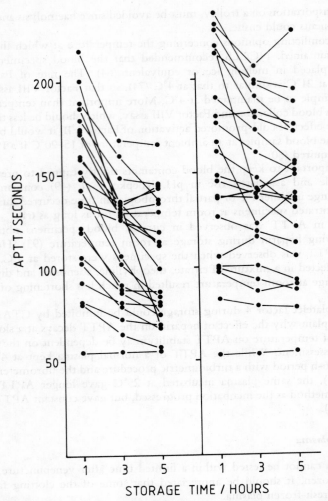

Fig. 6.2 APTT (Manchester Reagent) of individual patient samples as a function of storage time. Patients were monitored for treatment with heparin. Left panel: blood samples were collected in sodium citrate (in polystyrene tubes) and stored at room temperature. Right panel: blood samples were collected in a mixture of citrate, theophylline, adenosine, dipyridamole (in polystyrene tubes) and stored at room temperature. (From Ref. 93, with permission.)

Activated partial thromboplastin time (APTT)

The APTT test is widely used as a screening test for disorders of the intrinsic coagulation pathway. Furthermore, it is the most commonly used test to monitor the

Table 6.3 Effect of freezing and thawing of plasma on prothrombin time

	Mean PT (s)			
	Normals ($n=4$)		Patients ($n=10$)	
	Citrate	Plus HEPES	Citrate	Plus HEPES
Thromboplastin–FS	15.0	15.2	31.6	32.2
Thrombotest	36.0	37.7	113.3	116.5
BCT/099	15.0	15.3	43.1	43.6

Plasma specimens described in Table 6.2 were centrifuged at 20,000 **g** for 30 min at 4°C and then were frozen at −70°C and stored for 20 h. After thawing in a waterbath at 37°C for 3 min, PTs were determined as described in Table 6.2.

level of anticoagulation in patients receiving heparin therapy. It is also used to detect acquired inhibitors of coagulation, e.g. lupus–like inhibitors and Factor VIII inhibitors.

There is a wide diversity of APTT reagents and techniques in use. Many of these differ in sensitivity and responsiveness to the clotting factors of the intrinsic pathway, to heparin, or to the acquired inhibitors. There is now urgent need for standardization of reagents and techniques, as stressed by Thomson and Poller (82).

The first step towards standardization is the adoption of a set of guidelines for the acceptable performance of APTT testing in clinical laboratories, taking into account the needs for the clinical care of the patient (47). Comparative studies of different APTT-systems have been reported (79).

Reference (normal) ranges

One of the first steps in the introduction of an APTT technique must be to determine the range of normality. This range must be established using fresh plasma samples from subjects who should be taking no medication and have no known illnesses. Sufficient plasma samples must be included for adequate statistical analysis to establish mean and ±2 SD as the normal range. According to Koepke (47) at least 40 different individuals are necessary for this, although Thomson and Poller (82) suggest that at least 50 samples should be tested over a wide age range as the APTT progressively shortens from childhood to old age. Each laboratory should develop its own reference range. Once this is reliably established, it should not be necessary to have to change the stated normal range but frequent checks are advised to control any inter-batch variations of reagents or changes in technique. If the distribution of the normal values is non-Gaussian by examination of coefficients of skewness and kurtosis, the data require transformation to obtain a corrected normal range (79).

Requirements for precision and responsiveness

Within-run precision may be calculated by performing ten replicate analyses on one normal plasma and one abnormal patient plasma. The within-run coefficient of variation should be less than 3%. Between-run precision (same day) should be better than 4% (CV).

Between-day variation may be assessed by analysing appropriate lyophilized plasmas in the normal range daily for 20 days. The between-day precision should be better than 5% CV. Lyophilized plasmas are available from some commercial manufacturers. These are valuable in assessing day-to-day variation. The slope of the line relating the APTT to the logarithm of the Factor VIII concentration is linear over a wide range. Acceptable tolerance limits for the APTT as a function of Factor VIII concentration have been proposed (47).

Prothrombin time (PT)

The PT originally described by Quick *et al.* (72) should be regarded as a misnomer. Quick thought it was specific for prothrombin (Factor II) but later work showed that it was prolonged also by deficiencies of Factors V, VII and X. Lack of fibrinogen and excess heparin in the blood also prolong the PT but this is of academic interest only since both conditions are rare and, when they do occur, they are readily recognized and easily differentiated from depression of Factors II, V, VII and X.

The PT is the most frequently used assay in the coagulation laboratory because it serves two important purposes: screening of the extrinsic coagulation system and control of oral anticoagulant treatment.

Many modifications have been introduced to the test described by Quick. In addition to rabbit brain as a source of tissue thromboplastin, other material has been used, e.g. rabbit lung, porcine lung, human brain, human placenta, monkey brain, ox brain. Extracts of all these tissues, with the exception of human brain, are commercially available. Some thromboplastin preparations are supplemented with adsorbed plasma as a source of fibrinogen and Factor V, e.g. Thrombotest (69). Such combined reagents were developed specifically to control oral anticoagulant treatment.

In addition to the wide variety of thromboplastin preparations, there are many techniques and instruments (coagulometers) available to determine the clotting time in the PT test. Depending on the principle of clot detection, different clotting times may be obtained in a given specimen–thromboplastin mixture; and to further complicate PT testing, different methods of expressing the results are still in use, e.g. clotting time in seconds, clotting time ratio, activity and index.

Due to all these variables, comparability of results obtained by different centres has been poor. Several methods were proposed to standardize the prothrombin test. In some countries, the practice has been to use a single reagent or technique. In other countries, standardization by means of lyophilized plasma standards was proposed (24, 50, 91).

One of the first steps leading to the establishment of a reference method for the one-stage PT test was the recommendation of a standardized test procedure (36). Although this is now of historical interest, many of the recommended conditions of testing have been maintained in the test procedures of reagents which are now commercially available. Despite these efforts many years passed before international agreement was achieved on a universal system for PT standardization and a uniform scale for expressing of results (39). It is hoped that careful application of this system will resolve the confusion about the optimal therapeutic range for oral anticoagulant (53, 55).

International standardization

International standardization of the PT can be achieved by relating any given test system to an established primary standard reference method. In 1977, a research standard prepared by ICTH in collaboration with the National Institute of Biological Standards and Control (NIBSC), London, was established by the World Health Organization (WHO) as the primary international reference preparation (IRP) for thromboplastin (97). This material, coded 67/40, was prepared from human brain supplemented with adsorbed bovine plasma (combined reagent), to be used according to meticulously defined instructions (1).

WHO calibration model

A further advance in standardization was the development of a model for the calibration of any PT test system in terms of the primary IRP, as proposed by Kirkwood (44). In this model, a linear relationship was hypothesized between the logarithms of PTs obtained with the primary IRP method and the logarithms of PTs obtained with the test system (Fig. 6.3). Furthermore, the model required that a single relationship be valid for fresh plasma specimens of normal individuals and fresh specimens of patients on stabilized oral anticoagulant treatment:

$$\log \mathrm{PT}_{67/40} = a + c. \log \mathrm{PT}_{\mathrm{test}}$$

in which a and c are the intercept and slope of the calibration line, respectively. The model leads to a simple equation to transform a PT ratio R ($=$ patient PT : mean normal PT) obtained with a working PT system into the PT ratio which would have been obtained had the primary IRP 67/40 been used:

$$R_{67/40} = R^{\mathrm{ISI}}$$

in which ISI is the *international sensitivity index*. The ISI is equal to the slope c. $R_{67/40}$ is usually called the *international normalized ratio* (INR). The INR is the universal scale to express the PT for oral anticoagulant control. This calibration model was tested successfully in an international collaborative exercise organized by the European Community Bureau of Reference (BCR) and ICSH (33). Consequently, this model was adopted by WHO (98).

Calibrations of other thromboplastins have been carried out in accordance with the WHO model (14, 70, 83, 84, 92). However, the WHO model is empirical and for a particular combination of thromboplastins, a significant deviation from the model has

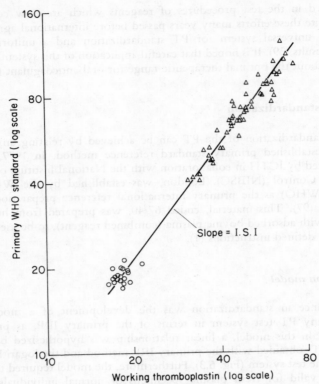

Fig. 6.3 Calibration of a working thromboplastin system against the primary WHO Standard (Preparation coded 67/40). The working thromboplastin PTs are plotted along the horizontal axis and the primary Standard PTs along the vertical axis. PTs of normal individuals (circles) and of patients on stabilized oral anticoagulant treatment (triangles) are plotted on double-logarithmic scales. The calibration line is calculated by orthogonal regression analysis. The slope of the line is the designated ISI of the working thromboplastin system.

been observed although a modified model could account for the experimental calibration data (27).

Generally speaking, it is the thromboplastin manufacturer's responsibility to provide the calibration data for each batch of their material (39). This can be done in several ways, i.e. reporting of ISI-value or providing a table in which the relationship between clotting time (ratio), percentage activity and INR is given.

In some countries, e.g. the Netherlands, national reference laboratories are involved in the determination of calibration data for thromboplastins being used in that country.

Selection of thromboplastin standards

The WHO model for thromboplastin calibration requires a hierarchy of standardization (Fig. 6.4). The secondary standards have been calibrated against the primary IRP in international collaborative exercises. The calibration of a thromboplastin is, in general, more precise when comparisons are made between similar preparations from the same species. The secondary standards represent different species and types of reagents commercially available. It is suggested that laboratories and manufacturers use the secondary standard of the same species for the calibration of their materials (98). Furthermore, the composition of the thromboplastin reagent has been shown to have considerable effect on the precision of calibration (85, 86). Plain reagents (i.e. without addition of adsorbed plasma) should be calibrated against a plain secondary standard; combined reagents should be calibrated against a combined standard. At present only one combined standard (OBT/79) is available, as the primary IRP 67/40 has been discontinued (99).

The WHO standards are intended only for the calibration of national reference preparations. A supply is available to a limited number of national control laboratories (98).

Secondary standards are also available from the BCR. These reference materials are intended to be more widely available to manufacturers of commercial or non-commercial thromboplastins. The BCR reference materials have been certified in terms of the primary WHO IRP 67/40. Manufacturers of thromboplastin are being urged to introduce a house standard or working reference preparation which is a batch of thromboplastin set aside for the calibration of individual production batches. The calibration of the house standard should be performed by comparison with a (BCR) secondary standard. The calibrated house standard may then be used for the calibration of subsequent batches of the same production line. Batch-to-batch calibration may be carried out with pooled plasmas (either deep-frozen or lyophilized) instead of fresh plasmas.

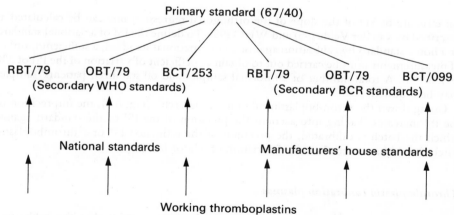

Fig. 6.4 Hierarchy of thromboplastin calibration. The first international reference preparation, coded 67/40 (primary standard), was a human-brain thromboplastin with added adsorbed bovine plasma (combined preparation). This was replaced in 1984 by a human-brain preparation, plain (coded BCT/253). The secondary standards BCT/099 (human, plain), RBT/79 (rabbit, plain) and OBT/79 (bovine, combined) are available from the BCR. RBT/79 and OBT/79 are also available from WHO to national control laboratories.

Requirements for fresh patients' samples

According to the recommendations of WHO (98), plasmas for calibrating thromboplastin should come from patients who have been on oral anticoagulants for at least 6 weeks and have been stabilized. In the calibration of the secondary thromboplastin standards (33), it was required that the patients' INR values were between 1.5 and 5. Some investigators have suggested that the WHO calibration model is not completely appropriate for some thromboplastins (77). For those thromboplastins, the ISI determination could be dependent on the intensity of anticoagulation in the patient group used for calibration and patients with high INR values could introduce a bias. The accuracy of the ISI may be improved by a slightly narrower range (INR 1.5–4.5) and by homogeneous distribution of patients' samples over this range.

Orthogonal regression equation

The parameters a and c may be estimated by orthogonal regression analysis. Ordinary linear regression is not appropriate because the errors of the quantities along both axes are of the same magnitude (95). In the orthogonal regression analysis the orthogonal distances of the measurement points to the line are used for calculation of the line. Furthermore, this analysis allows calculation of the standard deviation about the line. It was recommended to remove measurement points whose orthogonal distance to the line is larger than 3 SD (33).

Statistical evaluation

An estimate of SD of the slope of the orthogonal regression line can be calculated as described by van der Velde (95) and WHO (98). To define the ISI of a national standard or a house standard by calibration against an international standard, a sufficient number of measurements must be carried out to obtain a coefficient of variation of the ISI of 3% or less (98). A total number of 20 normal samples and 60 stabilized patients' samples may be required.

Going down the thromboplastin calibration hierarchy (Fig. 6.4), the imprecision of the ISI increases. Taking into account the precision of the ISI of the standard against which the batch is calibrated, the precision of the estimated ISI of a thromboplastin batch should have a coefficient of variation of 5% or less (98).

Thromboplastin calibration plasmas

Any plasma which is used in thromboplastin calibration is referred to as a calibration plasma. As described before, the calibration of a thromboplastin system in terms of a reference system is carried out primarily by using a series of fresh plasmas of normals and patients stabilized on oral anticoagulant therapy.

There are three obstacles in the implementation of the WHO system for thromboplastin calibration. Firstly, manufacturers of commercial thromboplastins have difficulties in obtaining the required number of fresh plasmas for calibration of each batch of their material. Secondly, it is practically impossible to provide calibration data (i.e. ISI) for each combination of thromboplastin and instrument based on fresh plasmas. Thirdly, for determination of a PT–ratio, each laboratory should have a value for the mean PT of a sufficient number of normals, which is not always available. These obstacles could be overcome if fresh plasmas could be replaced by lyophilized plasmas without loss of accuracy.

Calibration plasmas 'normal'. Several thromboplastin calibration studies have been published in which the calibration slopes obtained with fresh plasmas were compared with the slopes based on lyophilized pooled plasmas (1, 38, 56).

From the published data, the effect of replacement of fresh normal plasmas by lyophilized normal plasmas cannot be assessed directly, because the fresh patient plasmas were replaced by lyophilized plasmas as well. Experience with batch-to-batch calibration of Thrombotest has shown that the slopes obtained with freshly prepared normal plasma may differ systematically from those obtained with lyophilized normal plasma (58). According to these authors, the difference is probably the result of changes in the clottability of normal fibrinogen caused by the lyophilization process.

Another study has shown that there can be differences in calibration slopes between lyophilized normal plasmas from different manufacturers (89), which may be due to different levels of contact activation of the plasmas.

Calibration plasmas 'abnormal'. Calibration plasmas designed to mimic the coagulation defect induced by oral anticoagulants can be prepared by adsorption of vitamin K-dependent coagulation factors to barium sulphate or aluminium hydroxide. Many studies were performed to investigate whether or not such artificially depleted plasmas could replace patient plasmas.

In one study, lyophilized artificially depleted plasmas were compared with lyophilized pooled patient plasmas and with freshly prepared patient plasmas (1). The study showed that it is possible to obtain similar calibration slopes with fresh and freeze-dried patient plasma for all thromboplastins in that study except one. The calibration slopes obtained with artificially prepared plasmas were different from the fresh-plasma slopes for all thromboplastins except one. The authors concluded that artificially prepared abnormal plasmas appear to have little use in the calibration of thromboplastins for control of anticoagulant therapy.

This conclusion was confirmed by a large collaborative study (38). Values obtained from freeze-dried coumarin plasmas gave generally similar results to those from fresh plasmas for all thromboplastins, whereas values from artificial plasmas agreed with those from fresh plasmas only when similar thromboplastins were being compared. Loeliger and Van Halem-Visser (57) concluded that all types of lyophilized plasmas included in the ICTH/ICSH collaborative study were to some degree distinguishable from fresh patient plasmas. Primary calibration of a thromboplastin must therefore still be performed with freshly prepared normal as well as patient plasmas.

Even though lyophilized plasmas may not be suitable for the calibration of unlike thromboplastins, they might be useful for batch-to-batch calibration of thromboplastins. Successive batches of a given brand are expected to be very similar and slight differences in response to the coumarin–induced defect might be reflected accurately by lyophilized plasmas. A recent study showed that for three brands of rabbit tissue thromboplastins, batch–to–batch calibration could be performed accurately using three lyophilized plasmas: one pooled normal and two pooled patient ('coumarin') plasmas (92). For two brands, however. a significant difference between fresh plasmas and lyophilized plasmas was observed (92). For another brand of thromboplastin, freeze–dried artificially depleted plasma was equally good as fresh coumarin plasma for calibration of production batch against a house standard (15). However, if the buffering capacity of a batch is different from that of the house standard, e.g. by addition of phenol, inaccurate estimates of the calibration slope may be obtained by using lyophilized or artificial plasmas (15).

Control plasmas

The term control plasma refers to plasma used in internal quality control. It serves the purpose of checking the day–to–day consistency of an assay system. If the plasma is used for precision control only, the 'true value' of the assayed parameter is not of interest. Both normal and abnormal control plasmas should be used. Fresh and frozen control plasmas may be prepared by the laboratory itself. Lyophilized control plasmas can be obtained also from commercial sources. The use and limitation of artificially depleted plasma for calibration has been described above (p. 133). This applies also to its use in external quality assessment. In proficiency testing surveys in the US, the estimated effects of thromboplastins on the PT measured in lyophilized pooled patient plasmas were different from those in lyophilized artificially depleted plasmas, even though all thromboplastins were prepared from rabbit tissues (91). Organs of the same species may be prepared in different ways, for example, brain tissue may be extracted freshly, after deep freezing or after acetone drying, and these preparations will react differently to the various types of plasma which may be used for calibration or proficiency testing.

The all–important property of a control plasma is its stability. Stability should be determined before use in internal quality control (see below).

Stability of lyophilized plasma

The reliability of a lyophilized control plasma or a calibration plasma is determined by its stability. Commercially available, artificially prepared abnormal plasmas are claimed to be stable for at least 18 months at 4°C (62). Lyophilized normal and coumarin plasmas stored for 4 years at −20°C did not show signs of deterioration (59).

However, the stability of lyophilized plasmas is monitored by using thromboplastins which may not be stable themselves (35); this problem may be avoided by predicting the stability from accelerated degradation studies (40, 43). This method has been used for the prothrombin time in lyophilized coumarin plasmas by Lang and Kleindel (52), who showed that the Arrhenius equation could be used for the prediction of plasma stability and that the stability could be improved by reducing the residual moisture in the lyophilized plasmas. The drying of biological materials by sublimation of ice *in vacuo* is not a single, simple process. The final product obtained is a function of the chemical and physical nature of the macromolecules present, the kinds and amounts of water molecules and their relation to the types and kinds of macromolecules, the influence of water on the conformation of the macromolecules, the gaseous environment in which dried preparations are placed and the physical principles regulating the process of lyophilization. Accelerated degradation studies of dried influenza virus showed that an optimum content of residual moisture is associated with greatly increased stabilities (31).

Studies in our laboratory suggest that the stability of lyophilized plasma is decreased at residual moisture contents below approximately 1.5%.

The stability of reconstituted plasma depends on several factors. Firstly, the treatment of plasma before lyophilization determines the level of activation of clotting factors (56, 89). The vials containing the plasma should be well-siliconized. If not, the plasma will be activated. The plasma should be buffered (e.g. with HEPES) to avoid a pH increase and a concomitant decrease of Factor V activity (100).

Secondly, the change in clotting time depends on the reagent used. Thrombotest, a bovine thromboplastin, is very sensitive to activation of Factor VII. In several studies, shortening of the Thrombotest clotting times was observed (12, 56, 89).

Thirdly, the temperature at which the reconstituted plasma is stored affects the stability. According to Brozovic *et al.* (12), storage at 4°C is the optimal condition for stability of reconstituted plasma. Activation of Factor VII did not occur at 4°C, but was significant at 20°C and 37°C.

A small but significant change in PT (rabbit-brain thromboplastin) of reconstituted plasmas stored at room temperature was observed in the ICTH/ICSH study (38). In that study, storage for about 6 h resulted in a PT increase of 6% for one plasma, but in a PT decrease of 3 and 5% respectively for two other plasmas.

Therapeutic control of oral anticoagulation

An important part of internal quality control in the anticoagulation clinic is the assessment of therapeutic control achieved in the patients under treatment. This type of self-audit has demonstrated that the quality of oral anticoagulant therapy may require considerable improvement, particularly in short-term patients (61). In some hospitals, under-anticoagulation is the main deficiency in the therapeutic control, most probably due to excessively cautious prescribing by junior staff concerned to avoid the risk of bleeding problems (32).

There are two types of therapeutic control which are complementary. The proportion of time spent in the therapeutic range is an overall view of the clinic's performance and information is provided as to whether there is over- or under-treatment. The second type of control is the number of patients achieving a stated degree of therapeutic control, as a measure of the individual's control (13). For example, under-anticoagulation for 10% of the time could be due to many patients being under-treated for a short time, or alternatively a few patients over a prolonged period.

Different methods have been advocated for assessing the proportion of time spent in the therapeutic range. Duxbury (19) and Raper (73) used the time interval between the midpoints of successive tests to calculate the duration of satisfactory control. This method has been criticized by Majumdar and Payne (61), arguing that when dose changes are made, correction of the prothrombin time would usually be expected sooner than the midpoint of the interval between successive tests. Copplestone and Roath (13) assumed that the prothrombin time remained stable between clinic visits, and the weeks between were counted as the same as the succeeding clinic visit.

Another method of therapeutic control is the assessment of the number of satisfactory tests expressed as the percentage of total tests either in the individual patient or in the whole patient population (32, 61). However, in the latter method the frequency of unsatisfactory control is overestimated because tests are usually performed more frequently during unstable periods, thereby increasing the number of unsatisfactory results in relation to the total number of tests. This bias can be avoided by considering only the latest tests for all patients under treatment (11). In this method, called the 'cross-section through the files' approach (54), each patient is assessed with equal weight. It provides an overall view of the clinic's performance (Fig. 6.5). The Federation of Dutch Thrombosis Centres requests its members to perform such assessment of their patient populations twice a year. Loeliger (54) compared the 'cross-section through the files' approach with the proportion of time spent in the therapeutic range. Although the results obtained with the two methods were very similar, the frequency distribution of the proportion of time spent in range was broader than the distribution of the cross-section through the files, suggesting that therapeutic control is underestimated by the assessment of time spent in range (Fig. 6.6).

It is not difficult to find one reason for this phenomenon. When a patient is over-

CROSS-SECTION THROUGH THE FILES

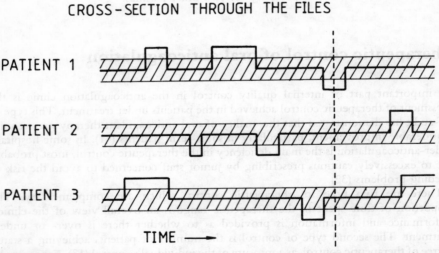

Fig. 6.5 Principle of assessment of a clinic's therapeutic control by taking a cross-section of all patients' files. For simplicity, only three patients are depicted. The hatched bar represents each patient's therapeutic range. The patient's actual anticoagulant level is represented by the thick line. The probability that a patient is within the therapeutic range at any moment (vertical stippled line) is equal to the proportion of time spent in the range.

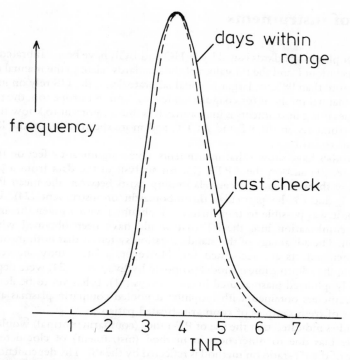

Fig. 6.6 Frequency distributions of anticoagulant intensity in patients with artificial heart valves on long-term treatment. All 180 patients of the Leiden Thrombosis Centre in the files on 15 October 1984 were assessed. The solid line represents, for the period between 15 July and 15 October 1984, the results calculated according to the method of Duxbury (19). The dashed line represents those from the 'cross-section through the files' approach. (From Ref. 54, with permission of author and S. Karger AG, Basel.)

anticoagulated at one clinic visit and under-anticoagulated at the next visit, the patient must have been in the therapeutic range for a proportion of time between the visits, but both the method of Duxbury (19) and that of Copplestone and Roath (13) neglect this proportion of time. The assumption that an unsatisfactory test result would reflect the whole period between successive tests may not be true.

For this reason, the 'cross-section through the files' approach is recommended for therapeutic control in the anticoagulant clinic. A random sample of 100 charts from the files can be expected to reflect the quality of the patients' adherence to the recommended ranges (54). One should be cautious in comparing the therapeutic control data of different clinics, especially if they do not use the same ranges. The difficulty of maintaining therapeutic control becomes increasingly greater with narrower and higher ranges (20, 21).

Effects of instruments

The thromboplastin standards issued by WHO and BCR have been calibrated by means of manual techniques, and the ISI values of the standards relate to the manual technique. However, more than 98% of larger hospital laboratories in the US rely on instruments rather than manual methods for coagulation testing, and in Europe too, the proportion of laboratories using instruments is increasing. It is thus important to know the effect of different instruments on the PT and APTT, and more specifically, on the ISI for oral anticoagulant control.

Several studies have shown that instruments have a significant effect on the PT (24, 38, 48, 50, 78, 91) and on the APTT (7). An analysis of the data from a proficiency testing survey showed that a linear relationship exists between the mean PT and the effect on PT due to the particular thromboplastin or instrument (24). Using that relationship, it was possible to transform a PT obtained with a given thromboplastin/ instrument combination into the PT that would have been obtained with another combination. The advantage of this standardization system is that both thromboplastin and instrument effects are accounted for. However, a later study showed that the parameters in the additive linear model proposed by Evatt *et al.* (24) were dependent on the type of lyophilized plasmas used in the surveys (91). It has yet to be demonstrated that the parameters obtained with lyophilized pooled coumarin plasmas are valid to convert PTs of fresh samples of coumarin-treated patients.

Some studies indicated that the use of PT-ratios (coumarin:normal) would eliminate some of the bias due to differences in method (instrument) of clot detection. The dependence of the PT-ratio on method is reflected by the ISI. The dependence of the ISI on method has been investigated in our laboratory. A batch of Thromboplastin-FS and of Thromboplastin-C were calibrated against the standard for rabbit thromboplastin (RBT/79) according to WHO procedure. RBT/79 was tested using the manual technique, but the other two thromboplastins by means of a number of other methods in addition to the manual technique (Table 6.4). For these thromboplastins, photo-optical instruments had higher ISI-values than mechanical instruments. This is partly due to longer PTs of normal samples in the photo-optical instruments than in the mechanical instruments. Our results imply that the thromboplastin manufacturer should indicate the instrument(s) for which the stated ISI is valid.

However, it is practically impossible to assess ISI-values for all instruments which are now used by clinical laboratories. A more practical approach would be for manufacturers of thromboplastin to provide lyophilized reference plasmas with an assigned INR. For this purpose it does not matter whether the plasma which the manufacturer provides has a coumarin-induced or artificial defect but it should only be tested against the manufacturer's own thromboplastin (59). We have calculated INR-equivalents for an artificial plasma (Citrol-2) using a mechanical and a photo-optical instrument (Table 6.5). The relative difference between the INR-equivalents is smaller than the difference between the PT-ratios. This suggests that the instrument-specific ISI-values can allow determination of INR-equivalents with acceptable precision on an artificial plasma sample. In principle, only two calibration plasmas are required by the clinical laboratory to establish the relationship between local PT and INR-scale (Fig. 6.7). Since the local mean normal PT has a fixed value, both PT and PT-ratio may be used for the

Table 6.4 ISI and control values for two rabbit-brain thromboplastins

	Thromboplastin-C lot no. 322			Thromboplastin-FS lot no. 23A		
	ISI	Fresh normals $\bar{x} \pm SD^a$ (s)	Citrol-1 lot no. 298B (s)	ISI	Fresh normals $\bar{x} \pm SD^a$ (s)	Citrol-1 lot no. 298B (s)
Mechanical (Schnitger & Gross, Amelung)	2.14	11.9 ± 0.6	12.5	1.28	14.2 ± 0.9	14.6
Mechanical (Fibrometer)	2.15	11.7 ± 0.5	11.8	1.27	13.9 ± 0.8	14.4
Photo-optical (MLA 700)	2.37	12.2 ± 0.5	12.6	1.48	15.2 ± 1.0	15.6

^{a}SD = standard deviation, including biological variation between normal individuals ($n = 20$).

Table 6.5 INR-equivalents for artificially depleted control plasma

	Thromboplastin-C			Thromboplastin-FS		
	Citrol-2 lot no. 276 (s)	PT-ratio^a	INR^b	Citrol-2 lot no. 276 (s)	PT-ratio^a	INR^b
Mechanical (Schnitger & Gross, Amelung)	20.9	1.75	3.33	34.1	2.40	3.07
Photo-optical (MLA-700)	19.6	1.61	3.09	33.1	2.18	3.17

^{a} PT-ratios were calculated using the mean PT of fresh normal samples (see Table 6.4).
^{b} INR-equivalents were calculated using the equation INR = (PT-ratio)^{ISI} and the ISI values given in Table 6.4.

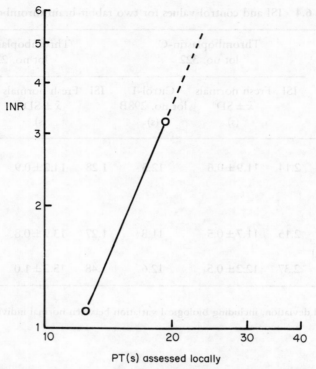

Fig. 6.7 Example of PT calibration line assessed locally by means of lyophilized calibration plasmas with assigned INR-values, for translation of PTs of patients on stable oral anticoagulation. Each calibration plasma is tested at least six times with the local PT system and the mean PT-values are plotted along the horizontal (logarithmic) scale. The assigned INR-values are to be provided by the manufacturer for the brand of thromboplastin used locally.

graph. Each calibration plasma should be tested on at least six occasions to obtain a precise mean value of the PT or PT-ratio. If one of the calibration plasmas has been prepared from normal plasmas without artificial depletion of clotting factors, lyophilization may affect the PT (see p. 133). Therefore, the manufacturer should indicate the relationship between such 'normal' calibration plasma and fresh pooled normal plasma. For the assessment of relationship or the INR-equivalent the manufacturer should use the mean PT of a sufficient number of fresh normal plasmas ($n \geqslant 10$) to eliminate the effect of biological variation (60).

Evaluation of duplicate PT and APTT assays

Proposed guidelines for coagulation assays require that all samples must be measured in duplicate (22, 64). Results of coagulation tests by manual methods have traditionally been reported as the mean of duplicate analyses on the same specimen as averaging of duplicate test results helped overcome lack of precision in these methods.

Advances in instrumentation have provided marked improvements in precision through the automation of the reagent-pipetting and clot-detection components of the assay. It has been shown that large-scale sample-pipetting errors are not detected by the performance of duplicate analyses, so that the use of duplicate analyses for that purpose may be unwarranted (75). As clinical laboratories are being challenged to cut operating expenses without significantly degrading the accuracy of test results, this emphasizes the need for re-evaluation of the requirements for duplicate PT and APTT assays.

To evaluate the utility or medical appropriateness for duplicate assays, it is necessary to determine the current level of duplicate assay precision under routine laboratory testing conditions. Clinical precision requirements must be related to the analytical precision in order to determine if elimination of duplicate assays would significantly affect the medical accuracy and the quality of patient care. A recent study showed that tolerance criteria based on percentage difference between duplicates provide more evaluation uniformity over all levels of PT and APTT values than does absolute difference (76).

In two clinical laboratories, fewer than 1% of the samples analysed for PT by either laboratory would require duplicates if a difference between duplicates of 5% or less is deemed analytically or clinically insignificant (76). Establishing a cut-off point, where all single PTs that exceed that value would be re-run in duplicate, affects the accuracy of reported results. As the cut-off value is set higher, the percentage of PT-values that would have to be re-run in duplicate decreases; however, the percentage of erroneous results obtained also increases. In one institution, only 5% of approximately 27,000 patient PTs per year are tested in duplicate (63). At a 25-second cut-off point chosen by the same institution to repeat PTs, probable case errors are only about 0.5%.

There is a greater degree of variation between duplicates in APTT testing than in PT testing (42, 76). According to Scheer *et al.* (76), a duplicate difference of 15% or less would probably be a realistic medically useful level for the APTT. Using such criterion, fewer than 2% of samples would exceed this limit for one laboratory, but 6.0% of samples from another laboratory exceeded this limit.

Based on these results, it was concluded that the decision as to whether or not to eliminate duplicate analyses should be made by each laboratory on the basis of data generated from the instruments, reagents, personnel and patient population of that institution relative to an acceptable level of clinical precision, particularly for APTT assays.

Coagulation factor assays

Apart from global screening tests like the PT, APTT and thrombin time, many laboratories regularly perform specific coagulation factor assays. In most situations the results of these analyses are used for the laboratory diagnosis of acquired or hereditary coagulation factor deficiencies. Also, the measurement of concentrations of individual coagulation factors may be used to confirm a medical diagnosis or to monitor progress of a disease or effectiveness of therapy.

In both situations it is important that the laboratory can provide the clinicians with precise values. The correctness of the values is especially important for the identification of patients with hereditary coagulation defects (mild and moderate defects; identification of heterozygotes) and for the monitoring of replacement therapy (safety of the patient). Therefore, internal quality control of coagulation factor assays should aim at both precision and correctness of the result. The first can be achieved by the critical evaluation of reagents, instruments and methods and the use of suitable control plasmas. Information on the correctness of assay results can be obtained by calibration of the local standards against international standards and by participation in external quality assessment schemes (see Chapter 7).

Selection of assay methods and reagents

In general, the concentration of an individual coagulation factor is measured with a one-stage coagulation assay. Dilutions of the test plasma are incubated with a plasma deficient of the relevant factor and clotted after addition of an activator (thromboplastin, APTT reagent, snake venom) and $CaCl_2$. The concentration of the coagulation factor is then calculated from the observed clotting times by interpolation in a calibration curve relating clotting time versus the concentration of the relevant coagulation factor (dilution of the pooled normal plasma).

The only exception on this general rule is the fibrinogen assay, in which deficient plasma is not required. Most laboratories now use the Clauss method for the fibrinogen assay. In this method dilutions of the test plasma are clotted with a fixed amount of thrombin, after which the clotting time is compared with those obtained with dilutions of plasma of known fibrinogen concentration.

Important for the final performance of the assay are the choice of the instrument, deficient plasma and the activator. In general, it is recommended that a laboratory first decides on the type of instrument from simple mechanical devices to fully automated autoanalysers, that would best fulfil the requirements of the laboratory. This largely depends on the daily workload, the size and degree of education of the laboratory staff, and the budget of the laboratory. With instruments which have the possibility of computerized data processing it is important to check whether the calculations are based on generally accepted procedures (see later). The method used for endpoint detection (mechanical; photo-optical; turbidimetric) may also have important implications for the applicability of different reagents and plasmas (i.e. lyophilized calibration and control plasmas).

Once the instrument has been selected, one should decide on the type and source of reagents. Formerly, commercial deficient plasmas were almost exclusively obtained from patients with isolated coagulation defects. However, the availability of commercial factor-deficiency plasmas is limited due to frequent transfusion of the patients, rarity of the disorder, and the risk of infectious disease (9). This might explain why other types of deficient plasma have been evaluated. These include artificially depleted or constructed plasmas (65) and also plasmas from (deficient) animals (28, 71). It is possible to prepare deficient plasmas by specific removal of the relevant coagulation factor with immuno-affinity procedures (6, 25, 29, 66, 87). Many of these plasmas are now commercially available and their use largely reduces the risk of transmittance of infectious diseases, a problem which became increasingly urgent during the past years with the use of congenital-deficiency plasmas (41).

The sensitivity of the assay is largely dependent on the residual amount of the relevant coagulation factor in the deficient plasma. This is of special importance for those coagulation factors where accurate results at levels below 10% of normal are required (e.g. Factor VIII, Factor IX) (8, 10). Also, the specificity of the test might depend on the selection of a deficient plasma, especially when the production procedure (chromatography; lyophilization) introduces a loss of activity of other coagulation factors (e.g. Factor V, fibrinogen) (9).

A clear advantage of the use of immune-depleted plasmas as deficient plasmas, is that these, in general, are better defined than the congenital-deficiency plasmas. It has been well established that many patients with a hereditary coagulation defect have a functionally defective molecule rather than a true molecular deficiency. This seems to be true especially for Factor VII and Factor IX deficiencies (5, 88). For most of the commercially available congenital-deficiency plasmas it is not known whether there is an abnormal molecule present or not and, if so, to what extent this abnormal molecule might interfere with the assay of the normal coagulation factor due to competition between normal and abnormal proteins, as for instance described for Factor IX-Bm and Factor X in the ox-brain thromboplastin time (67). Finally it is important to check whether the selected deficient plasma is sufficiently stable (especially after reconstitution) for efficient use in daily practice, and whether batch-to-batch variation is acceptably low.

The selection of a suitable activator requires several decisions to be made. For the assay of the extrinsic coagulation factors (Factors II, V, VII and X) a large number of thromboplastin preparations are commercially available. Some of these thromboplastins contain $CaCl_2$ and therefore it should be checked whether such a thromboplastin will comply with the assay design (especially important for automated instruments). Secondly, it should be checked whether the thromboplastin preparation is sufficiently stable for practical use (especially lyophilized preparations requiring reconstitution). Finally, special attention should be given to its application in the Factor VII assay. As the thromboplastin–Factor VII complex is the rate-limiting factor in determining the actual clotting time in this assay, it is important that the thromboplastin itself does not contain Factor VII, as this will result in a low sensitivity and less steep calibration curves. Further, it is important to check the interaction between the thromboplastin and the Factor VII-deficient plasma, especially if a congenital deficiency plasma has been selected. Brandt *et al.* (10) demonstrated that the residual Factor VII activity in this type of plasma largely varies with the type of thromboplastin used. On one hand this is due to the specificity of the thromboplastin–Factor VII interaction, on the other hand this might be related to abnormalities in the variant Factor VII of the patient, which are only detected with certain types of thromboplastin.

The different types of thromboplastin also differ in their ability to measure native and activated Factor VII. This may result in apparently discrepant results when changing from one type of thromboplastin to another.

For the assay of the intrinsic coagulation factors (Factors XII, XI, VIII, IX, V, X, II, prekallikrein and high molecular weight kininogen) both an activator (kaolin, silica, ellagic acid) and a phospholipid preparation need to be selected. Many commercial reagents can be considered as combined reagents, as they contain both the activator and the phospholipid. The stability of these reagents should be carefully checked, especially when they contain particulate material or are combined with locally prepared phospholipid preparations.

The type of activator and the source of phospholipid can have an important influence on the sensitivity of the assay and the steepness of the calibration curve (3). Together they have been found to contribute significantly to inter-laboratory variation for Factor VIII assays (46).

Calibration of assays

For the calibration of single-factor assays a pooled normal plasma is used. This can either be a locally prepared plasma pool, consisting of the plasmas of at least 20 healthy volunteers (no oral contraception users; rather wide age distribution) according to generally accepted guidelines and stored at $-20°C$ (for short-term use) or at $-70°C$ (for long-term use). By definition such a plasma pool will contain 1 unit/ml (or 100%) of each of the coagulation factors. However, subsequent pools may differ considerably with respect to the actual concentration of a specific coagulation factor. This is especially true for notoriously labile factors like Factors V and VIII (2). Therefore, it is recommended that subsequent pools be calibrated against each other or against a working or house standard to avoid a drift in the unity with time.

With respect to the measurement of the 'true value' for a specific coagulation factor it is important that the local pool has been calibrated (either directly or indirectly) against international standards as provided by WHO. In this way it will be possible to express the results in international units (IU). WHO has established standards for plasma Factor VIII (coded 80-5111) and for plasma Factor II, plasma Factor IX, plasma Factor X and plasma Factor VII (coded 84-665). In addition, it can provide standards for Factor VIII concentrate and Factor IX concentrate.

Many laboratories use commercial plasma pools, only some of which have been calibrated by the manufacturer against the relevant WHO standard. One should realize, however, that calibration has usually been performed by one laboratory using only one technique and type of reagents. In general, one should be careful in using a commercial lyophilized plasma pool as calibration plasma, because there always is the possibility that the production process has influenced the activity of the various coagulation factors in a different manner, thus introducing systematic deviations with respect to deep-frozen plasma pools.

Further criteria for the selection of a suitable commercial plasma pool should be its stability after reconstitution (18) and its availability in siliconized containers (to avoid contact activation during the production and after reconstitution).

Calculations

The calculation of the concentration of a single coagulation factor should be based on the principle of parallel dose–response curves (45). It is essential that the clotting times obtained at different dilutions of the calibration plasma and test plasma can be fitted in a linear dose–response curve. To achieve this it may be necessary to use log-transformed data. The coagulation factor concentration can then be calculated from the horizontal distance between the two parallel lines. If the dose–response curve for the test plasma is not parallel to that for the calibration plasma, it is impossible to calculate a potency for the test plasma. In practice this means that it is very important to check the parallelism, by testing at least two different dilutions of the plasma in duplicate in the assay. Non-parallelism is frequently observed when the unknown sample and the calibration plasma are unlike materials (for instance, coagulation factor concentrates). In such a situation one can either use a different standard (Factor IX or Factor VIII concentrate of known potency) or make an initial dilution of the concentrate in a plasma deficient of the relevant factor (4).

Control plasmas

To monitor the performance and precision of single-factor assays it is strongly recommended that one or two control plasmas be included in each run (68). The use of such control plasmas is extremely helpful to detect changes or drift in the assay performance.

Of course it is very important that such plasmas have a good and well documented stability. They can either be prepared locally and stored at $-20°C$ or purchased commercially. The use of these control plasmas will also allow the calculation of within-run, between-run and day-to-day variation and therefore will help in assessing the precision of the assay. Ideally, one should select one control plasma-normal (about 1 unit/ml of the relevant coagulation factor) and one control plasma-abnormal (containing the relevant coagulation factor at a critically lower level). It is important to include the control plasma-abnormal because it provides information on the performance of the assay at a coagulation factor level that is relevant for the decision-making of the clinician.

Chromogenic methods

For many of the coagulation factors and inhibitors specific chromogenic methods are commercially available or are being developed. The advantage of this type of assay is that it does not require deficient plasmas and can be easily automated. In most cases these assays are offered to the laboratory as complete kits; this has the obvious advantage of constant quality of the reagents. On the other hand, it is not always easy to modify the complicated design of the assay for use in a particular instrument. Moreover, different results might be obtained for the same patient samples when using kits from different manufacturers. This might be due to different sources and/or concentrations of the specific activators or enzymes used, but it also might be related to the use of different chromogenic substrates (different specificities). Therefore it is important to introduce chromogenic coagulation factor assays in the laboratory only after careful analysis of both the specificity and sensitivity of the various methods available. The internal quality control of such assays proceeds along the same lines as discussed for the coagulation assays.

Acknowledgements

The authors acknowledge the excellent technical assistance of Miss H. van Mansfeld. Mrs E. W. H. Vletter-Imanse prepared the typescript. This work was supported in part by the Netherlands Public Health Institute (Rijksinstituut voor Volksgezondheid and Milieuhygiene).

References

1. Bangham, D. R., Biggs, R., Brozovic, M. and Denson, K. W. E. (1973). Calibration of five different thromboplastins using fresh and freeze-dried plasma. *Thrombosis et Diathesis Haemorrhagica* **29:** 228–239.
2. Barrowcliffe, T. W. (1985). The use of standards in blood coagulation. In Thomson, J. M. (ed.) *Blood Coagulation and Haemostasis. A Practical Guide*, pp. 410–432. Edinburgh: Churchill Livingstone.
3. Barrowcliffe, T. W. and Gray, E. (1981). Studies of phospholipid reagents used in coagulation I: Some general properties and their sensitivity to factor VIII. *Thrombosis and Haemostasis* **46:** 629–633.
4. Barrowcliffe, T. W., Tydeman, M. S. and Kirkwood, T. B. L. (1979). Major effect of prediluent in factor IX clotting assay. *Lancet* **2:** 192.
5. Bertina, R. M. and Veltkamp, J. J. (1978). The abnormal factor IX of hemophilia B+ variants. *Thrombosis and Haemostasis* **40:** 335–349.
6. Bertina, R. M., Orlando, M. and Tiedemann Alderkamp, G. H. J. (1978). Preparation of a human factor VII deficient plasma. *Thrombosis Research* **13:** 537–541.
7. Brandt, J. T., and Triplett, D. A. (1981). Laboratory monitoring of heparin. Effect of reagents and instruments on the activated partial thromboplastin time. *American Journal of Clinical Pathology* **76:** 530–537.
8. Brandt, J. T., Carr, D. and Orr, C. A. (1986). Factor VIII assays: perspectives gained from monitoring intralaboratory quality control parameters. In Triplett, D. A. (ed.) *Advances in Coagulation Testing: Interpretation and Application*, pp. 33–46. Skokie, Illinois: College of American Pathologists.
9. Brandt, J. T., Triplett, D. A. and Fair, D. S. (1986). Characterization and comparison of immunodepleted and hereditary factor VII deficient plasma as substrate plasmas for factor VII assays. *American Journal of Clinical Pathology* **85:** 583–589.
10. Brandt, J. T., Triplett, D. A. and Fair, D. S. (1986). Choice of substrate plasma: the emerging role of immune-depleted substrate plasmas for one-stage coagulation factor assays. In Triplett, D. A. (ed.) *Advances in Coagulation Testing. Interpretation and Application*, pp. 1–8. Skokie, Illinois: College of American Pathologists.
11. Broekmans, A. W. and Loeliger, E. A. (1982). Therapeutic control of anticoagulant treatment. *British Medical Journal* **284:** 1330–1331.
12. Brozovic, M., Howarth, D. J., van Halem-Visser, L. P. and Loeliger, E. A. (1973). Stability of freeze-dried plasma prepared from patients on oral anticoagulants. *Journal of Clinical Pathology* **26:** 857–863.
13. Copplestone, A. and Roath, S. (1984). Assessment of therapeutic control of anticoagulation. *Acta Haematologica* **71:** 376–380.
14. Dati, F., Barthels, M., Conard, J., Flückiger, J., Girolami, A., Hänseler, E., Huber, J., Keller, F., Kolde, H. J., Müller-Berghaus, G., Samama, M. and Thiel, W. (1987). Multicenter evaluation of a chromogenic substrate method for photometric determination of prothrombin time. *Thrombosis and Haemostasis* **58:** 856–865.
15. Denson, K. W. E. (1986). Artificially depleted plasma for manufacturer international calibration of thromboplastin. *Clinical and Laboratory Haematology* **8:** 55–60.
16. DIN (1987). Einstufenmethode zur Bestimmung der Faktor VIII-Gerinnungsaktivität (F VIII:C). Deutsches Institut für Normung 58909 Teil 1, p. 2. Berlin: Beuth Verlag.

17. DIN (1987). Referenzplasma. Deutsches Institut für Normung 58939 Teil 1. Berlin: Beuth Verlag.
18. Dombrose, F. A., Barnes, C. C., Gaynor, J. J. and Elston, R. C. (1982). A lyophilized reference plasma for coagulation factors: evidence for stability of factors I, II, V and VII through XII. *American Journal of Clinical Pathology* **77**: 32–45.
19. Duxbury, B. McD. (1982). Therapeutic control of anticoagulant treatment. *British Medical Journal* **284**: 702–704.
20. Duxbury, B. McD. (1985). Assessment of therapeutic control of anticoagulation. *Acta Haematologica* **73**: 118.
21. Duxbury, B. McD. (1986). Therapeutic quality control leading to further clinical assessment of oral anticoagulation. *Acta Haematologica* **76**: 76–77.
22. ECCLS (1987). Standard for Quality Assurance. Part 4: Internal Quality Control in Haematology. ECCLS Document Vol. 4 No. 2, p. 10. Berlin: Beuth Verlag.
23. ECCLS (1987). Standard for Quality Assurance. Part 4: Internal Quality Control in Haematology. ECCLS Document Vol. 4, No. 2, p. 4. Berlin: Beuth Verlag.
24. Evatt, B. L., Brogan, D., Triplett, D. A. and Waters, G. (1981). Effect of thromboplastin and instrumentation on the prothrombin time test. *Clinical and Laboratory Haematology* **3**: 331–342.
25. Exner, T., Richard, K. A. and Speers, S. (1977). Factor VIII deficient plasma for laboratory tests prepared from normal plasma and a human antibody. *Haemostasis* **6**: 157–162.
26. Gilmer, P. R. (1982). Preanalytical variables in coagulation testing. In Triplett, D. A. (ed.) *Standardization of Coagulation Assays: An Overview*, pp. 1–8. Skokie, Illinois: College of American Pathologists.
27. Gogstad, G. O., Wadt, J., Smith, P. and Brynildsrud, T. (1986). Utility of a modified calibration model for reliable conversion of thromboplastin times to International Normalized Ratios. *Thrombosis and Haemostasis* **56**: 178–182.
28. Goldsmith, J. G., Chung, K. S. and Roberts, H. R. (1978). A simple assay for human factor IX: use of canine hemophilia B plasma as substrate. *Thrombosis Research* **12**: 497–502.
29. Goodall, A. H., Kemble, G., O'Brien, D. P., Rawlings, E., Rotblat, F., Russell, G. C., Janossy, G. and Tuddenheim, E. G. D. (1982). Preparation of factor IX deficient human plasma by immunoaffinity chromatography using a monoclonal antibody. *Blood* **59**: 664–670.
30. Gralnick, H. R., Kessler, C. R. and Palmer, R. (1982). The prothrombin time: variables affecting results. In Triplett, D. A. (ed.) *Standardization of Coagulation Assays: An Overview*, pp. 57–65. Skokie, Illinois: College of American Pathologists.
31. Greiff, D. (1971). Protein structure and freeze-drying: the effects of residual moisture and gases. *Cryobiology* **8**: 145–152.
32. Harries, A. D., Birtwell, A. J. and Jones, D. B. (1981). Anticoagulant control. *The Lancet* 1320.
33. Hermans, J., van den Besselaar, A. M. H. P., Loeliger, E. A. and van der Velde, E. A. (1983). A collaborative calibration study of reference materials for thromboplastins. *Thrombosis and Haemostasis* **50**: 712–717.
34. Hoak, D. R., Mammen, E. F., Banerjee, S. K. and Kaldor, G. (1985). A fully automated method for clot based coagulation panels using an MCA Multistat centrifugal analyzer. *Thrombosis Research* **39**: 485–499.
35. Ingram, G. I. C. (1979). The stability of the WHO Reference Thromboplastin NIBS & C 67/40. *Thrombosis and Haemostasis* **42**: 1135–1140.
36. Ingram, G. I. C. and Hills, M. (1976). Reference method for the one-stage prothrombin time test on human blood. *Thrombosis and Haemostasis* **36**: 237–238.
37. Ingram, G. I. C. and Hills, M. (1976). The prothrombin time test: Effect of varying citrate concentration. *Thrombosis and Haemostasis* **36**: 230–236.
38. ICTH/ICSH (1979). Prothrombin time standardization: report of the expert panel on oral anticoagulant control. *Thrombosis and Haemostasis* **42**: 1073–1114.
39. ICSH/ICTH (1985). ICSH/ICTH recommendations for reporting prothrombin time in oral anticoagulant control. *Thrombosis and Haemostasis* **53**: 155–156.
40. Jerne, N. K. and Perry, W. L. M. (1956). The stability of biological standards. *Bulletin of the World Health Organization* **14**: 167–182.
41. Jones, P., Hamilton, P. J., Oxley, A., Codd, A. and Tedder, R. (1985). Anti-HTLV-III positive laboratory reagents. *Lancet* **1**: 1458–1459.
42. Keshgegian, A. A., Mann, J. M. and Cooper, J. H. (1986). Is duplicate testing for prothrombin time and activated partial thromboplastins time necessary? *Archives of Pathology and Laboratory Medicine* **110**: 520–522.

43. Kirkwood, T. B. L. (1977). Predicting the stability of biological standards and products. *Biometrics* **33:** 736–742.
44. Kirkwood, T. B. L. (1983). Calibration of reference thromboplastins and standardization of the prothrombin time ratio. *Thrombosis and Haemostasis* **49:** 238–244.
45. Kirkwood, T. B. L. and Snape, T. J. (1980). Biometric principles in clotting and clot lysis assays. *Clinical and Laboratory Haematology* **2:** 155–167.
46. Kirkwood, T. B. L., Rizza, C. R., Snape, T. J., Rhymes, I. L. and Auster, D. E. G. (1977). Identification of sources of interlaboratory variation in factor VIII assay. *British Journal of Haematology* **37:** 559–568.
47. Koepke, J. A. (1986). Partial thromboplastin time test – Proposed performance guidelines. *Thrombosis and Haemostasis* **55:** 143–144.
48. Koepke, J. A. and Klee, G. G. (1979). Automated coagulation detection systems. *Clinical and Laboratory Haematology* **1:** 75–86.
49. Koepke, J. A., Rodgers, J. L. and Ollivier, M. J. (1975). Pre-instrumental variables in coagulation testing. *American Journal of Clinical Pathology* **64:** 591–596.
50. Koepke, J. A., Gilmer, P. R., Triplett, D. A. and O'Sullivan, M. B. (1977). The prediction of prothrombin time system performance using secondary standards. *American Journal of Clinical Pathology* **68:** 191–194.
51. Lämmle, B., Noll, G., Häuptli, W., Tran, T. H., Luengo, E., Lohri, A., Ritz, R. and Duckert, F. (1984). Ein häufiges Problem bei der LaborKontrolle der Heparinisierung: Kontamination der Blutproben mit exogenem Heparin. *Schweizerische medizinische Wochenschrift* **114:** 873–875.
52. Lang, H. and Kleindel, M. (1984). Prüfung der Lagerstabilität von lyophilisiertem AK-Plasma durch beschleunigte Degradation. *Berichte der Osterreichischen Gesellschaft für Klinische Chemie* **7:** 93–96.
53. Loeliger, E. A. (1979). The optimal therapeutic range in oral anticoagulation. History and proposal. *Thrombosis and Haemostasis* **42:** 1141–1152.
54. Loeliger, E. A. (1985). Laboratory control, optimal therapeutic ranges and therapeutic quality control in oral anticoagulation. *Acta Haematologica* **74:** 125–131.
55. Loeliger, E. A. and Lewis, S. M. (1982). Progress in Laboratory control of oral anticoagulants. *Lancet* **ii:** 318–320.
56. Loeliger, E. A. and van Halem-Visser, L. P. (1975). A simplified thromboplastin calibration procedure for standardization of anticoagulant control. *Thrombosis et Diathesis Haemorrhagica* **33:** 172–190.
57. Loeliger, E. A. and van Halem-Visser, L. P. (1979). Results of calibration by the Dutch national reference laboratory of the thromboplastins included in the ICTH/ICSH collaborative study of prothrombin time standardization. *Thrombosis and Haemostasis* **42:** 1128–1131.
58. Loeliger, E. A., van der Hoeff-van Halem, R. and van Halem, L. P. (1978). Thromboplastin calibration. Experience of the Dutch reference laboratory for anticoagulant control. *Thrombosis and Haemostasis* **40:** 272–287.
59. Loeliger, E. A., van den Besselaar, A. M. H. P. and Bertina, R. M. (1980). Critical appraisal, clinical usefulness and implementation of the thromboplastin concept of prothrombin time standardization. *Scandinavian Journal of Haematology* **25,** Suppl. 37: 34–48.
60. Loeliger, E. A., Poller, L., Samama, M., Thomson, J. M., van den Besselaar, A. M. H. P., Vermylen, J. and Verstraete, M. (1985). Questions and answers on prothrombin time standardization in oral anticoagulant control. *Thrombosis and Haemostasis* **54:** 515–517.
61. Majumdar, G. and Payne, R. W. (1985). Quality of oral anticoagulant therapy. *Clinical and Laboratory Haematology* **7:** 125–131.
62. Miale, J. B. and Kent, J. W. (1972). Standardization of the therapeutic range for oral anticoagulants based on standard reference plasmas. *American Journal of Clinical Pathology* **57:** 80–88.
63. Morris, M. W., Brooker, D. W., Miller, J. L. and Winkelman, J. W. (1987). Single versus duplicate prothrombin time assays. *Laboratory Medicine* **18:** 524–526.
64. NCCLS (1982). Tentative guidelines for the standardized collection, transport and preparation of blood specimens for coagulation testing and performance of coagulation assays. NCCLS Publication Vol. 2 No. 4, pp. 103–128, Villanova, PA.
65. Nemerson, Y. and Clyne, L. P. (1974). An assay for coagulation factor VII using factor VII-depleted bovine plasma. *Journal of Laboratory and Clinical Medicine* **83:** 301–303.
66. Ofosu, F., Cassidy, K., Blajchman, M. A. and Hirsh, J. (1980). Immunodepletion of human plasma factor VIII. *Blood* **56:** 604–607.
67. Østerud, B., Kasper, C. K., Lavine, K. K., Prodanos, C. and Rapaport, S. I. (1981). Purification and

properties of an abnormal blood coagulation factor IX (factor IX Bm)/kinetics of its inhibition of factor X activation by factor VII and bovine tissue factor. *Thrombosis and Haemostasis* **45:** 55–59.

68. Over, J. (1984). Quality control of the one-stage factor VIII (VIII:C) assay in the coagulation laboratory. *Scandinavian Journal of Haematology* **33,** Suppl. 41: 89–100.

69. Owren, P. A. (1959). Thrombotest. A new method for controlling anticoagulant therapy. *Lancet* **ii:** 754–758.

70. Palareti, G., Coccheri, S., Poggi, M., Bonetti, M., Cervi, V., Mazzuca, A., Savoia, M., Veri, L., Fiori, F., Gaspari, G. and Palareti, A. (1987). Oral anticoagulant therapy control: evidence that INR expression improves the inter-laboratory comparability of results – The Bologna oral anticoagulant control exercise. *Thrombosis and Haemostasis* **58:** 905–910.

71. Poller, L., Thomson, J. M., Sear, C. H. and Thomas, W. (1971). Identification of a congenital defect of factor VII in a colony of beagle dogs: the clinical use of the plasma. *Journal of Clinical Pathology* **24:** 626–632.

72. Quick, A. J., Stanley-Brown, M. and Bancroft, F. W. (1935). A study of the coagulation defect in hemophilia and in jaundice. *American Journal of the Medical Sciences* **190:** 501–511.

73. Raper, C. G. L. (1983). The therapeutic quality control of anticoagulant clinics. *Clinical and Laboratory Haematology* **5:** 325–327.

74. Rotblat, F. and Tuddenham, E. G. D. (1981). Immunologic studies of Factor VIII coagulant activity (VIII:C) assays based on a haemophilic and an acquired antibody to VIII:C. *Thrombosis Research* **21:** 431–445.

75. Sage-El, A., Burns, E. and Wenz, B. (1985). The unwarranted use of replicate analysis in routine coagulation studies. *American Journal of Clinical Pathology* **83:** 81–83.

76. Scheer, W. D., Catrou, P. G., Libscomb, G. E. and Boudreau, D. A. (1986). A comprehensive evaluation of the performance of duplicate prothrombin time and activated partial thromboplastin time assays. *American Journal of Clinical Pathology* **85:** 456–462.

77. Spaethe, R. and Dombrose, F. A. (1986). A manufacturer's viewpoint on the use of the ISI and INR: Calibration of two commercial rabbit brain thromboplastins that differ in their sensitivity to coagulation factors. In Triplett, D. A. (ed.) *Advances in Coagulation Testing: Interpretation and Application*, pp. 379–387. Skokie, Illinois: College of American Pathologists.

78. Starr, H., Rhoades, P., Lam-po-tang, P. R. L. C. and Archer, G. T. (1980). Prothrombin times: an evaluation of four thromboplastins and four machines. *Pathology* **12:** 567–573.

79. Stevenson, K. J., Easton, A. C., Curry, A., Thomson, J. M. and Poller, L. (1986). The reliability of activated partial thromboplastin time methods and the relationship to lipid composition and ultrastructure. *Thrombosis and Haemostasis* **55:** 250–258.

80. Thomson, J. M. (1984). Specimen collection for blood coagulation testing. In Koepke, J. A. (ed.) *Laboratory Hematology*, pp. 833–863. New York: Churchill Livingstone.

81. Thomson, J. M. (1985). Pre-test variables in blood coagulation testing. In Thomson, J. M. (ed.) *Blood Coagulation and Haemostasis. A Practical Guide*, pp. 340–369. Edinburgh: Churchill Livingstone.

82. Thomson, J. M. and Poller, L. (1985). The activated partial thromboplastin time. In Thomson, J. M. (ed.) *Blood Coagulation and Haemostasis. A Practical Guide*, pp. 301–339. Edinburgh: Churchill Livingstone.

83. Thomson, J. M., Tomenson, J. A. and Poller, L. (1984). The calibration of the second primary international reference preparation for thromboplastin (Thromboplastin, human, plain, coded BCT/253). *Thrombosis and Haemostasis* **52:** 336–342.

84. Thomson, J. M., Darby, K. V. and Poller, L. (1986). Calibration of BCT/441, the ICSH reference preparation for thromboplastin. *Thrombosis and Haemostasis* **55:** 379–382.

85. Tomenson, J. A. (1984). A statistician's independent evaluation. In van den Besselaar, A. M. H. P. (ed.) *Thromboplastin Calibration and Oral Anticoagulant Control*, pp. 87–108. The Hague: Martinus Nijhoff.

86. Tomenson, J. A. and Thomson, J. M. (1985). Standardization of the prothrombin time. In Thomson, J. M. (ed.) *Blood Coagulation and Haemostasis. A Practical Guide*, pp. 370–409. Edinburgh: Churchill Livingstone.

87. Tran, T. H. and Duckert, F. (1983). Preparation of factor VIII-free plasma by immunoaffinity chromatography on insolubilized antibodies against factor VIII related antigen. *Haemostasis* **13:** 73–77.

88. Triplett, D. A., Brandt, J. T., Fair, D. S., McGann, M. A. and Schaeffer, J. S. (1985). Factor VII deficiency: heterogeneity defined by combined functional and immunochemical analysis. *Blood* **66:** 1284–1287.

89. van den Besselaar, A. M. H. P., van Halem-Visser, L. P., Hoekstra-Schuman, M., van der Marel-van

Nieuwkoop, W. and Loeliger, E. A. (1980). Simplified thromboplastin calibration. Further experience of the Dutch reference laboratory for anticoagulant control. *Thrombosis and Haemostasis* **43**: 53–57.

90. van den Besselaar, A. M. H. P., van Halem-Visser, L. P. and Loeliger, E. A. (1983). The use of evacuated tubes for blood collection in oral anticoagulant control. *Thrombosis and Haemostasis* **50**: 676–677.

91. van den Besselaar, A. M. H. P., Evatt, B. L., Brogan, D. R. and Triplett, D. A. (1984). Proficiency testing and standardization of prothrombin time: effect of thromboplastin, instrumentation, and plasma. *American Journal of Clinical Pathology* **82**: 688–699.

92. van den Besselaar, A. M. H. P., Hermans, J., van der Velde, E. A., Bussemaker-Verduyn den Boer, E., van Halem-Visser, L. P., Jansen-Grüter, R. and Loeliger, E. A. (1986). The calibration of rabbit tissue thromboplastins: experience of the Dutch reference laboratory for anticoagulant control. *Journal of Biological Standardization* **14**: 305–317.

93. van den Besselaar, A. M. H. P., Meeuwisse-Braun, J., Jansen-Grüter, R. and Bertina, R. M. (1987). Monitoring heparin therapy by the activated partial thromboplastin time. The effect of pre-analytical conditions. *Thrombosis and Haemostasis* **57**: 226–231.

94. van den Besselaar, A. M. H. P., Hermans, J., Beeser, H. and Loeliger, E. A. (1988). Long-term stability of international reference preparations for thromboplastins. *British Journal of Haematology* **68**: 321–328.

95. van der Velde, E. A. (1984). Orthogonal regression equation. In van den Besselaar, A. M. H. P. (ed.) *Thromboplastin Calibration and Oral Anticoagulant Control*, pp. 25–39. The Hague: Martinus Nijhoff.

96. van Putten, J. J., van de Ruit, M., Beunis, M. and Hemker, H. C. (1984). Heparin neutralization during collection and processing of blood inhibited by Pyridoxal 5'-Phosphate. *Haemostasis* **14**: 253–261.

97. WHO Expert Committee on Biological Standardization (1977). Twenty-eighth Report. Technical Report Series 610, pp. 45–51. Geneva: WHO.

98. WHO Expert Committee on Biological Standardization (1983). Thirty-third Report. Technical Report Series 687, pp. 81–105. Geneva: WHO.

99. WHO Expert Committee on Biological Standardization (1984). Thirty-fourth Report. Technical Report Series 700, pp. 18–19. Geneva: WHO.

100. Zucker, S., Cathey, M. H. and West, B. (1970). Preparation of quality control specimens for coagulation. *American Journal of Clinical Pathology* **53**: 924–927.

7

External Quality Assessment

S M Lewis

Introduction

External quality assessment (EQA) is an important component of quality assurance. As described in Chapter 1, its essential purpose is to have an objective independent check of laboratory results in order to establish between–laboratory comparability. It also has other uses. It allows different instruments and methods for the same test to be compared and their reliability to be assessed. It is also possible to study new control materials and calibrants, and, by means of regular checks, to monitor batch products of reagents, control materials and kits. Performance in an EQA scheme should if possible be included in the evaluation of any new instrument. From EQA data the state of the art can be judged and selected methods can be recommended, whilst the standard of performance by the participants will indicate whether there is need for training by way of workshops and broadsheets.

EQA results will also reveal deficiencies which are the responsibility of the manufacturer. Thus, for example, a test kit which performs reliably in the hands of an expert may fail in a 'routine' laboratory if used by an inexperienced person unless it is accompanied by clear and unambiguous instructions for performing the test, reading the reaction, interpreting the results, use of controls, etc. When one laboratory fails to obtain the correct result for a test in an EQA survey it must be assumed that the fault lies with that laboratory; when a number of participants in the survey fail to get the correct answer with the same kit it is necessary to adjudicate between the reliability of the kit and the competence of the users. EQA data will usually help to resolve this question.

Principles

The principles by which EQA is organized for haematology are well established and have been set out in guidelines prepared jointly by ICHS and ECCLS (1). Schemes may, however, vary in practice, as described below.

(1) A scheme may be national (NEQAS), regional or organized only at a district

level. The type of scheme may depend on how health services are organized and administered in the country, the facilities and financial support available for the scheme, numbers of participants, geographic areas involved and the ease or difficulty in sending specimens and in communication between organizer and participants. Above all, the level of activity of a scheme will be determined by the enthusiasm and energy of its organizer and organizing committee. In order to apply statistical procedures for analysing results the number of participants in a scheme (or in any group within the scheme) should not be less than 20, but they may range from this minimal number to several thousand, provided that there is sufficient material available to distribute a representative aliquot to each participant.

National and regional (or district) schemes are not alternatives as each serves a different function. The advantages of a national scheme is that sufficient data may be obtained to provide an overview, taking account of all methods and instruments used. If all instruments used in one district have a similar bias this will be recognized by a national scheme but not by the district one. This might occur, for example, if one lot of a reagent or calibrant is defective and its distribution has been confined to one district. On the other hand, the advantage of a local scheme is that results are usually available more rapidly and personal contact can be monitored more easily between the participating laboratories and the organizer.

(2) The methods used in surveys depend on the different nature of the specimens to be tested (whole blood, lysate, plasma or serum, blood films, biopsy sections, etc), their stability and transit time between preparation and receipt of the material by the participants. Blood in EDTA anticoagulant is stable only for a few hours for a blood count whereas blood preserved in acid citrate dextrose (ACD) or citrate phosphate dextrose (CPD) can be used for 3–4 weeks. As preserved blood and EDTA blood react differently with some counters EQA surveys with preserved blood may be regarded as an artificial process if it is intended to assess performance in the laboratory where normally EDTA blood is used. However, tests on preserved blood will at least ensure precision and inter-laboratory comparability.

Blood films are an important component of any general haematology EQA, both for quantitative testing of differential leucocyte counts and for qualitative testing of identification of morphological abnormalities. All films from a single blood specimen should be near identical but there is no absolute guarantee that the distribution of different types of cells, and especially cells which are present only in small numbers, will be similar in every film. It is desirable that each film be screened before being sent to the participants, but this is impractical in schemes with several hundred or thousands of members. There is considerable debate on two aspects: (a) the amount of information that should be provided to the participants, and (b) whether haematological diagnosis should be requested as part of the assessment. Undoubtedly if clinical information is provided this may bias the morphological diagnosis, but it may be argued that this is the real-life situation, and that assessing morphology 'blind' without any guiding information is an artificial test. The present practice in the UK is to provide the films alone in the first instance for participants to return a report (Fig. 7.1) but to follow this up after 2–3 weeks with clinical details, a review of the film based on a consensus by a group of 8–10 referees; and other information from which the diagnosis has been established (Fig. 7.2). Thus, these surveys are used both for assessing competence and as an educative process. With increasing use of automated differential cell counting systems

UK NATIONAL EXTERNAL QUALITY ASSESSMENT SCHEME FOR HAEMATOLOGY

NEQUAS(H) FORM 6

BLOOD FILMS

Survey Number

Date of Receipt

Participant Reference Number

PLEASE READ INSTRUCTION SHEET CAREFULLY BEFORE COMPLETING THIS FORM

X   Y

Sample Number

Sample Quality 1 = Satisfactory
2 = Unsatisfactory

Morphology Codes
(Maximum 5 per film)

Possible Diagnosis

Comment:

Please return to: UK NEQAS(H)
Animal Health Trust
PO Box 5, Balaton Lodge
Snailwell Road
NEWMARKET Suffolk CB8 7DW

Signature ....   Date ....

Fig. 7.1 Blood-film report form in NEQAS surveys.

INTERNATIONAL EXTERNAL QUALITY ASSESSMENT SCHEME FOR HAEMATOLOGY

Survey 2786: Blood Films

The slides have been examined by a Referee Panel of seven members. The differential counts below represent a consensus of their results.

Film 278672 (Y)

Neutrophils	80 % 88%
Eosinophils	0 – 1%
Basophils	0 – 1%
Lymphocytes	8 – 14%
Monocytes	3 – 5%

The red cells showed anisocytosis with macrocytes and large oval poikilocytes; there were target cells and occasional schistocytes. There was also a minor population of hypochromic cells. The white cells showed a polymorph-leucocytosis with a few hypersegmented neutrophils. The platelet count was normal but there was platelet anisocytosis with some giant forms.

The diagnosis was liver disease with macrocytic anaemia: serum folate 1.7 ug/l, serum vitamin B_{12} 1476 ng/1. The bone marrow showed minor megaloblastic changes and iron utilisation defect with coarse iron deposits in the normoblasts.

Fig. 7.2 Report of blood film sent to NEQAS participants.

there is also need for a different type of survey to assess this aspect.

(3) Different procedures may be used to assess particular aspects of laboratory work, i.e. equipment, reagents, techniques, individual performance by each laboratory and overall performance by all participating laboratories. By contrast to internal quality control, where each test is controlled, EQA is not primarily a system for controlling specific tests, but it is desirable to include a range of tests which are undertaken by the laboratory so as to get a general impression of the standard of performance. Surveys should be carried out on a regular basis, the frequency being determined by the availability of materials as well as by their relevance and relative importance for clinical service.

(4) When a new investigation is introduced into EQA it is necessary to check the validity of the procedure used and the quality of the test materials before the performance by participating laboratories is assessed. These preliminary studies are referred to as 'trials' and the term 'surveys' is used only when they have been established in the programme.

(5) Tests in surveys may be quantitative, semi-quantitative or qualitative. Each requires an appropriate procedure for analysing results, assessing their closeness to the correct result and determining whether performance is satisfactory. This may be based on (a) statistical criteria, (b) comparison with performance by selected peer or referee laboratories, or (c) extent to which a discrepant result would influence clinical management.

There are three ways in which EQA may be organized:

(1) *Surveys*

As described above, identical specimens are sent to the participating laboratories where the requested tests are performed and the results are reported back to the EQA scheme organizer for analysis and assessment. Then either a general report is presented to all participants with the consensus result and/or assumed correct result based on referee testing, or individual reports are sent to each individual laboratory with appropriate comments on their performance (Fig. 7.3).

The specimens used in consecutive surveys should, if possible, include a range of other component(s) to be measured, and especially around the limits of normal reference and at critical levels for decision-making. Qualitative tests should include positive and negative samples.

Paired samples in a survey help to assess linearity; when a known amount of an analyte is added to one-half of the original specimen, difference in measurement between the two samples (i.e. with and without addition) gives an assessment of accuracy.

(2) *Physical inspection*

An inspector brings specimens to the laboratory and requests that they be investigated under his supervision by the routine procedures used in that laboratory. At the same time the inspector has the opportunity to observe working practices, the extent of internal quality control, record-keeping, instrument maintenance, etc. Results on the specific specimens are assessed by comparison with results obtained by a reference laboratory and/or by a reference method. This system is used when a scheme is linked to licensing of laboratories.

(3) *Pattern analysis*

Results of a test carried out on representative patients in one laboratory should not differ from the pattern of results in other laboratories serving a similar population. This has been used for EQA in histopathology on the assumption that the incidence of various abnormalities is constant throughout the country so that a statistically significant increase (or decrease) in a particular abnormality in one centre suggests error in diagnosis rather than a true population difference. A similar principle applies to various haematological diseases and also to the mean or median measurements of 'absolute values' (MCV, MCH, MCHC) as these should remain constant in each laboratory and between laboratories.

Selection of tests in an EQA scheme

Any or all tests carried out in the diagnostic laboratory might be included in the surveys, either regularly or occasionally. It has been argued that the least frequently performed tests require the greatest amount of assessment; but when the EQA surveys

UK NATIONAL EXTERNAL QUALITY ASSESSMENT SCHEME FOR HAEMATOLOGY 8/7/87

Results for Survey No. 8707   Participant Reference No. 236
                                                               System No. 2
Sample 1—Donkey ACD
Sample 2—Human CPDA—1+FCC

Instrument	Test		Result	DI	Median	SD	CV%	N	
Coulter Hb–Mter	HB		[g/1]						
		1	111	−1.35	113	1.48	1.3	762	all
				−0.90	113	2.22	2.0	189	group
		2	140	−1.80	144	2.22	1.5	761	all
				−1.80	144	2.22	1.5	189	group
Coulter ZF	RCC		[×10**12/1]						
		1	4.98	−0.93	5.07	0.096	1.9	680	all
				−0.39	5.03	0.130	2.6	115	group
		2	4.48	1.62	4.60	0.074	1.6	679	all
				−0.65	4.55	0.107	2.4	115	group
Coulter MCV/HCT Unit	PCV								
		1	0.338	−0.07	0.339	0.0133	3.9	720	all
				−0.18	0.340	0.0111	3.3	91	group
		2	0.420	−0.84	0.435	0.0178	4.1	719	all
				−0.67	0.430	0.0156	3.6	92	group
Coulter MCV/HCT Unit	MCV		[f1]						
		1	68.0	0.36	67.0	2.74	4.1	677	all
				0.00	68.0	1.48	2.2	88	group
		2	94.0	−0.12	94.4	3.45	3.7	676	all
				−0.11	94.3	2.74	2.9	89	group
Coulter Hb–Mter	MCH		[pg]						
		1	22.3	0.00	22.3	0.59	2.7	657	all
				−0.30	22.5	0.67	3.0	103	group
		2	31.2	0.00	31.2	0.67	2.1	658	all
				−0.28	31.5	1.07	3.4	104	group
Coulter Hb–Mter	MCHC		[%]						
		1	32.8	−0.63	33.6	1.26	3.8	658	all
				−0.25	33.1	1.19	3.6	109	group
		2	33.3	0.22	33.0	1.37	4.2	659	all
				0.00	33.3	1.11	3.3	110	group
Coulter ZF	WCC		[×10**9/1]						
		1	4.1	0.45	4.0	0.22	5.6	745	all
				0.34	4.0	0.30	7.4	168	group
		2	8.2	0.00	8.2	0.37	4.5	740	all
				0.54	8.0	0.37	4.6	168	group

Fig. 7.3 Blood count report to an individual NEQAS participant.
'All' refers to all participants; 'group' refers to the instrument or method used by the individual participant.

provide most of the specimens received in a laboratory for a particular test, the time has come for that laboratory to withdraw that test from its service.

As far as possible survey materials should resemble test specimens and, as already mentioned, should include both normal and abnormal results. For some tests human blood is necessary but for others animal or avian blood can be used with advantage in order to conserve limited human blood supplies and also to have specimens with features which parallel abnormalities in human blood. Thus, for example, equine (horse or donkey) red cells resemble human microcytes with an MCV of 50–60 fl; sheep blood is a source of G6PD deficiency; avian blood has nucleated red cells which are suitable as simulated leucocytes; artificially depleted animal plasma provides material for pro-thrombin time and other coagulation assays. When human blood is used it is essential to check that it is hepatitis-Bs-antigen and HIV-antibody negative.

Preparation of EQA material

In the following section methods for preparing material for EQA surveys will be described. These include Hb, RBC, PCV and other tests on preserved blood, Hb on lysate, WBC, platelet counts and blood films. Brief account will also be given of tests for analytes in plasma and serum, coagulation tests and blood group serology.

The methods for specimen preparation are intended for the organizers of EQA schemes, whether national or on a lesser scale. These preparations are, however, also suitable for internal quality control.

Preserved blood

This is suitable for Hb, blood count, Hb A_2 and Hb F assay, abnormal haemoglobins (from appropriate donors), G6PD.

Blood is collected into blood collection bags containing CPD or ACD.* One unit of blood as obtained from a Blood Transfusion Service will provide 500 ml of preserved blood. If a larger volume is required, blood from two or more donors of the same ABO group are pooled. Equine blood may be collected in bags of up to 2 litre capacity from each horse or donkey.

(1) Run the blood through blood administration sets directly into a round-bottom mixing flask and continue mixing for at least 20 min after the addition of the last unit of blood or other material.
(2) Cell levels may be adjusted, as follows:
   (a) To increase red cell count – sediment cells over exit vents of bag and run into the flask with minimum of plasma.
   (b) To lower red cell count – add solution of anticoagulant (CPD or ACD*) in 9 g/l NaCl; the anticoagulant:saline ratio must be the same as the usual anticoagulant:blood ratio.

*CPD: Trisodium citrate, dihydrate 26.3 g; citric acid, monohydrate 3.27 g; sodium dihydrogen phosphate, monohydrate 2.22 g; dextrose 25.5 g; water to 1 litre. The solution is sterilized by autoclaving at 121°C for 15 min. Its pH is 5.6–5.8. For use, 7 vols of blood are added to 1 vol. of solution.

ACD (NIH-A): The following formula was recommended by the US National Institute of Health; hence referred to as 'NIH-A' solution. Trisodium citrate, dihydrate 22 g; citric acid, monohydrate 8 g; dextrose 25 g; water to 1 litre. The solution is sterilized by autoclaving at 121°C for 15 min. Its pH is 5.4. For use, 10 vols of blood are added to 1.5 vol. of solution.

    (c) To lower white cell count – pass blood through a leucocyte filter (e.g. Sepacell R-500, Ashahi Medical Co. Ltd, Tokyo, Japan).

    (d) To increase white cell count – add fixed avian cells (see p. 159).

(3) Add antibiotics, e.g. 10^6 units of benzyl penicillin and 1 g of streptomycin sulphate per 500 ml.

(4) With *continuous mixing* dispense into sterile containers; cap and seal with a plastic seal (e.g. Viskrings, Viscose, Development Co. Ltd, Croydon, Surrey, UK). The importance of adequate mixing of whole-blood preparations cannot be overstated. It is a great advantage to use the Ward and Chappel mixing flask (10) which has been designed to ensure homogeneity in the dispensed blood (Fig. 7.4). Sealing the containers is necessary to prevent evaporation.

(5) When dispensing has been completed, refrigerate at 4°C until needed.

(6) For analysis, the sample should be brought to room temperature and gently mixed on a roller mixer or by hand before opening. Unopened vials of human blood keep in good condition for about 3 weeks at 4°C, and those of equine blood for up to 3 months.

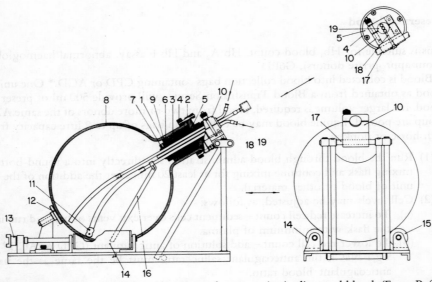

Fig. 7.4 Design of mixing flask used to ensure homogeneity in dispensed blood. (From Ref 10, with permission.) Supports for rotating flask: (1) PTFE washer; (2) polypropylene bearing housing; (3) Tufnol spacer; (4) Tufnol collar hinged to allow removal at autoclaving, with stainless steel studs, for clamping 4.2 in neck of flask; (5) stainless steel disc; (6) two PTFE bearings; (7) collar; (8) 10 or 20 litre bolthead flask; (9) stainless steel washer; (10) Dural coupling; (11) glass weight on output line; (12) Tufnol thrust plate for flask; (13) Dural coupling; (14) driven rubber-covered roller; (15) free-running covered roller; (16) stainless steel paddle; (17) stainless steel rod; (18) stainless steel pin; (19) stainless steel tube assembly containing three smaller tubes silver soldered into the end caps of main tube.

Haemolysate

This is suitable for haemoglobinometry. The starting point is blood collected into ACD or CPD (see p. 157, footnote).

(see p. 157, footnote)

(1) Centrifuge the anticoagulated blood in bottles of appropriate size (e.g. 30 ml screw-cap glass containers). Remove the plasma and buffer coat aseptically.

(2) Add to each red cell deposit an excess of physiological saline (9 g/l NaCl), mix well, and re-centrifuge. Discard the supernatant and any remaining 'buffy coat'.

(3) Repeat saline wash two times to ensure complete removal of plasma, white cells and platelets, each time removing the top layer of packed red cells.

(4) Add to the washed cells half their volume of carbon tetrachloride, cap the containers and shake vigorously on a mechanical shaker or vibrator for one hour. Refrigerate overnight to allow the lipid/cell debris to form a semi-solid interface between tetrachloride and lysate.

(5) On the following day centrifuge at *ca* 2500 × g for 20 min. Remove the upper lysate layers and pool them in a clean bottle.

(6) Using Whatman No. 1 filter paper in a Buchner funnel, filter the pooled lysate into a side-arm flask connected to gentle water-pump suction.

(7) Repeat filtration using Whatman No. 42 filter paper, changing the paper if filtration slows down. It is important not to overload the funnel with lysate.

(8) To each 70 ml of lysate add 30 ml of glycerol. Then add antibiotics (see p. 158). When yeasts or fungal infection is a problem, also add amphotericin (e.g. Fungizone, Squibb) 50 mg/l.

(9) If a lower concentration is required add an appropriate volume of 30% (v/v) glycerol in 9 g/l NaCl to the concentrated lysate. Mix well.

(10) Dispense aseptically into sterile containers. Cap and seal.

Fixed cells (pseudo-leucocytes)

Chicken and turkey red blood cells are nucleated and when fixed, their size, as recognized by electronic cell counters, is within the leucocyte size range for these counters. Thus, they are suitable to act as 'pseudo-white' cells in preserved whole bloods. For this purpose 25 ml of blood collected into ACD (NIH-A) is sufficient for many preparations, when an appropriate amount is added to a bulk of preserved blood.

Reagents

0.15 M iso-osmotic phosphate buffer (pH 7.4). (A) Sodium dihydrogen phosphate ($NaH_2PO_4.2H_2O$) 23.4 g/l. (B) Anhydrous disodium hydrogen phosphate (Na_2HPO_4) 21.3 g/l or $Na_2HPO_4.12H_2O$ 53.7 g/l. Both stock solutions keep well when refrigerated. For use, mix in proportion 18 ml A + 82 ml B. Check that the pH is 7.4.

0.25% Glutaraldehyde fixative. To 1 litre of phosphate buffer, add 5 ml 50% glutaraldehyde solution (commercially available), mix and use at once.

Glycerol : saline. Add 60 vol. glycerol to 40 vol. of 9 g/l NaCl. Mix well and store in a refrigerator.

Method

(1) Centrifuge the blood at $150 \times \boldsymbol{g}$ for 15 min. Remove the plasma, which contains the leucocytes and platelets.

(2) Add an excess of phosphate buffer to the red cells, mix and transfer to centrifuge bottle; re-centrifuge and discard supernatant.

(3) Repeat this wash centrifugation twice.

(4) Add to the washed cells 10 times their volume of 0.25% glutaraldehyde fixative, mix by vigorous shaking to ensure complete re-suspension and rotate slowly on a mechanical mixer for 1 h. Leave on bench for further 2 h with occasional shaking.

(5) Centrifuge the suspension at $1000 \times \boldsymbol{g}$ for 20 min and discard supernatant.

(6) Add distilled water to the fixed cell deposit, re-suspend and mix by stirring and shaking: again centrifuge and discard supernatant. Repeat twice.

(7) Re-suspend the washed fixed cells to approx 30% concentration in 0.1% sodium azide in 9 g/l NaCl. Mix well by vigorous shaking.

(8) If the material has been stored, re-suspend by vigorous hand shaking (or by a vortex mixer) until no clumps remain at the base of the container, then roller mix for at least 20 min. If available, sonication for 1–2 min should also be used.

(9) Carry out a rough count by routine method to determine the approximate concentration.

(10) Autoclave at 121°C for 15 min.

(11) For use, mix by vigorous hand shaking or by vortex mixer followed by roller mixing for at least 20 min.

(12) Transfer an appropriate amount to a volume of preserved blood (see p. 157) from which the leucocytes have been filtered.

(13) Alternatively dilute in glycerol–saline to the required concentration.

(14) Mix well for 20 min and with continuous mixing in a mixing flask (Fig. 7.4) dispense into sterile containers. Cap and seal.

(15) For measurement re-suspend blood by vigorous hand shaking followed by leaving on a mechanical mixer for at least 15 min before opening the tube.

Fixed platelets

Materials

EDTA solution. EDTA (100 g/l) in modified Alsever's buffer. This will keep at 4°C for up to 6 months.

Modified Alsever's buffer. (A) Trisodium citrate 16 g; NaCl 8.2 g. Make up to 1 litre with distilled H_2O. Keep at 4°C. (B) Dextrose 41 g. Make up to 1 litre with distilled H_2O. Keep at 4°C. Mix A + B immediately before use. Discard any remaining solution after use.

Fixative. Formaldehyde (40% v/v) 2 ml per 100 ml of Alsever's buffer.

Platelet-rich plasma. Collect one or more units of blood into plastic bags with ACD or CPD anticoagulant (see p. 157). Centrifuge the bags at $200 \times \boldsymbol{g}$ for 10 min; collect the platelet concentrate from each into a transfer pack or another plastic bag. When reconstituted (see below) one unit of normal blood should provide 500 ml with a platelet count of about 70–80×10^9 per litre or 250 ml with a platelet count of 150×10^9 per litre.

Method

(1) Add one unit of platelet-rich plasma into each of a series of 150 ml glass bottles containing 1 ml of EDTA solution. Leave at 37°C in a water-bath for 1 h to allow the platelets to disaggregate.

(2) If possible the disaggregation should be checked by passing a small sample from each bottle through a blood counting system set for platelet counts and with a facility for analysing size-distribution curves, or by visual inspection of a diluted sample in a haemocytometer chamber. If aggregation is still present leave in the water-bath for another hour.

(3) Dispense 200 ml of fixative into each of a series of plastic bottles, and into each add the solution from one of the glass bottles. Leave at room temperature (*ca* 20°C) for about 48 h.

(4) Centrifuge the bottles at *ca* $50 \times \boldsymbol{g}$ for 10 min at room temperature.

(5) Distribute the platelet-rich supernatants from the plastic bottles equally into two sterile 500 ml glass bottles. Fill the bottles with Alsever's buffer.

(6) Wash three times in Alsever's buffer, centrifuging between washes at *ca* $750 \times \boldsymbol{g}$ for 30 min at room temperature. After the third wash remove the buffer and re-suspend the platelets in 10 ml of fresh buffer. Mix well.

(7) Pool the contents of the two bottles into a glass container or mixing flask (Fig. 7.4). Add an appropriate volume (see above) of Isoton or similar diluent. Add antibiotic (see p. 158). With continuous mixing dispense into sterile containers. Cap and seal.

This preparation will be satisfactory for at least a year if stored at 4°C.

Blood films

Films are prepared in the usual way either as wedge-smears or by spread method; they are then methanol-fixed and stained by a Romanowsky–Giemsa stain. The standardized Azure B–Eosin method of ICSH (5) is recommended.

Serum

Serum is required for haematology EQA surveys of vitamin B$_{12}$, folate, iron, transferrin and ferritin. It should be sterile and free from cloudiness or particles. This is often difficult to achieve when the serum is a pooled collection from a large number of donor-samples. It may thus be necessary to subject the material to micropore filtration at 0.2 µm. This has the disadvantages of being time-consuming and expensive, and in addition 25–30% of the initial volume is lost by the filtration. Attempts have been made to overcome these difficulties by preceding the 0.2 µm–filtration by a series of coarse filtration, e.g. at 20, 8, 3, 1 and 0.45 µm successively. This process does not entirely resolve the problem and it is preferable, as far as possible, to obtain serum either from a single donor or from a small number of selected donors.

Blood coagulation

In blood coagulation, determination of prothrombin time (PT) or prothrombin ratio and activated partial thromplastin time (APTT) are the usual regular EQA survey tests, while plasma fibrinogen concentration, Factor VIIII:C assay and other tests might be included from time to time. Lyophilized plasma obtained by plasmapheresis from a patient receiving oral anticoagulant therapy provides material suitable for the pro-thrombin time; normal human lyophilized plasma and plasma obtained by plasmapher-esis from patients with mild haemophilia or von Willebrand's disease is used for APTT test and Factor VIII assay; human lyophilized plasma is suitable for fibrinogen assay. (See also p. 134.)

Although there are some difficulties in tests on the samples obtained by plasmaphere-sis of patients with coagulation defects (12) this has proved to be a valuable source of large volumes of material, at least for parts of the testing procedures. However, increased incidence of HIV antibody is making it more difficult to obtain suitable material from this source.

Blood group serology

Survey tests include compatibility testing, ABO/Rh blood grouping and antibody screening. Plasma is obtained from a selected donor by plasmapheresis, pooled if more than one donor is used, defibrinated with bovine thrombin, dialysed against saline, filtered under sterile conditions and then distributed in 1.5 ml aliquots (4). For the red cells, whole blood is collected in ACD or CPD anticoagulant (see p. 157) from donors of selected genotypes.

Data processing

Processing starts when results are received by the organizer. Except for small schemes, where a simple calculator will suffice, a computer facility is essential, especially for retrieving data for cumulative assessments and for retrospective studies of equipment performance etc.

The primary object of the assessment is to evaluate the performance of individual participants and to identify problems relating to methods, instruments, reagents, controls and calibrators which have been used by the participants. Statistical analysis is by fairly simple standard computer programs. It is, however, necessary to define a reference point which can be assumed to be the true numerical value or qualitative observation. Several methods are used to establish reference points. It is, however, important to appreciate that unless the true value is established by a definitive method all reference points are biased estimates.

Consensus mean

Consensus may be biased because a particular type of instrument or reagent or calibrator is used by a large majority of participants. To obtain statistically valid data for analysing a subgroup an adequate number of participants (at least 20) is necessary in the group. Thus a newly introduced method or instrument suffers a disadvantage until a sufficiently large number of participants register for that group. On the other hand comparison of mean values provides a measure of inter-method biases without necessarily identifying any as being the correct value.

For the analysis, first any obvious blunders are deleted, such as a result which differs by more than 100% from the overall mean. Then, assuming a Gaussian distribution, the mean ($\bar{x}$) and standard deviation (SD) are calculated by standard statistical procedures, and re-calculated from the residual data after excluding any outlier results falling outside ± 3 SD. The outliers are recorded as unsatisfactory performance (see later).

This method of excluding outliers is valid only if the SD is narrow. If it is wide it is preferable to trim the data by setting the data in numerical sequence and deleting an equal number of observations from both ends (3). When there are less than 16 data points, one should be deleted from each end; when there are 16 or more, 10% of the total sample should be deleted. Then the trimmed mean and SD are calculated in the usual way.

Consensus median

When the distribution is non-Gaussian or there are a large number of outliers it is usually more appropriate to use non-parametric statistics. In this case an estimate of the measure of dispersion about the *median* is obtained from the spread of the distribution of the data around the midpoint between 25th and 75th percentiles ($P25$ and $P75$, respectively). This central range which includes 50% of the results, is known as the H (or hinge) spread. It is used to estimate the standard deviation. Outliers are truncated if outside the range $P25 - 3H$ to $P75 + 3H$. This is equivalent to $\bar{x} \pm 4.7$ SD (8).

Expert laboratories

Results are obtained from a set of *appointed* reference laboratories (referees) who assay the specimens repeatedly by reference methods, thus establishing the inter-laboratory and intra-laboratory precision, as well as the standard deviation of the whole set (2). The main disadvantage with this method is that an unnoticed bias in performance in one laboratory in a small group will disproportionately affect the reference results; enlarging the group to compensate for this effect can quickly overburden the scheme.

For qualitative procedures, correct results may also be based on consensus of all participants or of a selected group of expert referees. In some instances, e.g. for sickle cell disease and G6PD deficiency, results which are to be expected in a qualitative screening test can be confirmed by means of a quantitative estimation on the same sample. For morphological haematology the referees may have the advantage of knowing the patient's subsequent clinical course and other data from which a diagnosis may have been made; however, whilst this is important from the educative viewpoint it does not give a fair yardstick for judging performance by the ordinary participant.

In scoring qualitative tests account must be taken of both positive and negative misleading information in a test interpretation. Thus, for example, if the test requires identification of the presence of an abnormal feature, a correct result should be scored as 2, missing the feature as 1 whilst interpreting it incorrectly as -1.

In analysing blood-film reports, weighted scores should be used to give higher credit for more important features, especially those which point to the specific diagnosis. Conversely, 'trivial' features such as anisocytosis should not earn a score point even if correctly identified, if there are other more important abnormalities which should have been seen.

Assessment of performance

For quantitative tests, blunders will have been detected in the initial stage of statistical analysis described above. Thereafter unsatisfactory performance can be identified by one of the following procedures.

Deviation index (DI)

This is a measure of how a test result (x) differs from the mean ($\bar{x}$) or median (m) value. When the mean is used it is a multiple of the truncated standard deviation (SD'), i.e. excluding results which are outside ± 3 SD in a preliminary calculation. When the median (m) value is used, standard deviation is taken as the 50 percentile, i.e. the central 50% of values. Thus

$$DI = \frac{x - m}{SD'} \text{ or } \frac{x - \bar{x}}{SD'}$$

The main advantage is that the index is independent of the value m or $\bar{x}$ so that it allows measurement for different samples and parameters to be readily compared (9). Performance is assessed in terms of the DI as follows: DI < 0.5 = excellent; DI 0.5–1.0 = good; DI 1.0–2.0 = satisfactory but borderline; DI > 2.0 unsatisfactory.

Variance index (11)

Participant reference is compared with the best performance obtainable with the particular method, expressed as the chosen coefficient of variation (CCV). This can refer either to the CV of the method performed under ideal conditions by expert laboratories or the CV for all results returned by the participants, truncated by exclusion of results outside ± 2 SD. First, the variation of the individual (V) is obtained as a percentage,

$$V = \frac{x - \bar{x}}{x} \times 100$$

Then

$$\text{Variation index} = \frac{V}{\text{CCV}} \times 100$$

To base acceptable limits of performance on statistical analysis alone is unrealistic. Thus, for example, the remarkably low CV for haemoglobin means that even a measurement at 3 SD from the mean will not result in an error of more than 10–15% and is unlikely to influence clinical decision, whereas platelet counts have a high CV such that 3 SD may represent an error of 50%. In the case of prothrombin time and calculation of prothrombin ratio a small difference may result in a dangerously incorrect level of therapy. In reality, therefore, poor performance should be defined as a result which might lead to inappropriate clinical action.

Some schemes, e.g. College of American Pathologists, have established an adjusted standard deviation which takes account of clinical needs alongside reasonable goals for precision and accuracy. Another method is to set the limit of deviation at 15% of the normal reference range for each parameter; alternatively, Tonks' formula (11) sets the limit of deviation as

$$\frac{\text{Normal reference range} \times 0.25}{\text{Mean normal value}} \times 100$$

In practice, a limit of ± 2 SD is reasonable for most parameters. A comparison of this criterion with the others mentioned above is given in Table 7.1.

Persistent poor performers

In some tests, especially qualitative tests such as screening for sickle cells, blood grouping and compatibility tests, even a single incorrect observation may be deemed to be hazardous and to require urgent corrective action by an appropriate authority. In

Table 7.1 Methods for defining limits of acceptable performance in EQA surveys

	UK NEQAS 3 SD	College of American Pathologists surveys	15% of normal reference range	Tonks' formula
Hb	4	5	5	8
RBC	6	6	5	9
PCV	6	6	5	8
MCV	6	6	4	5
WBC	12	10	14	23
Platelets	34	25	20	22

Values expressed as percentage deviation from referee or consensus mean values.

general, however, while participants would be expected to recognize problems as soon as any of their results fall outside acceptable limits, intervention by an authority is required only if the participant fails to rectify the fault within a reasonable interval. In the UK NEQAS criteria for persistent poor performance are a DI > 3* in three or more parameters on any one sample in a survey on three occasions in a 6-month period, or a DI > 3* in any one of the parameters on one or both samples in three consecutive surveys.

For less frequent quantitative surveys a DI > 3* or an incorrect interpretation of the measurement (i.e. 'high', 'low' or 'normal') for any of the samples in three successive surveys indicates persistent poor performance. Similarly, for qualitative tests, an incorrect result in three consecutive surveys is usually regarded as persistent poor performance.

Presentation of results

Analysis of surveys should be set out clearly in standard format. Four types of report are necessary:

(1) **Individual reports** (Fig. 7.3) give the following information:
   (a) survey and participant identification;
   (b) type of sample used in the survey;
   (c) instrument, kit or method used by the participant;
   (d) 'all method' mean or median and SD; analysis of participant's results and DI related to 'all methods';
   (e) similar analysis and assessment in the relevant group.

*Or DI > 2 if appropriate for any test.

(2) **General reports** (Fig. 7.5) give statistical analysis of mean or median and SD, both overall for all methods and by group analysis. The report may also include a summary of the participants' interpretation of their results as 'low', 'normal', or 'high' (Fig. 7.6).

(3) **Blood–film report** (Fig. 7.2) of differential leucocyte count, morphological features and review of clinical and haematological aspects.

(4) **Performance table** (Fig. 7.7) shows a cumulative summary of deviation indices for various parameters in last six surveys. It also shows when no results were returned by the participant.

Organization of a National External Quality Assessment Scheme (NEQAS)

The way in which a scheme is organized depends on a number of factors. These include the role in the scheme of government health authorities and of professional bodies, whether the scheme is a commercial undertaking or run from an academic or public health institute, whether participation is obligatory or voluntary, whether it is used as the basis for licensing of laboratories and/or for recognition of laboratories for training, and what action is taken with regard to unsatisfactory performance.

In the United States and in Canada there is a legal obligation to participate in an EQA scheme; in some European countries also (e.g. France and West Germany) participation is compulsory but in others it is voluntary. Where it is voluntary it is encouraged in different countries to varying degrees by health authorities, by professional bodies, and by health insurance agencies who are responsible for paying the fees for the services provided. The general public do not appear to be as alert to their rights to reliable laboratory tests as they are for other consumer services.

In a number of countries there are commercial schemes, in some cases organized by instrument manufacturers for users of their products. Commercial schemes may complement, supplement or even substitute for a national scheme. It is important, however, that a national scheme be independent of any undue pressures and that the organizer of such a scheme should not have a commercial interest in any particular reagent or instrument. It is acceptable practice for materials used in surveys to be prepared under contract by a manufacturer who may also be the manufacturer of material used routinely by participating laboratories, but the specifications of such survey materials must be set by the organizer and his committee.

In the United Kingdom participation in NEQAS is voluntary but strongly encouraged by the medical and technical professional bodies. Virtually every National Health Service (NHS) laboratory participates, as do the majority of laboratories in the private sector. The UK NEQAS is a good model and its organization will be described in detail. It is based on a committee structure which takes account of interrelated interests of the health authorities, professional societies and individual laboratories, and also the need to have co-ordination of different schemes concerned with various aspects of laboratory practice (Fig. 7.8).

The Government Health Authority, the Department of Health and Social Security

UK NATIONAL EXTERNAL QUALITY ASSESSMENT SCHEME FOR HAEMATOLOGY

Results for trial no. 8704   sample no. 2
Sample 2 – Human CPDA—1+FCC

Test		Class	Median	SD	CV%	N
HB	[g/dl]	all	14.1	0.22	1.6	831
	Fully automated Coulters	1	14.1	0.30	2.1	186
	Coulter S–Plus 1	2	13.9	0.37	2.7	37
	Coulter S–Plus 2 & Plus 3	3	14.0	0.30	2.1	21
	Coulter S–Plus 4	4	14.1	0.15	1.1	156
	Technicon H6000 & H6010	5	14.1	0.15	1.1	29
	Ortho ELT 8 & 800	6	14.2	0.22	1.6	33
	Coulter S880	7	14.0	0.15	1.1	58
	Technicon H1	8	14.2	0.22	1.6	40
	Semi automated instruments	10	14.2	0.22	1.6	228
RCC	[×10**12/1]	all	4.55	0.10	2.3	739
	Fully automated Coulters	1	4.51	0.13	3.0	184
	Coulter S–Plus 1	2	4.60	0.15	3.2	37
	Coulter S–Plus 2 & Plus 3	3	4.61	0.13	2.9	21
	Coulter S–Plus 4	4	4.56	0.07	1.5	155
	Technicon H6000 & H6010	5	4.55	0.16	3.4	29
	Ortho ELT 8 & 800	6	4.64	0.12	2.6	33
	Coulter S880	7	4.55	0.07	1.6	57
	Technicon H1	8	4.56	0.08	1.8	39
	Semi automated instruments	10	4.55	0.13	2.9	150
PCV		all	0.414	0.01	3.6	786
	Fully automated Coulters	1	0.417	0.01	3.2	181
	Coulter S–Plus1	2	0.420	0.01	2.6	37
	Coulter S–Plus 2 & Plus 3	3	0.414	0.02	4.1	21
	Coulter S–Plus 4	4	0.404	0.01	1.7	155
	Technicon H6000 & H6010	5	0.407	0.01	3.5	29
	Ortho ELT 8 & 800	6	0.442	0.01	3.2	33
	Coulter S880	7	0.415	0.02	3.9	57
	Technicon H1	8	0.424	0.01	2.8	40
	Spun PCV	10	0.419	0.01	1.8	75
	Computed PCV	11	0.415	0.02	4.3	119
MCV	[f1]	all	90.9	2.97	3.3	735
	Fully automated Coulters	1	92.0	1.48	1.6	181
	Coulter S–Plus 1	2	91.2	1.63	1.8	37
	Coulter S–Plus 2 & Plus 3	3	89.0	0.82	0.9	21
	Coulter S–Plus 4	4	88.8	1.26	1.4	155
	Technicon H6000 & H6010	5	89.7	0.96	1.1	29
	Ortho ELT 8 & 800	6	95.0	2.97	3.1	33
	Coulter S880	7	90.9	3.34	3.7	57
	Technicon H1	8	92.5	2.19	2.4	39
	Calculated MCV	10	91.0	3.15	3.5	23
	Computed MCV	11	91.0	2.45	2.7	117
MCH	[pg]	all	31.0	0.74	2.4	707
	Fully automated Coulters	1	31.3	0.82	2.6	171
	Coulter S–Plus 1	2	30.7	1.19	3.9	37
	Coulter S–Plus 2 & Plus 3	3	30.6	1.11	3.6	21
	Coulter S–Plus 4	4	30.9	0.52	1.7	155
	Technicon H6000 & H6010	5	30.9	0.74	2.4	29
	Ortho ELT 8 & 800	6	30.9	0.74	2.4	33
	Coulter S880	7	31.0	0.67	2.2	58
	Technicon H1	8	31.0	0.70	2.3	39
	Semi automated instruments	10	31.1	0.82	2.6	131

MCHC	[g/d1]	all	43.1	1.19	3.5	718
	Fully automated Coulters	1	33.8	0.93	2.7	171
	Coulter S–Plus 1	2	33.5	0.82	2.4	37
	Coulter S–Plus 2 & Plus 3	3	33.9	1.41	4.2	21
	Coulter S–Plus 4	4	34.9	0.67	1.9	155
	Technicon H6000 & H6010	5	34.6	0.70	2.0	28
	Ortho ELT 8 & 800	6	32.2	1.19	3.7	33
	Coulter S880	7	33.9	0.89	2.6	58
	Technicon H1	8	33.4	1.19	3.6	38
	Semi automated instruments	10	34.2	1.19	3.5	143
WCC	[×10**9/1]	all	19.1	0.96	5.0	811
	Fully automated Coulters	1	19.0	0.82	4.3	186
	Coulter S–Plus 1	2	18.8	1.07	5.7	36
	Coulter S–Plus 2 & Plus 3	3	19.5	0.59	3.0	21
	Coulter S–Plus 4	4	19.5	0.67	3.4	156
	Technicon H6000 & H6010	5	17.8	2.00	11.2	29
	Ortho ELT 8 & 800	6	14.5	1.11	7.7	17
	Coulter S880	7	19.6	0.59	3.0	58
	Technicon H1	8	18.8	1.22	6.5	40
	Semi automated instruments	10	19.0	0.82	6.5	40
	Haemocytometry	11	19.0	1.93	10.1	13

Fig. 7.5 Summary of blood count results in a NEQAS survey.

(DHSS) sponsors, and is responsible for financing the scheme along with parallel schemes in clinical chemistry, microbiology, histopathology and cytopathology, cytogenetics, autoimmune serology, immunochemistry, hormone assays and therapeutic drug monitoring (7).

Apart from this sponsorship, the DHSS maintains a low profile in the running of NEQAS as this is regarded as being primarily a matter for the professions. There is no system of laboratory registration and licensing so that poor performance is exclusively the concern of the professions. The DHSS does, however, have an important role in coordinating the activities of the various EQA schemes in different specialities. This is achieved by means of an interdisciplinary Advisory Committee on Assessment of Laboratory Standards (ACALS). Its members represent the professions and health authority, while the scheme organizers and chairmen of the steering committees report to the committee annually. The primary purpose of the committee is to advise the Government on the maintenance of laboratory standards. Its regular meetings ensure that the schemes in different specialities set similar standards and they provide cross-fertilization of ideas from experts involved with the various schemes.

Scheme organizers are, in general, university or public hospital consultants (specialists) within the NHS who are not paid specifically for their NEQAS activities. They are not appointed directly by the DHSS but facilities are provided in their institutions by contract from the DHSS.

Each scheme has a steering committee appointed by the DHSS chaired by an independent expert, and consisting of technical experts together with clinical advisers and representatives of the DHSS who sit on each committee as observers. The role of the steering committee is to advise the organizer on the overall operation of the scheme,

UK NEQAS (H) Survey 8752 JUNE 1987   Red cell G-6-PD

Sample 875251   Human Blood

Referee Analysis
(IU/gHb at 30°C)

n	12
mean	7.8
sd	0.57

Data Analysis

Qualitative Assessment	Code	Quantitation	No.	Low	Equivocal	Normal	Median	SD	CV%
Dye decoloration: Sigma 400	1	All methods	123	10	5	108	3.8	0.67	17
Other commercial	2		25	8	3	14	6.7	1.33	19
In-house	3		1	0	0	1	8.6	1.70	19
Fluorescent screening: Sigma 202	4		5	0	2	3			
Other Commercial	5		69	2	0	67			
In-house	6		0	0	0	0			
			23	0	0	23			

Quantitative

Temperature (C)	No
25	6
30	58
37	23

Median + 3sd

0.0   2.0   4.0   6.0   8.0   10.0   12.0   14.0

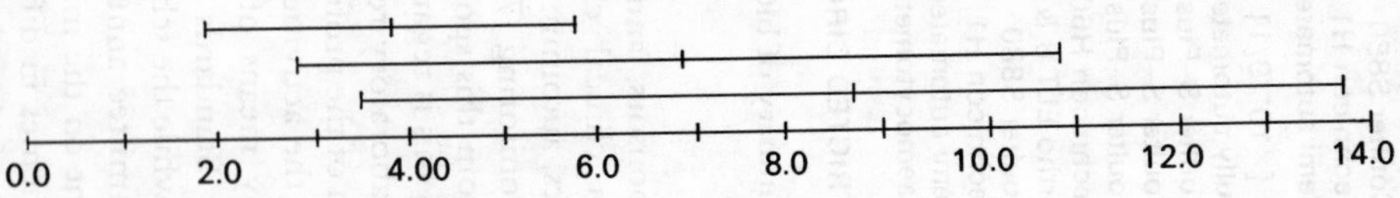

Fig. 7.6 Report of G6PD survey.

UK NATIONAL EXTERNAL QUALITY ASSESSMENT SCHEME FOR HAEMATOLOGY

PERFORMANCE TABLE FOR LAST 6 SURVEYS   17/9/87   Page 1

Survey	Method	Sample	HB	RCC	PCV	MCV	MCH	MCHC	WCC	Sample Quality	Results rec late
						DEVIATION INDICES					
8/03	all	1	2.02	0.45	0.27	0.52	−0.56	0.67	−4.27	GOOD	−
	group	1	2.02	0.11	0.00	0.41	−0.24	0.77	−3.66		
	all	2	1.35	−0.49	0.67	1.03	1.42	−0.08	0.00	GOOD	
	group	2	0.90	−0.30	0.67	1.30	0.98	−0.17	0.17		
8/04	all	1	**	**	**	**		**	**	**	**
	group	1	**	**	**	**		**	**		
	all	2	**	**	**	**		**	**	**	
	group	2	**	**	**	**		**	**		
8/05	all	1	1.80	0.90	0.34	0.00	0.84	0.63	0.00	GOOD	−
	group	1	2.70	0.78	0.34	−0.47	0.27	0.57	0.34		
	all	2	2.25	0.40	0.07	0.00	1.35	0.75	0.67	GOOD	−
	group	2	2.16	0.58	−0.79	−0.58	0.86	0.76	1.01		
8/06	all	1	4.05	1.23	1.28	0.61	2.19	0.48	−0.67	GOOD	−
	group	1	5.40	0.76	2.70	0.75	1.62	0.34	−0.42		
	all	2	4.95	0.83	3.17	3.19	2.70	−0.93	−0.86	GOOD	−
	group	2	4.50	0.81	5.40	2.67	1.57	−1.14	−0.67		
8/07	all	1	6.07	−2.91	0.82	2.55	5.40	0.95	0.45	GOOD	−
	group	1	4.05	−1.85	2.70	2.19	4.50	1.43	0.34		
	all	2	4.05	−1.75	0.28	1.04	4.50	1.24	0.27	GOOD	−
	group	2	4.05	−0.74	0.67	0.68	2.51	1.26	0.81		
8/08	all	1	6.74	0.37	−0.28	−0.26	3.15	2.02	−1.12	GOOD	−
	all	1	4.05	0.27	−1.23	−1.55	2.33	2.25	−0.67	GOOD	
	all	2	3.60	1.46	−0.63	−1.69	1.50	3.15	−0.45		
	group	2	2.36	1.45	−1.35	−1.18	0.74	2.41	0.22		

** − INFORMATION NOT SUPPLIED

Fig. 7.7 Cumulative report of blood count performance by a participant.

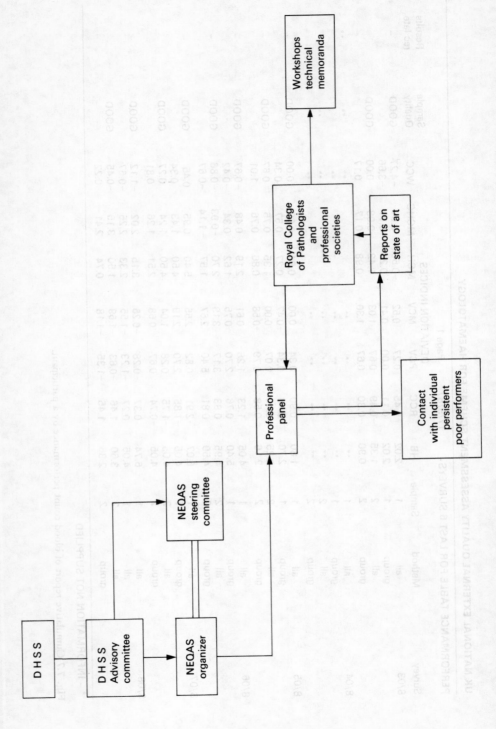

Fig. 7.8 Organization of NEQAS in UK.

including such aspects as the frequency of sample distribution, type of sample, tests to be undertaken, methods of statistical analysis of results, style of data presentation. The steering committee may discuss general performance as it relates to state of the art but it is not concerned with the performance of individual participating laboratories except

Review of individual participant performance is the function of an advisory panel consisting of representatives nominated by the appropriate professional bodies; in haematology these are the Royal College of Pathologists, British Society for Haematology, Association of Clinical Pathology and Institute of Medical Laboratory Sciences and the British Blood Transfusion Society. The scheme organizer attends the meetings of the panel *ex officio*.

The scheme has been established on the basis of confidentiality between organizer and individual participants. When there is a problem of persistent poor performance the organizer reports to the advisory panel, but the identity of the laboratory is known to the panel only by code number. Accordingly, when the chairman of the panel writes to enquire if assistance is required, this letter is passed to the coded participant by the organizer. Only if the discordance persists and no response has been received, will the identity of the participant be revealed to the panel chairman who writes directly to the head of the laboratory. In some cases members of the panel may then visit the laboratory to help resolve the problems. In the general haematology NEQAS less than ten participants per year require a chairman's letter, and only rarely has there been need for a panel visit. On the other hand, the organizer and his staff have relatively frequent direct contact by letter or telephone with participants whose problems are usually resolved by appropriate advice.

It should be emphasized that whilst a specific technical fault might be identified and corrected, persistent poor performance may be an indication of the general performance and reliability of that laboratory. Administrative problems are as likely to cause poor performance as technical errors. These include staff shortage, inadequate supervision in a branch (satellite) laboratory and use of obsolete equipment. In this context NEQAS can play a useful role in helping to influence authorities to provide funding to overcome such adverse conditions.

In attempting to identify the cause of technical errors, especially when a personal visit to the laboratory is not possible, an intensive survey should be offered. Thus, for example, for haemoglobinometry the survey would include the following:

(1) polycythaemic blood
(2) anaemia blood
(3) second sample of (1)
(4) second sample of (2)
(5) lysate
(6) haemiglobincyanide solution
(7) Thomson's grey solution

Discrepancies from the established values in one or other of the specimens might indicate imprecision, bias, non-linearity, dilution error, defective reagent, defective photometer, incorrect wavelength or filter, inadequate mixing of sample.

International EQA scheme

An international EQA scheme has also been established (6). Organized by World Health Organization in conjunction with the UK NEQAS (which serves as the WHO Collaborating Centre for Quality Assurance in Haematology), it was initiated in response to the recognized need to improve laboratory services (13). It is intended primarily to help the laboratory services in developing countries, but also to achieve reliability and harmonization of analytic tests worldwide. In each country, after consultation between the health authorities and WHO, one or more laboratory is invited to act as a reference centre for haematological standardization and to be responsible for the organization of EQA. Because of postal and customs delays, often under unfavourable climatic conditions, only stable materials can be sent from London. At present they are lysates for haemoglobin, stabilized white cells and platelets, sterile plasma for vitamin B_{12}, folate, iron and ferritin, films for reticulocytes, and Romanowsky-stained films for differential counts and blood cell morphology. The Collaborating Centre, with the help of the UK NEQAS consensus, provides the target values. From these the range of acceptable performance for the international EQA scheme is established. The reference centres are also provided with international reference standards by the ICSH.

Conclusion

External quality assessment is one aspect of the comprehensive programme of quality assurance which is essential in the diagnostic laboratory. It is an educational process by means of which good laboratory performance can be assured with inter-laboratory harmonization, and problems which prevent reliable laboratory tests can be identified. It should not be regarded as a chore but as a *professional* obligation whether or not it is a *legal* requirement. To question performance by skilled workers is not an impertinence. The questions and the challenge is to the state of the art and to the laboratory tests themselves, rather than to the individual worker, whose technical skills can be assessed more aptly in other ways.

References

1. ECCLS (1986). Standard for Quality Assurance. Part 5: External Quality Assessment in Haematology. ECCLS Document Vol. 3 No. 1. Berlin: Beuth Verlag.
2. Hansert, E. and Stamm, D. (1980). Determination of assigned values in control specimens for internal accuracy, control and for interlaboratory surveys. *Journal of Clinical Chemistry and Clinical Biochemistry* **18**: 461–490.
3. Healy, M. J. R. (1979). Outliers in clinical chemistry quality-control schemes. *Clinical Chemistry* **25**: 675–677.
4. Holburn, A. M. and England, J. M. (1982). The U.K. national external quality assessment scheme in blood group serology, 1979–1980. *Clinical and Laboratory Haematology* **4**: 3–12.

5. ICSH (1984). ICSH reference method for staining of blood and bone marrow films by Azure B and Eosin Y (Romanowsky stain). *British Journal of Haematology* **57:** 707–710.
6. Lewis, S. M. (1988). *Quality Assurance in the Haematology Laboratory.* World Health Forum.
7. Lewis, S. M. and Jennings, R. D. (1988). United Kingdom External Quality Assessment Schemes. Annual Report for 1987. London: Department of Health and Social Security.
8. Tukey, J. W. (1977). *Exploratory Data Analysis.* Boston: Addison-Wesley.
9. Ward, P. G. and Lewis, S. M. (1975). Interlaboratory trials: a national proficiency assessment scheme in Britain. In Lewis, S. M. and Coster, J. F. (eds) *Quality Control in Haematology*, pp. 37–51. London: Academic Press.
10. Ward, P. G., Chappel, D. A., Fox, J. G. C. and Allen, B. V. (1975). Mixing and bottling unit for preparing biological fluids used in quality control. *Laboratory Practice* **24:** 577–583.
11. Whitehead, T. P. (1977). *Quality Control in Clinical Chemistry.* London: Wiley.
12. Whitehead, T. P. and Woodford, F. P. (1981) External quality assessment of clinical laboratories in the United Kingdom. *Journal of Clinical Pathology* **34:** 947–957.
13. World Health Organization (1982). Seventh General Programme of Work. Geneva: WHO.

8

Choice of Analytic Methods

N K Shinton

Selection of the proper method and instrumentation to be used in the laboratory is an essential part of total quality control (8). Once the requirements of the method and instruments available to meet them have been reviewed, choice will depend upon precision and accuracy, practicality and cost-effectiveness provided safety has been assured. To obtain this information, a technical assessment and/or costing exercise may have to be carried out. The general principles of these procedures will be the same but details will vary for such specific methods as automated blood cell counting, coagulometry and use of kits for chemical analytes such as haemoglobins, ferritin and vitamin B_{12}.

Requirements of the method

When a new method is being introduced or an old method is replaced, consideration of the requirements of the new method should be made at the earliest stage. The choice may be limited by considerations of space and resources available such as manpower and capital. The workload for the method must be ascertained. It may be essential for the results to be compatible with other methods such as those used during emergency hours. The level of precision required will vary with the requirements, e.g. screening, monitoring, diagnosis or research.

Review of information

The choice of methods available can be obtained from a variety of sources including:

(1) published surveys in journals, textbooks, newsletters of societies both national and international;
(2) manufacturers' information data;
(3) directories of reagents;
(4) organizations of external quality assessment schemes;

(5) health agencies; and

(6) other laboratory workers.

From this information review the following details can be assembled which will be of value in reaching a decision:

(1) equipment and reagents required including calibrators and controls;

(2) methodology and principles of method;

(3) degree of mechanization or automation;

(4) sample requirements and method of identification;

(5) safety aspects;

(6) alarm system for instrument failure;

(7) dimensions and weight of instruments;

(8) service requirements – electrical supply, water pressure, water quality, vacuum or compressed air, drainage;

(9) effect on environment:

(a) needs of instrument or method,

(b) heat production, noise, vibration of instruments;

(10) data presentation and expression of values;

(11) maintenance arrangements;

(12) use of method by other laboratories;

(13) costs – capital, consumables, labour.

When this has been assembled and considered against the requirements, a number of methods should be selected as suitable. It may be necessary for some of these methods to be compared by obtaining further information on their precision, accuracy and cost-effectiveness. ICSH (9), Shinton *et al.* (23) and ECCLS (5) give details of recommended procedures.

General principles of method evaluation

Preliminary planning

Sites of assessment

Methods, particularly those requiring an instrument, need to be evaluated by the manufacturer of the instrument or reagent, by consumer organizations either in association with the manufacturer or independently, and by the individual user. It follows that there will be a variety of levels of evaluation. The manufacturer will want to type-test engineering prototypes, and also pre-production and production models, possibly on multiple sites. A consumer organization will wish to type-test, possibly again on multiple sites, followed by publication of the results. The individual user will only wish to test an individual instrument or evaluate a method in a specific laboratory.

Evaluation of a method on multiple sites has the advantages of using multiple instruments, possible increased variety of reagent material, wider spread of pathological samples, environmental variation and greater objectivity. It also avoids the disadvantage of excessive burdening of workload on a single site. The disadvantages are the difficulties of data comparability requiring greater time for co-ordination with its inherent delays (6).

Planning

A realistic estimate of the time required to achieve a technical assessment of the method must be made initially. If an instrument has to be borrowed or leased from a manufacturer his agreement to the planned time scale must be guaranteed. If the assessment requires reagents, calibrators or control materials, similar assessments and arrangements must be made to ensure sufficient quantities of single lots of these materials and of multiple lots to assess lot-to-lot reproducibility.

The evaluator must ensure that the local arrangements to service and maintain the instrument in an operational state are adequate. If this is not the case, the manufacturer must be asked to guarantee the ready availability of an appropriately trained engineer. In the case of a leased instrument, any financial implications associated with the engineering back-up should be agreed before the start of the evaluation.

Internal resource planning

The necessary arrangements for availability of appropriate grades and categories of staff must be made. These must include instrument operation, obtaining and handling special samples, maintaining detailed records and the writing of an evaluation report. Depending on the circumstances of the evaluation, a decision will have to be made whether to test only those claims made by the manufacturer or to investigate areas for which claims have not been made. For example, a paediatric haematology laboratory may wish to test the effects of pre-dilution (micro-samples) on precision although the manufacturer has not made any claims on this aspect.

Reagents, calibrators and control materials

Reagents and calibrators should conform with the recommendations of the manufacturers, especially where an instrument is being evaluated. Some manufacturers may not wish to be responsible for the performance of an instrument unless their recommended reagents and consumables are used. The storage criteria and shelf-life of all reagents used throughout the evaluation must receive careful consideration and the manufacturer's recommendations followed strictly. Reagent labelling should be checked for its content and clarity and should include, as a minimum, the product name, lot number, storage requirements and shelf-life, both opened and unopened. The product literature should contain clear and unambiguous statements regarding the use of the product and details of interferents and conditions for use.

Reagents should be checked for suitability during the calibration process, e.g. background counts to detect any contamination. Sufficient reagent must be available to complete tests from a single supply lot. At a later stage, various lots of reagents should be assessed to determine whether or not lot-to-lot variation exists. Calibration should be assessed in accordance with the method specified by the manufacturer. Where calibration materials are supplied or recommended by the manufacturer, the validity of their assigned values must be confirmed by the investigator. A calibrator may be a single or multiple parameter material and, in the case of the latter, each measurement must be verified.

It may be necessary to consider prior biological safety checking of any material used.

Samples

Arrangements must be made for the collection of appropriate samples for testing the method. This should include selection of appropriate patients, details on method of collection, needle, anticoagulant and its final concentration which should be recorded. If samples have to be specifically obtained from volunteer donors or from patients, informed consent should be obtained. This must include permission for any biological safety checking that has to be carried out. Consideration must be given to the inclusion of samples which reflect the various abnormalities in quality or quantity of the methods under test. When comparing with reference methods, the sample distributions should approximate to one-third in the normal range, one-third in the low range and one-third in the high range. Fresh human blood samples will normally be used which have been collected from healthy donors or patients who have recently been shown to be hepatitis-Bs-Ag negative and HIV-antibody negative. The blood may be collected either by syringe or into an evacuated container using a 19 SWG needle (4, 20). The volume of blood collected will depend upon requirements but should not exceed 30 ml at any one time.

Transport and storage of samples should be under conditions which satisfy appropriate safety codes of practice. The following samples should be rejected as unsuitable for the blood count: clotted or with microclots, visibly haemolysed, collected in the wrong container or containing less than 90% of the nominal volume of blood.

Mixing of samples should be by rotary rather than by rocker mixer to prevent layering of formed elements. Samples should be tested on all instrument operational modes (e.g. whole blood, pre-dilute, etc.). Where a sample is divided into aliquots, each aliquot should be allocated a number and the order of sample presentation to the instrument be regulated by a set of random numbers. Samples for within-day testing should be kept at room temperature (22°C) and for between-day testing at 4°C. Time-lapse studies should be performed on a series of unselected blood samples (both normal and abnormal) to mimic the effect of transport: (a) within hospital measurements made every 30 min for 4-h period; (b) post-measurement at time of sampling and subsequently at 24, 48 and 72 h.

A comment should be made on the minimum size of sample and the practicability of using the instrument for pre-diluted micro-samples.

Programmes of testing

A day-to-day programme of testing must be prepared so that as much information as possible can be obtained from each patient sample.

Records

A detailed record should be kept. This can be simplified by preparing, before the start of the programme of testing, a series of appropriate work-sheets which can be used to record results of each section of the evaluation as it is undertaken. This will simplify both statistical analysis and the preparation of a final report.

In addition to recording results, a daily record should be kept of instrument performance and this should include:

(a) all instrument down-time, with causes, engineer response time and action taken;
(b) details of routine maintenance;
(c) details of any instrument upgrading during the evaluation;
(d) an operator roster;
(e) changes of lots of reagents and control materials;
(f) details of reagents and control material consumption;
(g) details of several timing studies to assess instrument throughput rate;
(h) ambient temperature and humidity;
(i) electrical supply and interferences.

Training

If training is available, this should be undertaken before the evaluation starts. Assessment should be made of its effectiveness and of the facilities provided by the manufacturer, e.g. manuals and training aids.

Safety assessment

Electrical. Instruments should be examined by a competent authority to ensure that they comply with the relevant National Safety Codes.

Mechanical. Checks should be made for hazards which might cause injury to the operator, e.g. moving parts, sharp edges.

Microbiological. Instruments should be tested for the production during normal operation, of potentially infected droplets of aerosol. The most sensitive method requires the use of suspensions of bacterial spores, such as *Bacillus subtilis* var. *globigii*, and for this, the service of an experienced microbiologist will be needed. However, in the case of serum or plasma samples an estimate of the degree of microbiological hazard can be obtained by putting fluorescent chemical markers, such as fluorescein, into the samples, placing clean, white absorbent paper over possible areas of contamination and then running the instrument. Droplet formation will be demonstrated by the presence of fluorescence under ultra-violet light. Comment should be made on the possibility of the user's hand becoming soiled with potentially infected material or the production of potentially infected effluent and on the need to dispose of potentially infected consumables.

Chemical. Consideration should be given to whether reagents are corrosive, carcinogenic or toxic. The evaluation report should note whether appropriate warning notices are provided in literature and on packaging.

Radiation. If the use of a source of non-ionizing radiation is involved, e.g. laser light, the advice of a radiation expert should be sought and any comments incorporated in the report.

Familiarization

Before the technical assessment procedure can commence there has to be a period of familiarization with the method. During this period the effect of prolonged storage or various forms of transport necessary to obtain some samples should be determined. The means and coefficients of variation (CV) of both the test and comparative methods may also be assessed as a pilot study. The familiarization period terminates when the staff are able to perform the method with routine patient samples.

In any report, comment must be made on the duration of the familiarization period and any difficulties which are encountered.

Technical assessment

Precision

Precision, or more correctly, degree of imprecision is a measure of repeatability of the method. Its components can be estimated by:

(a) replicate testing within the same batch;
(b) replicate testing between batches;
(c) dilution testing for linearity;
(d) instrument carry-over experiments; and
(e) overall reproducibility.

It is desirable that these studies are made over as wide a range as possible and at least over the physiological and usually encountered pathological range. It is better to assay more samples over a wide range fewer times than to assay a few samples more times, though the final decision may be a compromise determined by availability of material. Sample storage and stability characterization require consideration when designing the study. Results should be analysed separately for each part of the range – high, mid and low.

Within-batch precision

Samples for testing will be divided into aliquots, each specimen container being given a number and the order of sampling being regulated by use of a table of random numbers in order to minimize sampling errors. The results should be quantified by determining the CV for high, mid and low range.

Between-batch precision

These experiments can be combined with the within-batch precision testing but include the effects of calibration and drifts where an instrument is involved.

Between-calibration. Experiments should be included where runs are separated by standard calibration procedures. This may involve a total re-calibration of some instruments whereas for others this may only be necessary if the instrument fails a pre-defined check.

Effect of drift. Several batches should be run separated by an interval but without re-calibration between.

Effect of sample ageing. To allow interpretation of any differences between batches due to storage effects, samples should be tested at intervals of $\frac{1}{2}$, 1, $1\frac{1}{2}$, 5, 7, 8, 24, 48 and 72 h. The results for each experiment should be analysed statistically by an analysis of variance in the high, mid and low range.

Effect of dilution

It is desirable for an analytical method to give a linear relationship over as large a range as possible and at least over the physiological and usually encountered pathological range. The linear relationship should also pass through the origin. These experiments require considerable technical expertise which may not always be available. Grades of testing are:

(a) Replicate tests of ten dilutions evenly spaced, i.e. 100, 90, 80 ... 20% values where meticulous diluting technique has been carried out using only well-calibrated displacement pipettes. Ideally, the concentration of each dilution should also be determined by a reference method to check the accuracy of the diluting technique.
(b) Replicate tests as in (a), using arbitrary dilutions which are determined by a reference or other method.
(c) Replicate tests of three control materials from the high, mid and low range.

This latter method allows a rough assessment by graphical means but for reliable assessment the results should be analysed statistically either by comparing how the data correspond with parabolic and linear functions (23) or by a complex analysis of variance (14). This latter method of analysis will show non-linearity unless the dilution technique has been meticulous in performance.

Carry-over assessment

This should be done according to the method of Broughton *et al.* (1) ensuring that sufficient samples are run before and after the carry-over to achieve instrument stability. Three high-level samples (a_1, a_2, a_3) are measured, followed immediately by testing consecutively three low-level samples (b_1, b_2, b_3). The carry-over percentage is then

$$\frac{b_1 - b_3}{a_1 - a_3} \times 100\%$$

Overall reproducibility

Whilst an estimate of overall reproducibility can be obtained from the above experiments it is also useful to make a practical check. Replicates of a large range of samples should be located randomly amongst samples being tested over a period of several hours. The overall reproducibility can be assessed by a one-way analysis of variance (14) (see p. 70). Sample storage and stability characteristics may affect the study if it is extended over an excessively long time period.

Accuracy

Accuracy has been defined as 'agreement between the best estimate of a quantity and its true value' (25). A true value must be obtained by a definitive or reference method, of which there are few in haematology. Where a reference or definitive method is not available for a method, resource has to be made to comparison with a selected method generally used for routine procedures. As many unselected samples as possible should be studied. If the unselected series does not give sufficient information about samples at the extremes of the range such samples should be selected and studied separately. The results are analysed by plotting the difference between method under test from the true value against the true value and a paired *t*-test carried out over the whole range of tests.

It may happen that accuracy or comparability studies using selected samples have not included certain specific abnormalities or known interferents. If this occurs special studies should be set up. In addition, comparison should be made where possible with material obtained from an external quality assessment scheme (see Chapter 7).

Recovery experiments

Known amounts of a parameter to be measured may be added to replicate samples of a substrate either free or with a very low concentration of the specific material or substance under test, and the level determined (2, 3). At least three different concentrates should be used so that the results span the clinically relevant range. Percentage recovery (R) can be determined by:

$$R = \frac{B - A}{C} \times 100$$

where B = measured concentration of material, A = measured concentration in untreated substance, and C = known concentration of added material.

Detection limit

Assays should be carried out where applicable using a reagent blank or other analyte-free specimens. Three determinations should be used with calibration of the mean and SD. The mean plus 2 SD is an estimate of the detection limit.

Efficiency assessment

Operational timing

A time–motion study must be carried out in order to measure throughput especially if an instrument is used. This operational timing must include standards or controls, dwell-time, start-up time, shut-down time, the percentage of samples processed without repeating or re-checking, the frequency and dilution of re-calibration. The optimum number of samples that can be tested in a normal working day (i.e. 8 h) should be determined. The start-up time for emergency testing should also be determined.

Data presentation

The clarity, format and ease of interface with a computer should be assessed.

Training

The ability of staff available to be able to carry out the method is necessarily important. The required level of staff for the method must be considered.

Reliability and maintenance

From the records kept during the evaluation period, the 'down-time' can be calculated. The response-time of the manufacturer for service and replacement must be considered where instruments are involved.

Laboratory staff acceptability

The impact of the methods on laboratory organization is a vital component of assessment.

Clinical usefulness

The value of a method for clinical diagnosis, screening or monitoring of therapy should be assessed. This can be done by a questionnaire of a sample of clinical users (21). At the time of request the user should be asked the reason for the request e.g. screening, pre-operation, post-operation, monitoring of therapy, diagnosis. This should be followed up by a second questionnaire on whether or not the results have been of clinical or research use. The effect on management should be assessed with particular reference to the start of new treatment, change of existing management indicating change of drug dosage. The requirement for further investigation is important additional information.

Cost evaluation

The determination of cost of a method is most easily calculated on an annual basis (21). It can be broken down under:

Fixed costs: Capital cost, amortization and maintenance.
Variable costs: Cost of reagents/consumables and labour costs.

The total annual cost (AC) can be determined from:

$$AC = LX + CX + A + M$$

where X = throughput, L = labour cost/specimens, C = consumable cost of specimens, A = annual capital cost, and M = maintenance costs.

The annual capital cost (A) must allow for amortization and replacement cost: A = replacement cost × mortgage factor, the mortgage factor (MF) being determined from:

$$MF = \frac{r}{1 - (1 + r)^{-n}}$$

where r = treasury discount rate and n = amortization (years).

These figures can be determined from the manufacturer's capital cost, revenue cost of reagents and other consumables and the treasury discount rate from a bank.

Automated blood cell counters

All automated blood cell counters measure a variety of values. These must be determined initially from the manufacturer and considered individually when planning an evaluation. Particular attention must be paid to the use of a calibrator which may be single- or multiple-value material (25). Details of an evaluation method are described by ICSH (14).

Samples

These must be of fresh human blood collected into EDTA and tested within 4 h of collection. Anticipated ranges for study are shown in Table 8.1; however, it must be stressed that evaluation throughout these ranges must be undertaken and this entails the use of multiple intermediate levels to assess uniformity of instrument performance throughout these ranges.

Precision

When testing the effect of dilution, consideration has to be given to parameters whose magnitude should be unaffected by dilution, e.g. red cell indices. Such data can be plotted out as the result against the concentration when a horizontal line with zero slope should be obtained.

Where the variable is expected to be proportional (e.g. red cell count) dilution of cells in autologous platelet-poor plasma is the usual method for obtaining the various concentrations. Checks should be made to ensure that the plasma is free of red and white cells. If there are small numbers of residual platelets in the plasma, an appropriate mathematical correction should be made to the results at the various concentrations.

Accuracy

The only relevant parameters that can be estimated accurately by reference methods are haemoglobin (10) and packed cell volume (11). Assessment therefore largely depends upon comparability studies. When this study exposes discrepant results, the samples should be re-tested by methods which the evaluator considers sufficiently accurate and precise. Examples of such methods are given in Table 8.2. Instrument evaluation can be

Table 8.1   Ranges for study

Haemoglobin (g/l)	35–210
Red cell count ($\times 10^{12}$ per litre)	1.5–6.5
PCV (litre per litre)	0.15–0.60
MCV (fl)	55–120
Total WBC ($\times 10^9$ per litre)	0.1–80.0
Neutrophils ($\times 10^9$ per litre)	0.1–80.0
Lymphocytes ($\times 10^9$ per litre)	0.1–80.0
Monocytes ($\times 10^9$ per litre)	0.1–20.0
Eosinophils ($\times 10^9$ per litre)	0.1–20.0
Basophils ($\times 10^9$ per litre)	0.1–1.0
Platelets ($\times 10^9$ per litre)	20–900
MPV (fl)	5.5–12.5

Table 8.2   Methods to be used to resolve discrepancies noted between the results obtained by the counter under test and those obtained by routine procedures.

Measurement	Reference or selected method
Haemoglobin	ICSH Reference Method (10)
Packed cell volume	ICSH Reference Method (11) or less ideally micro–haematocrit (12, 13)
Red cell count	Counter metering fixed sample volume
MCV, MCH, MCHC	Calculation from above measurements
Total white cell count	Counter metering fixed sample volume
Differential white cell count	NCCLS Method (17)
Platelet count	Visual haemocytometry using ammonium oxalate diluent (19)

badly affected by this limitation since it is difficult to decide whether a blood counter is working 'incorrectly' or has been calibrated with a preserved blood whose assumed values are 'incorrect'. For example if counter A always gave values 10% greater than counter B, this could be quite acceptable since the 'difference' could easily have been eliminated by correct calibration. It would be unacceptable, however, if counter A gave answers 5% higher on some samples and 50% higher on others: in this instance there would be serious variation which could not be attributed to calibration.

Distribution of the measurements will not be normal unless their logarithms are taken, e.g. white cell and platelet counts; if so, the logarithm of the results should be analysed rather than the results themselves. For differential white cell counting the absolute value should be used rather than results expressed as percentage.

The presence of abnormal cells and interferents is of particular concern when assessing automated blood cell counters and appropriate specimens should be incorporated in an evaluation (Table 8.3). The effect of microcytosis on platelet counts and of leucocytosis on haemoglobin determination should be studied.

Cost evaluation

The differences in the number of parameters measured complicates any comparison, particularly the marked difference between automated and labour-intensive manual differential counts. A cost analysis exercise on manual differential cell counting may have to be carried out (27).

Automated coagulometers

These instruments add test plasma and reagents, mix, detect and measure the time taken

Table 8.3 Abnormal samples and interferents requiring study

Abnormal samples	Interferents
Haemoglobin S and C	Haemolysis *in vitro*
Nucleated red blood cells	Microclots
Heinz and Howell–Jolly bodies	Cold agglutinins
Malarial parasites	Paraproteinaemia
Red cell fragments	Hyperbilirubinaemia
Atypical lymphocytes	Lipaemia
Immature white blood cells	Uraemia
Giant platelets	Non-ketotic hyperosmolarity

for clot formation and print out the results. Instruments in use are based on different principles as reviewed by Koepke and Klee (18). They are used mainly for large workloads such as prothrombin times but can be used for activated partial thromboplastin times and coagulation factor assays. A complete evaluation will require a protocol for each method but the general principles are similar (22). This must be prepared in such a way as to evaluate the instrument rather than the reagent. It is therefore essential that if a manufacturer bases his claims on the use of specific reagents these must be used in an evaluation exercise. In each exercise of testing, the reference method should be used alongside the instrument (15). Results should be expressed as raw data estimated in seconds, but in addition it may be useful to calculate results so that data can be compared in a clinically relevant context.

Samples

These must be plasmas obtained by collecting, with clean venepuncture, 9.0 ml blood from persons known to be free of coagulation inhibitors and those with a known abnormality such as those receiving oral anticoagulants or haemophiliacs and covering the whole range of abnormalities.

The blood must be added to 1.0 ml of 109 mM sodium citrate solution which is contained in a plastic or siliconized glass tube. After stoppering and mixing, the tube must be centrifuged within 10 min of collection at $1200 \times \boldsymbol{g}$ for 10 min. If the test cannot be carried out immediately, the plasma must be stored in aliquots in a stoppered container at $+4°C$ before rapid freezing within 2 h of collection. Frozen plasma should be stored at $-70°C$. Reconstituted lyophilized plasma samples may be used if available. Sufficient of the different plasma specimens should be available to carry out all the necessary tests. Where appropriate viscous, lipaemic, icteric and haemolysed plasma should be tested.

Reagents

(a) Calcium chloride ($CaCl_2$) 25 mM.

(b) Thromboplastin, this should be that specified by the manufacturer of the coagulometer or, if different, that which it is intended for use in the laboratory. Sufficient of the same batch should be available to carry out all the necessary tests.

Precision

Within-day (batch) replicated testing should be completed within as short a time as possible, preferably within 1 h to ensure that samples and reagents do not deteriorate at different rates. Between-day (batch) precision is best determined by repeating replicate testing on 20 days over a period of 4 weeks, testing on each day being completed within 1 h using reagents from the same batch, lyophilized if possible or preserved by freezing.

Accuracy

This can only be by comparison with the reference method. At least 40 fresh samples of plasma or reconstituted lyophilized plasma spanning the range from normal to very abnormal. Every tenth sample should be plasma from a healthy normal adult donor.

Thromboplastins

The principles of coagulometer evaluation are applicable using both normal and abnormal samples. The testing must be of the same batch of thromboplastin and the reference method for one-stage prothrombin times must be used. The methodology of evaluation can be adapted from that used for the determination of the international sensitivity index (16, 24), see also p. 129.

Kit evaluation

Here the method is a package containing some or all of the matched reagents and other materials required for use in the measurement and identification of one or more specified parameters. The form of packaging and its convenience are likely to influence choice. An initial consideration will be the information or 'package insert' which must be capable of being clearly interpreted (26).

In particular, storage information with regard to temperature, humidity and liquid solubility may influence choice, as well as expiry dates for opened and unopened constituents. Reagents may be in the form of cartridges, slides, strips, etc. or contained in vials which may require the addition of water or suitable dilution before use. These components are prepared by the manufacturer in batches which are distinguished by a batch and lot number. Variation may arise from differences between vials, packs, sizes and batches which must be taken into account when planning an evaluation. Testing a few vials may not be representative of the whole product. Planning the total number of vials to be used must be carefully calculated with a few extra being added in case of wastage. Allowance for wastage becomes an important factor in cost evaluation, remembering that each kit has a limiting shelf-life.

The technical assessment of a kit is the same as any other method, apart from the point made above in planning, and is described in an ECCLS document (7), and in chapter 9.

Reaching a decision

In arriving at a conclusion on whether or not to introduce a particular method, the decision would depend upon:

(a) clinical usefulness;
(b) safety assessment;
(c) reliability measured by precision experiments;
(d) accuracy and comparability with existing methods;
(e) cost-efficiency measured as cost per test over a year;
(f) maintenance; and
(g) staff acceptability.

A method that gives no useful information or is unsafe should be discounted without further consideration. In the technical assessment different weight of decision will be placed by an individual laboratory on each experiment. In general, the method giving the lowest CV for each parameter is to be preferred but the expected level of precision and degree of accuracy should be decided before the evaluation starts, together with acceptance limits. A system could therefore be introduced both for each characteristic tested and for its weighting. This is particularly helpful when comparing kits of similar type and cost.

For methods found to be technically acceptable a marked difference in annual cost and cost per test may lead to a decision, but with similar costings, choice will depend upon modes of maintenance, convenience and, finally, personal prejudices.

References

1. Broughton, P. M. G., Gowenlock, A. N., McCormack, J. J. and Neill, D. W. (1974). A revised scheme for the evaluation of automated instruments for use in clinical chemistry. *Annals of Clinical Biochemistry* **11:** 207–218.
2. Buttner, J., Borth, R., Bentwell, J. H., Broughton, P. M. G. and Bowyer, R. C. (1979a). Approved (IFCC) recommendations (1978) on quality control in clinical chemistry. Part 1, General principles and terminology. *Clinica Chimica Acta* **98:** 129F–143F.
3. Buttner, J., Borth, R., Bentwell, J. H., Broughton, P. M. G. and Bowyer, R. C. (1979b). Approved (IFCC) recommendations (1978) on quality control in clinical chemistry. Part 2, Assessment of analytical methods for routine use. *Clinica Chimica Acta* **98:** 145F–162F.
4. ECCLS (1984). Standards for Specimen Collection. Part 1: Blood Containers. ECCLS Document Vol.1 No. 1, pp. 1–6. Berlin: Beuth Verlag.

5. ECCLS (1985). Standards for the Labelling of Clinical Laboratory Materials. ECCLS Document Vol. 2 No. 3. Berlin: Beuth Verlag.
6. ECCLS (1986). Guidelines for the Evaluation of Analysis in Clinical Chemistry. ECCLS Document Vol. 3 No. 2. Berlin: Beuth Verlag.
7. ECCLS (1986). Guidelines for the User Laboratory to Evaluate and Select a Kit for its Own Use. Part 1: Quantitative Tests. ECCLS Document Vol. 3 No. 3. Berlin: Beuth Verlag.
8. Eilers, R. J. (1975). Principles of total quality control. In Lewis, S. M. and Coster, J. F. (eds) *Quality Control in Haematology*, pp. 1–12. London: Academic Press.
9 ICSH (1978a). Protocol for type testing equipment and apparatus used for haematological analysis. *Journal of Clinical Pathology* **31**: 275–279.
10. ICSH (1978b). Recommendations for reference method for haemoglobinometry in human blood (ICSH Standard EP 6/2:1977) and specifications for international haemoglobincyanide reference preparation (ICSH Standard EP 6/3:1977). *Journal of Clinical Pathology* **31**: 139–143.
11. ICSH (1980) Recommendations for reference methods for determination by centrifugation of packed cell volume of blood. *Journal of Clinical Pathology* **33**: 1–2.
12. ICSH (1980). *Recommended Methods for the Determination of Packed Cell Volume*. LAB/80.4 pp. 1–8. Geneva: WHO.
13. ICSH (1982) Selected methods for the determination of packed cell volume. In van Assendelft, O. W. and England, J. M. (eds) *Advances in Haematological Methods: The Blood Count*, pp. 93–98. Boca Raton, Florida: CRC Press.
14. ICSH (1984) Protocol for evaluation of automated blood cell counters. *Clinical and Laboratory Haematology* **6**: 69–84.
15. ICTH/ICSH (1979). Prothrombin time standardization: report of the expert panel on oral anticoagulant control. *Thrombosis Haemostasis* **43**: 1135–1140.
16. Kirkwood, T. B. L. (1983). Calibration of reference thromboplastins. *Thrombosis Haemostasis* **50**(3): 712–717.
17. Koepke, J. A. (1982). Differential white cell counting and the NCCLS methods. In van Assendelft, O. W. and England, J. M. (eds) *Advances in Haematological Methods: The Blood Count*, pp. 99–106. Boca Raton, Florida: CRC Press.
18. Koepke, J. A. and Klee, G. E. (1979). Automated coagulation detection systems. *Clinical Laboratory Haematology* **1**: 75–86.
19. Lewis, S. M., Wardle, J., Cousins, S. and Skelly, J. V. (1979). Platelet counting. Development of a reference method and a reference preparation. *Clinical and Laboratory Haematology* **1**: 227–237.
20. NCCLS (1980). *Standard for Evacuated Tubes for Blood Specimen Collection* (2nd edn), pp. 1–12. Villanova, PA: NCCLS.
21. Shinton, N. K. and Szezepura, A. (1988). In J. P. Ashby (ed). Current developments for improving laboratory economics and working practise, pp. 65–87. European Committee for Clinical Laboratory Standards, Lund, Sweden.
22. Shinton, N. K., Bloom, A. L., Colvin, B. T., Flute, P. T., Preston, F. E. and Kennedy, D. A. (1981). Tentative protocol for the evaluation of coagulameters based on one-stage prothrombin time. *Clinical and Laboratory Haematology* **3**: 71–76.
23. Shinton, N. K., England, J. M. and Kennedy, D. A. (1982). Guidelines for the evaluation of instruments used in haematology laboratories. *Journal of Clinical Pathology* **35**: 1095–1102.
24. Thomson, J. M., Darby, K. U. and Poller, L. (1984). The calibration of the second primary international reference preparation for thromboplastin. *Thrombosis Haemostasis* **52**: 336–342.
25. van Assendelft O. W. and England, J. M. (1982). Terms, quantities and units. In van Assendelft, O. W. and England, J. M. (eds) *Advances in Haematological Methods: The Blood Count*, pp. 1–9. Boca Raton, Florida: CRC Press.
26. WHO Expert Committee on Biological Standardization (1981). Requirements for Immuno-assay Kits. WHO Technical Report Series, No. 658.
27. West Midland Regional Health Authority Management Services Division (1982). Internal Report for DHSS. Scientific and Technical Branch Supply Division, pp. 1–13.

9

The Standardization of Calibration and Control of Instruments and Kits

R M Rowan

Introduction

The primary function of laboratory testing is the production of results which assist the clinician in the process of diagnostic decisions and patient management. Routine measurement of cell count and size are performed on instruments specifically for this purpose and although various technologies may be used by different manufacturers, it is essential for the reliable performance of these clinical tests that some degree of standardization be achieved at manufacturer level.

In addition, most modern diagnostic systems are linear comparators rather than absolute measurement devices and depend on satisfactory calibration procedures to perform correctly. All diagnostic systems require quality assurance procedures to ensure reliability of test results. Accurate measurement results can therefore be obtained if the analytical process has been carefully calibrated, the accuracy of calibration verified over the full range of anticipated values (normal and abnormal) and the process controlled to verify the constancy of calibration. In order to achieve these requirements for calibration and quality assurance there is also need for standardization of procedures at operational level. The existence of standards is a prerequisite for the calibration and control of instruments and kits. It is thus important to define standardization in the context of laboratory medicine.

A standard is defined variously as 'an established measure of extent, quantity, quality or value; any type, model or example for comparison; a criterion of excellence'. A standard can therefore define specifications for systems of nomenclature or classification, for biological or chemical reagents, reference preparations, reference methods, operating methods, calibrators and controls for equipment and test procedures. The process of standardization in a laboratory sense is, therefore, the description of uniform and reproducible systems of measurement to ensure precision, accuracy, specificity and harmonization of test results.

Precision is concerned with consistency of result each time the measurement is made on a particular specimen. Accuracy is concerned with the truth of a result or the closest approximation to truth which can be achieved. The term specificity implies that the measurement is restricted to the substance being measured without interference by other substances. Harmonization implies that blood specimens will give the same measured results wherever the test is performed, regardless of the type of instrument used.

Standards and standardization

Definitions

Definition of the word 'standard' can vary according to circumstance. ICSH (19) has produced a number of definitions as follows:

Proposed ICSH Standard: A specification which has been developed and/or evaluated by an Expert Panel on behalf of ICSH, submitted to the Secretariat where it has been reviewed for format, assigned a document number and forwarded to the Board (of ICSH) as a proposal for a tentative standard. In this context the term standard relates to materials, including biological and chemical substances and physical devices, to methods and procedures, to controls and calibrators for equipment and test procedures, to systems of nomenclature and classification and to modes of practice.

Tentative ICSH Standard: A proposed standard which has been reviewed and accepted by the Board (of ICSH) as a standard relevant to haematology and in a form which is suitable.

ICSH Standard: A tentative standard which has been subject to consensus review for at least one year and approved by a mail ballot of the Committee (the membership) as an international standard.

Reference Standard: A substance or device, one or more properties of which are sufficiently well established to be used for calibration of an apparatus, the assessment of a measurement method or for assigning values to a material. Where possible it must be based on or traceable to exactly defined physical or chemical measurement.

International Biological Standards: These are reference standards which cannot be determined by exactly defined physical or chemical measurement, but to which have been assigned international units of activity as defined by the World Health Organization. These materials are not intended to be used in the laboratory working procedures but serve as the means by which national and commercial reference materials and calibrators can be controlled.

Development of a standard

The need for development of a standard may be perceived by the standardizing body itself or may be suggested by an affiliated organization. Thereafter the procedures adopted by all standardization committees are very similar in operation. The ICSH approach will be described here.

Task force

When a proposal for a standard has been made the management board may consider that expert advice is necessary. A task force will then be appointed to make recommendations. Such a task force will have representatives from the professions, industry and health agencies as appropriate, selected for their special competence and interest in the subject area. The responsibility of a task force is to study the specific subject area to assess the need for and feasibility of establishing and maintaining standards. The task force report to the board should detail specific existing needs, deficiencies in present standards and names of persons capable of developing standards pertaining to the subject under review.

Expert panel

Following acceptance of a task force report, an expert panel is established by the board. The chairholder of the expert panel is selected by the board and he or she in turn proposes the membership of the panel for ratification by the board. As with task force membership, appropriate representation from the professions, industry and health agencies is necessary. In addition, collaborating laboratories may be selected by an expert panel to assist its work directly or the activities of any of its working groups. The expert panel is then responsible for a number of activities:

(a) critical appraisal of existing standards in its subject area;
(b) literature and data compilation on existing standards;
(c) performance of any developmental and validating work necessary for the preparation of proposed standards (in association with collaborating laboratories);
(d) preparation and submission of proposed standard to the board; and
(e) regular review and update of standard as necessary.

Consensus procedure

Transition from proposed standard to tentative standard is achieved by obtaining consensus from the membership of the standardizing organization and from peer groups. Members are encouraged to respond with comment on proposed standards when invited. This is considered a very important stage in the preparation of standards. Comments received are submitted to the appropriate expert panel for consideration and any revision of the proposed standard is re-submitted to the board for the consensus procedure to be repeated. Tentative standards can then be published.

Publishing policy varies with different organizations. ICSH publish in the scientific literature, whereas both NCCLS and ECCLS publish privately with a restricted circulation. A period of at least one year after publication is allowed for public review and challenge of a tentative standard. If at the end of that period no valid objection has been submitted, adoption as a formal standard can occur.

Cell counter calibration

Improvement in the performance of laboratory measurements is primarily a matter of education and understanding of the types of errors which may arise and methods for their prevention. One of the most common causes of error lies in faulty instrument calibration. The concepts of instrument calibration and control appear to pose difficulties for many laboratories. The processes of calibration and control are frequently confused, instruments being mistakenly calibrated using control materials. This erroneous practice is avoidable following careful consideration of the definitions of the frequently abused terms – calibration, calibrator and quality control material.

Definitions

The following definitions have been proposed by ICSH (19) to describe calibration and control:

Calibration: The determination of a bias conversion factor of an analytical process under specified conditions, in order to obtain accurate measurement results. The accuracy over the operating range must be established by appropriate use of reference methods, reference materials and/or calibrators.

Bias is defined as a systematic factor resulting in inaccuracy.

Calibrator: A substance or device used to calibrate, graduate or adjust a measurement. It must be traceable to a reference standard.

The calibrator is then used in conjunction with a calibration procedure to perform one or a sequence of adjustments on all or part of an analytical process or instrument. The calibrator has a value assigned by the use of a definitive or reference method.

Quality control material: A substance used in routine practice for checking the concurrent performance of an analytical process (or instrument). It must be similar in properties to and be analysed along with patient specimens. It may or may not have a pre-assigned value.

Methods for preparation of calibration and control materials are described in Chapter 5 (p. 114–117).

Quality control material is used exclusively to check the performance of the analytical process or instrument to detect and determine the amount of drift in the course of time. Before using a quality control material the analytical process or instrument must be calibrated. Comparison of the definitions of calibrator and quality control material reveals that while the former may be used as a quality control material, the latter must never be used as a calibrator. Within the definitions of calibration, calibrator and quality control material several other commonly used and relevant terms have been introduced, such as reference method, reference preparation and reference material. These too are often incorrectly used and will therefore now be defined (19):

Reference method: A clearly and exactly described technique for a particular determination which, in the opinion of a defined authority, provides sufficiently accurate and precise laboratory data for it to be used to assess the validity of other laboratory methods for this determination. The accuracy of the reference method must be established by comparison with a definitive method where one exists, and the degree of inaccuracy must be stated. The degree of imprecision must also be stated.

Definitive method: A method which after exhaustive investigation is found to have no known source of inaccuracy or ambiguity as judged by defined authority. It will however have a degree of imprecision which should be stated.

Reference material: A substance or physical device, one or more properties of which have been defined by a definitive or reference method. It is to be used for the verification of the accuracy of an analytical process (measurement system) used in routine practice. Reference materials should be based on or traceable to a national certified reference material or an international (certified) reference preparation. (24)

Specifications for reference material characteristics are more stringent than those for either calibrators or quality control materials. Not only must they be compatible with reference and test methods and have values assigned to them by competent authority, but they must also be stable over a reasonably long period of time. Reference materials are used to verify the accuracy of a calibrated analytical process or instrument, a procedure accomplished by comparing results on the reference material with the method under test with those obtained on the same material using the reference method. Reference materials may be primary or secondary. A primary reference material is one certified by a recognized national or international authority, e.g. WHO, ICSH, Bureau Communautaire de Reference (BCR) of the European Community, USA National Bureau of Standards (NBS). Secondary reference materials may be produced commercially or by individual laboratories and are used to calibrate instruments in routine laboratory practice. Their concentration is determined by an analytical process of known and specified precision and accuracy (reference method). Secondary reference preparations should be traceable to the primary or certified reference preparation. The term calibrator has been suggested for these materials.

Calibration procedures for automated cell counters

As previously stated, most blood cell counters are comparators and not absolute measurement devices. They therefore require careful calibration to ensure accuracy to match their high precision. Instrument calibration ultimately depends on the existence of reference materials to which values must be assigned and this process requires reference methods to determine 'true' blood cell values. Each laboratory requires well-documented calibration procedures for its automated instruments.

Prior to calibration, the automated cell counter must be checked to ensure proper operation. Manufacturers usually provide detailed procedures for checking electronic and hydraulic processes within the instrument. Once these have been verified, instrument precision should be assessed by replicate counting to ensure that tolerances lie within the manufacturers' claims (18). Only then can the instrument be assumed to be functioning optimally and be ready for calibration. While this may be a lengthy process it is a necessary prelude to the calibration procedure itself.

Some automated cell counters cannot be calibrated, but even such instruments require the use of control materials to demonstrate satisfactory function.

Calibrators may be produced from fresh blood, preserved blood or artificial materials, e.g. latex particles; the method for assigning a value to the calibrator depends on its nature and the system which is to be calibrated.

Fresh blood calibrators

Use of fresh blood is the preferred method for calibration of multichannel haematology instruments; however, this ideally requires the use of reference methods, and at this time there are few components of the blood count which can be measured by reference methods which satisfy the ICSH definition. Currently reference methods are available only for haemoglobin (15, 20) and packed cell volume (16, 17). High-grade standardized techniques have, however, been described by ICSH (21) which fulfil the definition of 'selected' method and these can be used for assigning values directly to fresh blood for use as a calibrator. Although not a simple procedure, use of these methods (see p. 200) will enable the average laboratory to perform a fresh blood calibration procedure for a multichannel analyser.

A selected method has been defined by ICSH (19) as:

> a procedure, the reliability of which has been validated by a collaborative study and which is recommended by defined authority for routine use in a laboratory analysis, having been selected on the grounds of its accuracy and precision, the intended scope of the test, economy of labour and materials and ease of operation. The degree of inaccuracy and imprecision must be stated.

When fresh blood is used as a calibrator it must be remembered that there are differences in packed cell volume (PCV) when the tripotassium salt of EDTA is used rather than the dipotassium salt. Use of K_3-EDTA produces shrinkage of red cells which results in a 2% decrease of PCV value. This obviously produces an effect on the observed MCV and MCHC values.

Preserved blood or artificial materials

It is some 17 years since the first report was published on the use of glutaraldehyde-fixed non-human red cells as a reference in blood counting (1).

Materials falling into these categories include glutaraldehyde-fixed animal blood cells as well as a number of artificial materials. The latter include pollens, mould spores, yeasts, polystyrene latex and other plastic polymers. Although most have proved disappointing, recent work with latex particles is promising both as a count and as a size standard. Haematological techniques cannot necessarily be applied directly to preserved blood or artificial materials. Under such circumstances values have to be assigned indirectly and the principles and procedures have been described previously (3, 7, 8). This involves two steps: (a) direct determination of fresh blood measurements using selected methods (WBC, RBC, Hb, PCV), and (b) use of an automated blood cell counter to make the same measurements for fresh blood and the surrogate material. Knowing the ratio of fresh blood to surrogate on the automated counter, it is possible to assign values to the preserved blood material. The calculation is simple:

$$\text{Assigned value} = \frac{\text{Direct value}}{\text{Ratio (fresh blood/surrogate)}}$$

Characteristics of a calibrator

Calibrators are used with a particular analytical process or instrument and therefore they need only be compatible with that system. Unlike control materials, calibrators do not require to share the characteristics of the blood sample. The calibrator must, however, possess one particular characteristic. It must possess an assigned value, established either by a reference or more usually a selected method. This value must be stable for the period between the assignment procedure and the time that the material is used for calibration.

A calibrator is used in conjunction with a calibration procedure to adjust the instrument. In performing this adjustment, a calibration factor may be necessary. For example, latex spheres (a mono-dispersed suspension of rigid spheres) may be used to calibrate an electronic impedance counter which in turn will be employed to measure the size of erythrocytes. This counter will, in fact, be calibrated with reference to latex particles and not red blood cells. For accurate calibration with reference to red cells, account must be made of the difference in shape factor between a deformable red cell and a rigid latex sphere. Shape factor is defined by the quotient of perceived volume to true volume and is typically 1.5 for rigid spheres. The assigned value of the calibrator must indicate the true size, such as might be obtained by diffraction or by microscopy; however, the labelling should also include the calibration factor. Application of the calibration factor remains a part of the calibration procedure. Resistivity and deformability of the cell are of primary concern in calibrating aperture-impedance instruments while index of refraction and shape may be more important in light-scatter instruments. If fresh blood is used for calibration purposes, shape factor conversion is not required.

An *ad hoc* task force of the ICSH Expert Panel on the Blood Count has formulated preliminary recommendations regarding the characteristics of materials used for calibration (12) on the assumption that these materials consist of suspensions of particles which may be described by their size, size distribution, concentration and purity.

For both count and size calibration >99% of the pulse characteristics produced by the calibrator must fall within the discriminant function of the instrument when set for a specified cell class. Calibration should be achieved at two or more points within the operating range of the instrument and these points should be spaced sufficiently far apart to ensure calibration over the anticipated range of the instrument. If artificial materials are used their size distribution should be symmetrical and as narrow as possible, the coefficient of variation not exceeding 10%. Adventitious and ambiguous particles possess physical characteristics sufficiently close to those of the calibrator to risk inclusion in the measurement. For count these should be <0.1% and for size <1.0% of the concentration of calibrator particles. Unambiguous particles, on the other hand, have sufficiently different physical characteristics to pose less of a problem. They should comprise <1.0% of the concentration of calibrator particles both for count and size. Clumping of calibrator particles should account for <0.5% of the particles present. Inaccuracy in labelling the concentration of calibrator particles should not be greater than the CV for reproducibility of the instrument for the parameter measured.

Assignment of values to fresh blood calibrators

The ICSH (21) guidelines for the assignment of values to fresh blood used for calibrating automated blood cell counters will be of value to diagnostic laboratories wishing to calibrate their automated counters without resort to preserved blood or surrogate calibrators from commercial sources.

Correct glassware is important. Use of micro-sampler pipettes with disposable tips (e.g. Eppendorf, Labora, Oxford, Scientific Manufacturing Industries) designed to dispense fluid automatically is not recommended. While such devices demonstrate good reproducibility, the volume dispensed by those pipettes tends to be lower than the stated volume and this varies with the nature of the fluid being dispensed. The recommended pipettes should be officially tested Class A glassware, calibration being checked by a gravimetric method using certified weights before they are put into service. Once the calibration check has been undertaken, pipettes should then never be heated above 50°C. White shell-back blood pipettes and volumetric pipettes with controlled draining time and prescribed waiting time are recommended for the assignment of values procedure; however, disposable glass pipettes may be used as an alternative provided they satisfy the specifications of a national standards body. Volumetric flasks should be of borosilicate glass and have a stated volume traceable to a national standards body or, failing that, checked gravimetrically by the individual user. Counting vials for use with the semi-automated single-channel instruments may be of plastic or glass but should be checked to ensure that blood cells do not adhere to the internal surface.

The following methods are recommended:

Haemoglobin

Haemoglobin measurement should be performed using the ICSH reference method (20). It should be noted that occasionally samples will be turbid and in such circumstances filtration is necessary through a low-protein-binding membrane filter.

Packed cell volume

Packed cell volume measurement should be carried out using the ICSH selected method for microhaematocrit determination without correction for trapped plasma (16, 17).

Red cell count

The red cell count should be performed using a semi-automated single-channel instrument which counts by electronic means all cells in a known displaced volume of diluted blood sample (within an accuracy of 1% as checked by reference to a primary metrological standard). At present, the only commonly available instruments which fulfil these requirements are aperture-impedance counters without sheathed flow. Instrument design should ensure that trapped air bubbles and turbulence do not occur and that recirculating of cells inside the orifice tube is an insignificant factor. Additionally, sample flow lines should not change volume when fluid pressure alters, nor should the materials from which they are composed cause adherence of blood cells. Coincidence correction may be provided automatically into the counter or be obtained from coincidence correction charts. Coincidence correction should be verified on installation of the counter or following aperture or major component change. The instrument must be able to discriminate red blood cells (35 fl–∞) and the threshold should be verified on each sample.

Potential sources of error in red cell counting by this method include sampling error (insufficient sample or unrepresentative sample of original whole-blood specimen); transport error in which cell count observed does not indicate every cell in the known volume of diluted blood (caused by sedimentation, cell loss, inaccuracy and imprecision of displaced volume); and counting error arising when the final count is distorted due to incorrect discrimination, spurious counts or inaccurate correction for coincidence loss.

Red cell indices

These are calculated from the primary measurements already made.

White cell count

The instrument principles and general specifications are the same as for red cell counting. The lytic agent must completely lyse the red cells and leave no material which contributes to the white cell count. The threshold settings are 45 fl–∞ verified on each sample. Verification of coincidence loss follows the same principles described for red cells.

Platelet count

Haemocytometer platelet counts are considered to have too many errors to be sufficiently reliable for use in assignment of values. The use of semi-automated single-channel instruments for counts on platelet-rich plasma (PRP) is also limited due to biases which occur during PRP preparation. There is no blood counter available which aspirates a known volume of diluted blood and directly counts platelets in the presence of red cells.

For these reasons an instrument capable of determining the ratio of red cell to platelet count is attractive, since when the red cell count is known the platelet count can be calculated. The instrument used must be capable of electronically discriminating platelets from other blood cells and from debris, sorting the platelet and red cell signals and totalling them in separate registers. The registers then contain counts obtained from the same, but unknown volume of blood and thus the ratio of the red cell count to the platelet count is available. This procedure prevents errors arising during a dilution step and by variations in sample flow rate. When more than one cell type is being enumerated by the same detector a more complex coincidence correction is required (13).

This method is not commonly available and in most laboratories, for the present, calibration of automated instrument platelet counting must rely on carefully performed haemocytometer counts using the ammonium oxalate method and phase-contrast microscopy (4, 21).

Control of diagnostic kits

Definition

A diagnostic kit has been defined by ICSH (19) as 'a package containing two or more reagents and/or other material and a method protocol for performance of a specified analytic procedure'. While such kits are often expensive they provide a convenient method of performing special assays. A wide variety of kits now exists encompassing many areas of chemistry and haematology.

The concept has been developed to incorporate instrumentation as well as reagents to form diagnostic systems. The latter are particularly relevant to chemistry where dry reagent carriers or special test packs are used together with microprocessor controlled analysers, mostly of the absorption or reflection spectrometry type. The reagent carriers can be either of solid phase impregnated with reagents mounted in plastic supports or based on the use of a multichambered plastic test pack containing liquid or dry reagents. These systems provide accurate pipetting, automatic wavelength selection, highly stable electronics requiring only infrequent calibration, automatic timing of incubation and automatic calculation and printing of test results. However, although these analysers are 'automatic' they still require electronic and hydraulic function monitoring, internal quality control of the process and external quality assessment. The demand for such systems is increasing, particularly for use in decentralized laboratories.

Haemoglobinometry is one of the analytes measured by this process but except for small blood counting devices, mainly of the semi-automated variety, such systems are not yet available for haematology. However, technological advance allied to clinical demand could change this, particularly for measurements of acute phase reaction, red cell enzymes and coagulation studies.

Analytical procedure

Clinical requirements for analytical procedures may vary depending on whether a test is used for screening or definitive purposes. Thus, even if analytical reliability is unsatisfactory a kit may be acceptable for a particular clinical purpose. The user, however, must be fully aware of the limitations of such an analytical system in order to decide whether or not to select the method for a given diagnostic problem and subsequently how to interpret the test result. The performance claims must be stated clearly by the manufacturer but should also be validated by the user.

Qualitative (coarse-graduated) tests

These simply yield a yes/no result if a particular property is present in a certain degree or not.

Semi-quantitative (coarse-graduated) tests

With this type of test the scale is no longer binary (yes/no) but has more points, e.g. negative, weakly positive, positive or strongly positive, thus allowing an estimate of concentration. This may be achieved by comparing a reaction product colour to a scale of colours representing different concentration ranges. It should be remembered that the correct use of such a test requires colour balancing of artificial illumination if natural light is not available. Some measurements are expressed in units which become logarithmic when serial dilutions are used. In this case the result is expressed as the number of tubes showing the effect.

All coarse-graduated scale tests should be designed in such a way that the analytical discrimination limit is close to the clinically relevant decision level. In addition, since the incidence of false-positive and false-negative test results is high in this type of procedure, design should be such that discrimination levels minimize the clinical consequences of false-positive and false-negative results (22). The discrimination limit is defined by statistical evaluation of a large number of test results according to approved evaluation procedures and the diagnostic 'cut-off' points are then specified as those concentrations at which 95% of the results are positive or negative depending on whether a criterion should be accepted or rejected (14).

Quantitative (fine-graduated) tests

These measurements are expressed as units of time or as ratios and include such data as weight and volume. Where possible such tests are generally preferred because of their greater potential precision.

Introduction of kit

A major component in the quality control of diagnostic kits lies in their manufacture. The manufacturer has the responsibility for ensuring the quality of reagents and for the reliability and traceability of the control materials included. In spite of this manufacturer obligation, however, no kit should be introduced into routine use without careful evaluation (see Chapter 8). Before adopting any diagnostic kit for routine use in the laboratory, the purpose for which it is intended requires review, the principle of the assay requires analysis and, if multiple kits are available for the same diagnostic procedure, these should be carefully compared to decide which performance characteristics are acceptable and which are not (9, 25).

If the diagnostic kit replaces an existing technique, careful comparison of the two methods over a wide range of values is mandatory. It may be necessary to exchange and simultaneously analyse samples with a reference laboratory. Test performance is generally expressed in terms of analytical imprecision and bias; however, analytical disturbances such as systematic shifts in baseline, increases in random error or interference can adversely influence the quality of test results.

The need for comprehensive quality control is determined by the frequency and the magnitude of analytical disturbances. If these occur infrequently or not at all, or their magnitude is negligible when compared to permissible analytical error, the need for quality control is minimal. Unfortunately, when dealing with biological systems, analytical disturbances tend to be frequent and their nature is often obscure and unpredictable. Under such circumstances the need for comprehensive and well-designed quality control is great. These principles apply no less to the performance of tests using diagnostic kits than to tests performed on automated multiparameter analysers.

Design of quality assurance procedures

As with all laboratory tests the introduction of a new diagnostic kit requires appropriate quality assurance procedures. Meaningful quality assurance is divided into non-analytical and analytical components. The large number of tasks on the non-analytical side of the programme often results in many being ignored or being considered mundane and not requiring attention. What is frequently forgotten is that criteria for patient preparation and specimen collection, specimen transportation, sample preparation and finally, recording and distribution of results are important components of quality assurance.

The components of analytical quality assurance are better recognized and more attention is paid to these. Included in the latter are assessment and maintenance of method reliability, equipment dependability and reagent quality, together with use of biological controls and participation in proficiency testing schemes.

Method reliability

A basic operational requirement for any laboratory is that it possesses well-conceived programmes for the evaluation and selection of test methods. Parameters of precision, accuracy, sensitivity and specificity must be assessed to determine the overall quality and reliability of any given procedure. Only by this means can consistent and objective evaluations be conducted and poor selections eliminated. Standardizing bodies such as ICSH, ECCLS and IFCC have produced evaluation protocols both for instruments and kits (5, 6, 18, 22). When carefully performed and documented, such evaluations provide the analyst with an awareness of both the strengths and the weaknesses of each test and also provide rigid standards for comparing alternative methodology.

Equipment dependability

Ensuring dependability of equipment is an essential part of every analytical quality assurance programme and depends on the care and maintenance provided both by laboratory personnel and the manufacturer as part of a preventive maintenance scheme.

Reagent quality

Procedures for ensuring reliable reagents are of major importance in test quality control. This must never be assumed and reagents must be checked regularly to ensure that they are without contamination or deterioration.

Biological controls

This is the best recognized aspect of quality assurance. The definition of quality control material has already been stated (p. 196). Achievement of the assigned values for these controls provides increased confidence in laboratory results.

Performance goals

Laboratory tests are performed to assist the physician to make clinical decisions. The best measure of the true value of a test is how well it performs in clinical practice. Clinical interpretation of tests results depends on a combination of factors including calibration, precision, biological variation within an individual and inherent difference between individuals. Analysis of these sources of variation can be used to set tolerance limits for test performance. Such tolerance limits can then be used as boundary levels within which variation has no clinical meaning.

The analytical quality of most laboratory tests is well documented. The clinical pathologist is aware of the degree of precision currently achievable in clinical laboratories from data gathered from national surveys and quality control programmes. Over the years steady improvement in test precision has occurred. Further improvements may be achievable but there is growing concern that this will be expensive and meaningless if not matched by improvement in the diagnostic value of a test, i.e. on the degree of precision required for optimal patient care. Pre-analytical variables now frequently lead to greater imprecision than the analytical procedure itself.

Clinical goals

Skendzel *et al.* (23) attempted to establish medically useful guidelines for the optimal precision of commonly used clinical laboratory procedures following a postal survey of randomly selected physicians. These physicians were asked to review a number of clinical problems and select that change in test results which would alter their diagnosis or treatment or prompt further analysis of the patient's condition. The responses obtained were used to calculate goals for laboratory precision sufficient to meet the requirements of the average physician. Three major findings emerged from this survey. First, most physicians required a substantial change in test results before they altered their diagnosis or treatment; current standards of laboratory precision fell well within these limits. Secondly, the physician response to what constituted significant change in test values depended to some degree on the clinical setting. For example, in asymptomatic patients, the change necessary to create physician concern was greater than in patients with acute illness or in therapeutic monitoring regimes. Finally there were only minor differences in selection among physicians from different specialities.

Clearly the physician makes a complex judgement when analysing test results, based on the degree of abnormality, the likelihood that further investigation will affect the therapy, and the cost associated with further investigation. To be effective this judgement must be based on knowledge of factors which affect test results, including inherent biological variation, pre-analytical factors (position of patient while collecting specimens, diet, collection technique, time from venous sampling to processing and handling of specimen prior to analysis) and analytical variability. To these must be added knowledge of the sensitivity, specificity and predictive value of a particular test.

The establishment of medically useful criteria for laboratory precision helps to place laboratory precision and the use of tests in proper perspective. This does not infer that laboratories should abandon current practices of quality control, but when the average laboratory achieves precision in testing which exceeds medically useful limits by several fold, additional efforts to improve performance will not increase diagnostic usefulness. The resources of the laboratory might be better directed to the study and control of pre-analytical factors affecting a test and to the development of more appropriate tests for diagnosis and treatment.

Laboratory goals

Limits of permissible error are determined by the complexity of test methodology. The test situations relating to diagnostic kits are identified in Table 9.1. Measurements of

Table 9.1 Test situations relating to diagnostic kits

Kit type	Measurement scale	Permissible error limit
Haematology	Ratio	±2 SD
Chemistry	Ratio	±2 SD
Coagulation	Time	±2 SD
Blood bank	Identity	None (+ or −)
Serology	Identity	None (+ or −)
Serology	If logarithmic	±1 dilution
Radioimmunoassay	Ratio	±2 SD

identity are restricted to the stated presence or absence of a given constituent. Measurements expressed in logarithmic function are assigned limits of ±1 dilution (tube). Time and ratio measurements are allowed ±2 SD.

The relative complexity of time and ratio measurements has resulted in a number of statistical treatments for expressing amount of permissible error. The most commonly used measurements are the standard deviation (SD) or the coefficient of variation (CV), both of which assess the ability to reproduce a measurement and are calculated from replicate determinations on the same specimen. For quality control purposes replicate assays (≥ 20) are performed on multiple aliquots of the same control material and the following formulae used:

$$SD = \sqrt{\left(\frac{\Sigma\, (x - \bar{x})^2}{n - 1}\right)}$$

$$CV = \frac{SD}{x} \times 100\%$$

where x is the value for each measurement, $\bar{x}$ is the mean of all the measurements, and n is the total number of aliquots. The allowable variation, used for subsequent assessment of daily control results, is taken as 2 SD. This means that if a single result is drawn at random from a series of assays on the same sample, the odds are 20 to 1 that the value will not be further removed from the mean than twice the SD; or, should this value exceed the limits of 2 SD, there is a 95% chance that this has resulted from avoidable error. It is important to appreciate that the numerical value of a standard deviation for the same method can vary from one laboratory to another because of different policies and techniques.

Although many different procedures have been recommended or are used in individual laboratories, it is usually considered good practice with time or ratio scales of measurement to select three quality control materials with levels at different clinical decision-making points (9):

(1) Where the analysis has a lower and upper medically significant decision level, the low, medium and high level materials should have analyte concentrations at the lower decision level, mid-point of the reference interval and upper decision level.

(2) Where the analyte does not have a lower medically significant decision level, the low, medium and high level materials should have analyte concentrations at the upper limit of the reference interval, the decision level and near the extreme upper range capability of the method.

(3) Where the analyte does not have an upper medically significant level the three materials should have analyte concentrations at the lower limit of the reference range, the decision level and near the lower range capability of the method.

Target values should be assigned by analysis of at least 20 replicates and the mean value and dispersion calculated. As a minimum, action limits of the mean ± 3 SD are set as the criteria for acceptance or rejection of the analytical batches, with warning limits at ± 2 SD of the means.

Since quality control materials of appropriate types and levels of analyte are likely to have been used during the formal evaluation of precision, the data for internal quality assurance procedures may be thought to be already available. It must be appreciated however, that the performance characteristics derived from formal evaluation studies will be those achieved under the best possible conditions. When a kit is used in routine practice, the performance characteristics will deteriorate since different analysts will perform the tests using different batches of reagents and other consumables. Under these circumstances the performance characteristics require re-assessment and often some down-grading, otherwise there will be false rejection of too many batches. It is extremely important to remember that optimal and routine conditions of variance differ.

Internal quality control

The function of internal quality control is to monitor the various aspects of the test procedure including measurement on specially prepared materials, repeated measurements on patient samples and statistical analysis day by day of the data obtained from routine tests. These measures achieve optimal precision but not necessarily accuracy. Internal quality control will identify analytical runs with unacceptable systematic or random error. Systematic error increases or decreases all the test results by the same amount and therefore causes the entire error distribution to be shifted in one direction. Random error causes the test results to have larger variation, thus widening the error distribution and increasing the size of the errors.

Controls

With tests using a measurement scale based on identity, ideally positive and negative controls should be used on each occasion. For time- or ratio-based tests the requirements are more complex and are determined by the number of specimens in each analytical run. Generally, using diagnostic tests, analytical runs contain a small number of individual tests. Under these circumstances it may be unrealistic to demand more than one of each control material available, i.e. high, normal and low. If, however, there is a trend to increasing inaccuracy or imprecision, the number of controls processed should be increased to speed up the decision of acceptance or rejection. Normally, control specimens should be equally distributed within the run. Statistical analysis is described in detail in Chapter 4.

Patient specimens

Duplicate or check tests on patients' specimens are easily carried out. Duplicate testing is ideal for diagnostic kit procedures. Ideally every specimen should be tested in duplicate. The standard deviation is calculated as follows:

$$SD = \sqrt{\frac{\Sigma d^2}{2n}}$$

where d^2 = difference between duplicates squared and n = number of specimens tested in duplicate.

None of the duplicate tests should differ from each other by more than $\pm 2\,SD$. This procedure identifies any isolated error in a specimen. Clearly, however, if the test performance is always poor, the SD will be wide and insensitive to individual tests.

Check tests are similar to duplicate tests but use specimens originally measured in an earlier batch. Again the tests should agree with each other within $\pm 2\,SD$. This procedure detects deterioration in apparatus and/or reagents which has occurred between tests, provided the specimens have not altered. It can be advantageous to use the same specimens both for check tests and duplicate tests. The SD can be established on the basis of technical competence from duplicate tests and if the SD for check tests is greater this provides indication of deteriorating equipment and/or reagents, provided again that the specimens have not altered.

Statistical analysis

The use of statistics, control charts and cumulative (CUSUM) charts is described in Chapters 4 and 5.

Correlation checks

Any unexpected test result must be checked to establish whether or not it can be explained on clinical grounds or whether it correlates with other tests. This is a very important aspect of internal quality control.

External quality assessment

This procedure denotes the objective evaluation by an external agency of laboratory performance on material supplied specially for this purpose. External quality assessment is described in Chapter 7. A check on accuracy can also be achieved providing the material supplied has been assayed by a reference laboratory using methods of defined precision alongside a reference preparation of stated value. The performance of diagnostic kits, particularly for ferritin, vitamin B_{12} and folate estimations and certain red cell enzymes, is regularly monitored in many external quality assessment schemes. This serves as an invaluable check, not only on individual laboratory performance but also on the reliability of the diagnostic kits.

Reference values

If the new diagnostic kit has performance characteristics identical to the method that it is replacing, then reference values are transferable without significant problems. However, if imprecision and inaccuracy have changed, for better or for worse, then the reference values will have changed and require to be re-defined. The generation of reference values is a complex subject which has been intensively studied during the past few years. This is described in detail in Chapter 3.

Communication with users

Non-analytical quality control has been discussed previously (see p. 204). Communication of results to clinical users is an important component of this. As the final step before the introduction of a new diagnostic kit, communication with all users of the laboratory service must be undertaken if any of the following have occurred:

(1) specimen requirements such as type and volume have changed;
(2) the frequency with which analyses are done has been changed, with consequent alteration of the turnaround time between obtaining the specimen and reporting of result;
(3) the imprecision and inaccuracy of the tests have changed to such a degree that interpretation of result is significantly different; or
(4) the performance characteristics have changed, leading to an alteration in the report format.

Diagnostic kits in decentralized clinical laboratories

There has been a growing tendency in recent years to perform analytical procedures in a decentralized setting. Decentralized clinical laboratory testing is performed in locations removed from the administrative control, standards and regulatory forces which apply in the centralized laboratory. Such sites include high–utility clinical areas in hospital and the physicians' office. The most important justification for decentralized testing is clinical requirement for an immediate result. This may arise because of the urgency of a clinical situation or for the convenience of the patient or the clinician.

Industry has been quick to appreciate that an enormous potential market exists and has responded by producing an ever-increasing selection of diagnostic kits and diagnostic systems accompanied by glossy brochures which often imply that their operation does not require any laboratory training. Undoubtedly many of these tests are or will be performed by individuals untrained in laboratory practice. However, although many of these systems are automated they still require adequately trained operators to provide the analytical service and internal quality control.

This subject has been reviewed by Grayson (11) who found an unacceptable degree of imprecision with results derived by untrained operators in the physician's office showing variability for most analytes ranging from 50% to 250% larger than for central laboratories. Similar differences have been reported by others (2, 10). When variability is correlated with the level of training of the individuals performing the test, there is clear evidence that those untrained in laboratory technology produce more variable results than the adequately trained operator. Technical complexity of testing will always be a limiting factor and automation, no matter how 'user friendly' is not necessarily an answer since most automated devices require considerable expertise to keep them operational.

The implication is clear. While it would be undesirable and inappropriate to attempt to prevent the development of decentralized testing, its proliferation must be under the advisory and supervisory control of a central, well-managed and well-equipped laboratory. Only in this way can good laboratory practice be transferred to the decentralized site. To achieve this the central laboratory requires additional resources of personnel and funds.

References

1. Archer, R. K. (1982). Available animals bloods and their potential uses. In van Assendelft, O. W. and England, J. M. (eds) *Advances in Haematological Methods: The Blood Count*, pp. 207–216. Boca Raton, Florida: CRC Press.
2. Crawley, R., Belsey, R., Brock, D. and Baer, D. (1986). Regulations of physician's office laboratories. The Idaho experience. *Journal of the American Medical Association* 255: 374–382.
3. Crosland-Taylor, P. J., Allen, R. W. B., England, J. M., Fielding, J. F., Lewis, S. M., Shinton, N. K. and White, J. M. (1979). Draft protocol for testing calibration and quality control material used with automatic blood-counting apparatus. *Clinical and Laboratory Haematology* 1: 61–64.
4. Dacie, J. V. and Lewis, S. M. (1984). *Practical Haematology* (6th edn), pp. 43–44. Edinburgh: Churchill Livingstone.
5. ECCLS (1982). 1st Draft Protocol for the Evaluation of Analytical Instruments. ECCLS Document Vol. 2 No. 4, pp. 53–97.
6. ECCLS (1985). 2nd Draft Guidelines for Kit Evaluation Guidelines for a User Laboratory to Evaluate and Select a Kit for its Own Use. ECCLS Document Vol. 5 No. 1, pp. 1–45.
7. England, J. M., Chetty, M. C., Garvey, B., Crosland-Taylor, P. J., Barnard, D., Lewis, S. M. and Wardle, J. (1982). Value assignment to quality control materials using the draft protocol published by the British Committee for Standards in Haematology. In van Assendelft, O. W. and England, J. M. (eds) *Advances in Haematological Methods: The Blood Count*, pp. 239–247. Boca Raton, Florida: CRC Press.

8. England, J. M., Chetty, M. C., Garvey, B., Lewis, S. M., Wardle, J., Cousins, S., Crosland-Taylor, P. J. and Syndercombe-Court (1983). Testing of calibration and quality control material used with automatic blood apparatus: application of the protocol devised by the British Committee for Standardisation in Haematology. *Clinical and Laboratory Haematology* **5:** 83–92.

9. Fraser, C. G. and Wilde, C. E. (1985). Introduction of a reagent kit into regular use in the clinical laboratory. *Communications in Laboratory Medicine* **2:** 71–75.

10. Gilbert, R. K. (1975). Progress and analytical goals in clinical chemistry. *American Journal of Clinical Pathology* **63:** 960–973.

11. Grayson, R. T. (1984). Effects of regulatory controls on the accuracy of clinical laboratory tests. *Journal of Medical Technology* **1:** 632–637.

12. Groner, W. (1982). Specifications of calibration, control and reference materials of cell counting and sizing apparatus. In van Assendelft, O. W. and England, J. M. (eds) *Advances in Haematological Methods: The Blood Count*, pp. 185–193. Boca Raton, Florida: CRC Press.

13. Groner, W. and Epstein, E. (1982). Counting and sizing of blood cells using light scatter. In van Assendelft, O. W. and England, J. M. (eds) *Advances in Haematological Methods: The Blood Count*, pp. 73–84. Boca Raton: Florida: CRC Press.

14. Haeckel, R., Bonini, P., Ceriotti, G., Kutter, D. and Vonderschmitt, D. J. (1985). Multi-centre evaluation of the Urine Test Strip Analyzer Rapimat. *Journal of Clinical Chemistry and Clinical Biochemistry* **23:** 473–492.

15. ICSH (1978). Recommendations for reference method for haemoglobinometry in human blood (ICHS Standard EP 6/2: 1977) and specifications for international haemiglobincyanide reference preparation (ICSH Standard EP 6/3: 1977). *Journal of Clinical Pathology* **31:** 139–143.

16. ICSH (1980). Recommended Methods for the Determination of Packed Cell Volume, LAB/80.4. Geneva: WHO.

17. ICSH (1980). Recommendation for reference method for determination by centrifugation of packed cell volume of blood. *Journal of Clinical Pathology* **33:** 1–2.

18. ICSH (1984). Protocol for evaluation of automated blood cell counters. *Clinical and Laboratory Haematology* **6:** 69–84.

19. ICSH (1986). *Handbook*, pp. 1–39. ICSH.

20. ICSH (1987). Recommendations for reference method for haemoglobinometry in human blood (ICSH Standard 1986) and specification for international haemoglincyanide reference preparation (3rd edn). *Clinical and Laboratory Haematology* **9:** 73–79.

21. ICSH Cytometry Panel (1988). The assignment of values to fresh blood used for calibrating automated blood cell counters. *Clinical and Laboratory Haematology.* **10:** 203–212.

22. IFCC (1983). Scientific Committee, Analytical Section: Expert Group on Diagnostic kits and Reagents. Revised recommendation (1983) on evaluation of clinical chemistry kits. *Journal of Clinical Chemistry and Clinical Biochemistry* **21:** 899–902.

23. Skendzel, L. P., Barnett, R. N. and Platt, R. (1985). Medically useful criteria for analytic performance of laboratory tests. *American Journal of Clinical Pathology* **85:** 200–205.

24. Van Assendelft, O. W. and England, J. M. (1982). Terms quantities and units. In van Assendelft, O. W. and England, J. M. (eds) *Advances in Haematological Methods: The Blood Count*, pp. 2–9. Boca Raton, Florida: CRC Press.

25. Wilde, C. E. (1985). The selection of a reagent kit for regular use in the clinical laboratory. *Communications in Laboratory Medicine* **2:** 5–7.

10

Organization and Management of the Laboratory

N K Shinton

Introduction

Organization and management are an integral part of providing a quality laboratory service and therefore of total quality assurance (13). The function of laboratory management is to co-ordinate resources so that an efficient and effective service is provided. This administrative process includes planning, decision-making, organizing, directing and controlling.

The initial planning function is to prepare a management structure with delegation downwards and accountability upwards. The system of management adopted must make provision for overall policy decision-making, laboratory operational procedures, implementation procedures and, finally, bench techniques or rules. Ways of introducing variations, when these are necessary, must be included. Successful management will depend upon knowledge of workload matched by available resources which includes capital building, equipment and revenue. Appropriate deployment may require a work-study to determine the best means of using the resources available. Built into the management system there must be means for maintaining a good standard of work with appropriate evaluation.

Management structure

A haematology department will vary with its workload and geographical position. The commonest variations would be either:

    (a)   totally independent organization within a large hospital or clinic;
    (b)   a section of another hospital department, e.g. clinical chemistry;
    (c)   a section of pathology department within a small hospital; or
    (d)   a private laboratory or clinic outside a hospital organization.

Head of department (director)

Whatever the size of organization there must be a head of department or director with clear lines of responsibility upwards and downwards. This appointment will vary with local arrangements of the employing authority which must be one which has respect of colleagues in other departments. It is desirable that the appointee has received basic training in management and essential to have received accredited training in the speciality. It is usual for the person to be medically qualified, often having associated clinical responsibilities.

The duties of the head of department are to determine broad policies and establish priorities and not necessarily to supervise directly or manage. (26). The person must, however, be the budget holder, although detailed accounting can be seconded to a manager. The head of department must be ultimately responsible for discipline of staff, with direct involvement at the dismissal stage. He or she must also be responsible for training, maintenance of standards, research and development, with delegation as appropriate.

The head of department must appoint a deputy to cover absence and must arrange a working relationship with colleagues of similar status within the department, i.e. other consultants. Rotation of headship can be arranged; the post should not change more frequently than every 3 years and requires notification to any employing authority.

Relations must be established with other heads of scientific departments who may meet together as a scientific group. The chairman of such a group may be the overall budget holder, i.e. pathology department. The head of a haematology department will also need to liaise and meet with other local or regional haematologists to discuss funding for major equipment and future developments.

Laboratory manager

If the head of department decides to appoint a manager the relationship between them and the division of functions must be laid down. It is not uncommon for the manager of a haematology laboratory to be a scientist or a medical laboratory scientific officer (MLSO) or technologist with responsibility for ordering of supplies, accounting, and appointment and training of junior staff. The function of the manager will be to achieve goals agreed with the head of department using the resources available. The laboratory manager requires to be a sound leader and to have skill in organization with the ability to motivate or instil motivation in subordinates (25). It requires an appreciation of human behaviour in a variety of circumstances. The person must be involved in disciplining procedures which must be agreed with the head of department.

As an alternative to appointing a laboratory manager, the head of department may appoint a laboratory administrator who will usually be a non-scientist who organizes the department within the framework and policies of the head of department. In these circumstances the head of department will combine the role with that of manager.

Line-management

A staffing structure with line-management must be determined with numbers and grading dependent upon workload. The level of delegation with functional appropriateness must be appreciated. This is particularly important in a haematology laboratory where both technical and medical decisions will be made. It is usual for the manager to have a number of supervisors who will oversee the activities of other staff to perform specific skills efficiently, focusing attention on operational provision. (Fig. 10.1) The relationship of these staff with unskilled laboratory aides, with ancillary staff responsible for cleaning and with secretarial staff must be laid down and organized.

The relation in line-management of other medical consultant staff must be considered and understood. Apart from deputizing on a clinical level and given specific responsibilities, they may have little involvement in laboratory management other than that of a user.

The administrative process

The administrative process includes planning, decision-making, organizing, directing and controlling (26).

Planning is a key function of all managers and includes both long-term and short-term plans. The long-term plans will derive from policy decisions made by the head of department but will require discussion with other appropriate members of staff, especially the manager and supervisors of sections. Short-term planning may only involve the manager with appropriate supervisors.

Decision-making is a part of all other aspects of the administrative process. It must depend upon the proper assessment of information and not rely on intuition, although this may well be a final factor. The commitment to a particular decision must be appreciated and understood in advance. Timing of implementation must obviously be considered. All decisions involve a value judgement of what is beneficial/non-beneficial, important/non-important in projecting the probable outcomes of the decision. The financial cost must be assessed and taken into consideration (27).

The style of decision-making can vary. It may be authoritarian, democratic with involvement of several members of staff in a voting procedure or by consensus. The chosen mode will to some extent depend upon procedures in vogue within the particular service to which the specific haematology department belongs. Whatever approach is chosen, a *laissez-faire* manner can only indicate that the head of department has abdicated from any administrative responsibility. The procedure may vary from one set of decisions to another, largely depending upon the time factor. Consensus is slow and authoritarian management quick, with an inverse effect on staff reaction, which itself is a value judgement. When time permits, an opportunity to discuss decisions with appropriate staff is desirable. Senior staff should meet regularly (e.g. monthly) with larger meetings of all staff from time to time. At such a meeting the objectives of the department must be clearly set out and ways of carrying out the chosen policy determined. Such meetings act as a feed-back in the day-to-day efficiency of communications within the department. Organization of such transmission of information within the laboratory and outside is a function of good administration. Interpersonal communication is essential to maintain good staff relationships.

Organizing the work of the department involves developing a working structure to

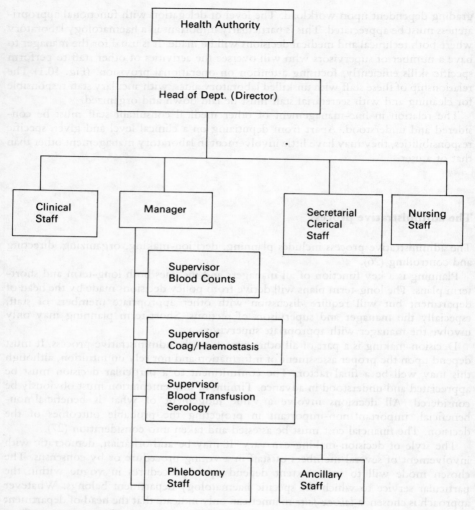

Fig. 10.1 Organization chart for haematology laboratory.

facilitate the co-ordination of resources to achieve completion of both long-term and short-term plans.

Directing the department requires leadership and involves the human element of management. Both the head of department and the manager must make themselves available to other members of staff to discuss individual and personal problems. This may be time consuming but can, in the longer term, save wasted hours of sub-standard work. The human needs of an individual member of staff have to be appreciated and seen to be understood for efficient management of a laboratory.

A particular relationship has to be established with the department's secretarial office. This will vary with the degree of involvement of the office in reporting of results. In some circumstances the office staff may not be managerially responsible to the head of department, in which case agreement on duties and disciplinary arrangements can be made with the appropriate administrative body.

Finally, the administrative process must include control to ensure that end–product of a decision conforms to the policies planned.

Workload

Information on predicted workload is an essential requirement for laboratory planning. A crude estimate can be made by recording the number of requests received over a defined period, but this takes no account of their nature (14). In haematology there is a vast difference in the capital and revenue resources required for a haemoglobin estimation compared with a bone marrow biopsy. An attempt to assess workload more closely was developed by the Canadian Association of Pathologists and further refined by the College of American Pathologists (7). This is a unit system in which a specific test is awarded a five–digit number of points based upon the level of resources required. It is based on the presumption of the use of classic time–engineering techniques and of a standard format for all procedures. The assuming of new workload values as procedures change results in an inevitable time–lag of introduction. Unit values are based upon the time required for initial handling of the specimen, specimen testing, recording and reporting, daily or routine preparation for a batch of tests, maintenance and repair, solution preparation, glassware washing and technical supervision. It does not include time for performance of quality assurance techniques.

With the introduction of laboratory data computerization, a program can be prepared for calculating the workload either as a raw count or by a unit system. It will probably be convenient for the data to be divided into sections such as blood counting, coagulation and haemostasis, blood transfusion serology, haematological biochemistry, and/or haemato–immunology. A breakdown between requests during normal working hours and emergency hours will be necessary and it may be of help to know the origin of requests, i.e. in–patients, out–patients, general practitioner (primary care) and screening clinics.

Resources

Capital

This may be a building with equipment or money available for them. This will come from Health Authorities, a private company or other funding body. In any case a detailed bid will have to be made based upon the estimated workload, number of staff to be employed and appropriate safety regulations. The financing agency may allot money for building to the head of department, with the manager having to determine the level of workload that can be encompassed. Where the capital is inadequate for the workload, the head of department must prepare the case for allocation of more capital money.

Revenue

An annual revenue allocation is usually made as a budget agreed with the funding authority (12). This budget will be broken down into revenue for staff and consumables with further divisions usually based on a coding arrangement. A laboratory may receive revenue from a number of sources but an annual income for each must be determined. Apart from budgetary agreements, revenue may arrive from the performance of specific work such as a research project, private requests on an individual basis, screening for safety measures in industry and donated gifts.

Use of resources

Building

Planning a new building or renovating an existing one requires the advice of an architect. The head of department must indicate the floor area for the whole project that will be necessary for the particular workload with breakdown into specific rooms of certain size for blood counting, coagulation, transfusion serology, haematological biochemistry and immunology, and research and development. Special rooms or areas must be set aside for 24-h emergency work, radioactive procedures and handling specimens with a biological hazard. An early decision must be made between an open-plan laboratory giving flexibility for change and easy movement, compared with separate rooms for sections which reduces noise and gives some privacy for work. A work flow-plan must be designed with a layout flow–chart (Fig. 10.2). Allowance must be made for circulation, and offices provided for senior staff with administrative duties and for secretaries. In addition, there must be rooms or areas for washing-up, stores, cloakrooms and toilets. Where there is a clinical function added to the laboratory, consulting rooms, waiting area and reception must be included in the plans, together with their own toilet facilities. These clinical facilities will probably be shared with other laboratory or hospital departments.

Once the outline plans have been agreed, a room-by-room schedule of work must be drawn up. The choice of methods to be used must be considered, especially in respect of automated blood counting where size and services of the instruments vary. Arrangements for reporting, particularly in respect of computer housing, must also be an early policy decision. Each room will require a detailed plan in respect of water, electrical and gas supply, lighting, heating, ventilation and drainage.

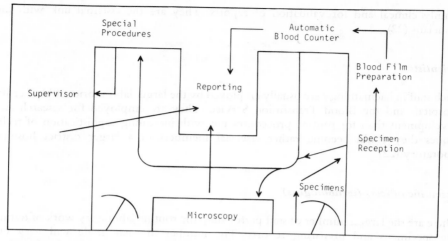

Fig. 10.2 Flow diagram for blood counting procedure.

Equipment

With a new building a costed equipment schedule must be prepared but in the case of transfer of an existing laboratory an inventory should already be available to which only new or replacement items require to be added.

Decision on purchase of new or replacement equipment will depend upon choice of methods. Reference to evaluation studies and cost analysis including maintenance are essential, especially where a committee has to be persuaded to make funding available (24).

Following delivery the new items must be added to the laboratory equipment inventory, which may be held by a computer.

Staffing

A haematology laboratory usually requires a range of staff, the number of each depending upon workload.

Medical

These will be consultants usually having associated clinical responsibilities for in-patients and out-patients; one will be head of department. A number of junior medical staff in training posts may be employed or alternatively general practitioners in the grade of hospital practitioner or clinical assistant. Their involvement in the laboratory is mainly clinical and for validation of reports. They are the essential link with the clinicians (22).

Scientists

Such staff in haematology are usually employed by the larger laboratories of University Hospitals and the Blood Transfusion Service. They are employed for research and development than for routine procedures but with increasing sophistication of techniques they could become rather essential members of a larger district hospital laboratory (22).

Scientific officers (technologists)

These are the largest number of staff performing the routine laboratory work of testing the specimens and preparing reports. The number in each grade will vary but managerially there will be a senior, usually the laboratory manager, heads of sections such as blood counting, coagulation and transfusion serology, and lower grade technologists.

Laboratory aides (laboratory assistants)

These persons will be performing unskilled or repetitive work such as feeding machines and preliminary setting up tubes for testing. Their training will be in-service for the particular task they are undertaking. A special group may be employed as phlebotomists for the collection of specimens.

Secretarial staff

A number of people are necessary to handle reports, arrange despatch, type orders and letters.

Nurses

These may be attached to an out-patient department or help with clinical care of haemophiliacs or patients receiving cytotoxic drugs. They are usually responsible managerially to the nursing administration.

Ancillary staff

These are employed as porters and cleaners but may carry out washing up of bottles and tubes. In this respect they will be responsible to members of the laboratory staff, particularly in respect of safety measures and discipline.

Consumables

These can broadly be divided into reagents, calibrators, quality control material and reporting paper. With the introduction of laboratory computers the stock information can be held at all times.

Reagents

The choice depends upon the method being used but their quality must be assured by reference to evaluation either from the literature or by testing. It is essential that they are compatible with any associated instrument. Attention must be given to the requirements for storage and their shelf-life.

Calibrators and quality control material

Calibrators must be those compatible with the instrument to be used and to have been tried and tested. Quality control material will be required daily and arrangements must be made for purchase or local collection. In either case it must be biologically safe and suitably tested. External assessment is best arranged by joining a scheme which will provide regular surveys.

Reporting paper

This has become an item of expenditure requiring a budget as a result of the widespread introduction of computerized reporting to the haematology laboratory.

Operational planning

Detailed operational planning must be decided upon with clear rules prepared for staff. This is particularly relevant with regard to blood counting with policy decisions on the indications for blood-film microscopy based upon clinical indicators given on the request form and on laboratory indications when the automated count result is available. Both primary and secondary indicators must be listed and this should be readily available at the bench (Fig. 10.3 and Table 10.1).

An important aspect of operational planning is the preparation of a properly designated request form acceptable to the users. This must be designed to meet the specific needs of the haematology laboratory for the particular group of tests.

Similarly, an agreed method of reporting must be instituted. This may be prepared by an analysing instrument, by a computer or written. Guidance on use of computers in haematology laboratories are available (5, 6) and larger texts on computing can be consulted (e.g. Ref. 4). The arrangements for verbal transmission must be agreed. The

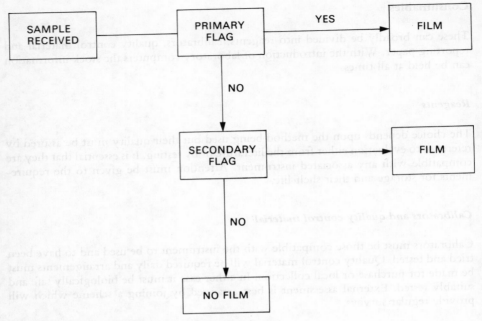

Fig. 10.3 Haematology flow chart for the blood count.

future storing of data both inside and outside the laboratory must be considered with particular reference to any legal requirements such as for blood transfusion compatibility results.

Financial accounting

From a basis of planning policy and resources the laboratory manager must be able to prepare a budget at least annually. This must be divided between capital (including equipment) and revenue. The latter should be divided between labour costs (staff) and consumables. With the aid of a computer, a cost-accounting system can be introduced so that the actual expenditure either monthly or quarterly can be seen in comparison with the budget. This should allow adjustment in policy as an on-going management procedure. Control of the budget must remain with the head of department.

Maintenance of good standards

Having developed a laboratory of good standard it is necessary to introduce into management means by which this can be maintained.

Table 10.1   Flags for blood count

Primary flags:

        Specific request by clinician

        Clinical diagnosis – glandular fever

                          anaemia

                          leukaemia, lymphoma

                          PUO

      Recent visit to Asia or Africa

Secondary flags:

        Blood count levels outside 'reference' range

Staff recruitment or replacement

The regular turnover of staff, which itself is a form of maintaining a good standard, requires a mechanism for replacement. Good recruitment is inevitably tied to good training for which the laboratory is both officially recognized and of good repute. It may be necessary to advertise and visit schools for a regular supply of trainees for technology posts. In times of difficulty an invitation to careers guidance teachers to visit the laboratory can be of great value. A system for interviewing must be documented, preceded by the preparation of a job description. The level of staff involved in the interview will vary with the grade of interviewee. When a person is selected by the interviewing panel, the terms and conditions of service must be agreed verbally and subsequently in writing. Claimed qualifications should be checked at this time.

Training

Induction

A short period of induction to the laboratory is necessary for all new staff. They must be told how the laboratory is organized and given any documents on general procedure, particularly with regard to safety matters. During this period they should be introduced to any occupational health department relevant to the laboratory. They should also attend any formal induction lectures applicable to hospital staff.

In-service training

For members of staff in training, arrangements should be made for regular in-service training each week. In a busy service department this may be difficult but it must be made part of the laboratory procedures. This type of training will also be necessary when new developments or methods are introduced.

Qualification training

All trainees in haematology require a qualification which may be medical, technical, or scientific. The laboratory will be recognized as suitable by the qualifying body for a particular form of training and the laboratory manager must make appropriate arrangements for staff, including recognized periods of study leave. Access to an adequate library either within the department or in a hospital centre is essential. Training programmes have been published for medical staff (20) and for technical staff (8).

Continuing education

This is necessary for all staff including the managers themselves. It may be arranged locally, regionally, nationally or internationally. Again, the laboratory manager must ensure that this is being carried out and allow sufficient time for staff to attend. A balance must be struck between service requirements and training which may have to be argued with the administrative hierarchy.

Promotion

This depends upon the system of grading in the staff group concerned and revenue available, apart from unexpected vacancies for established posts. The manager must be aware of deviations for job descriptions that result in greater responsibility being undertaken without recognition. With an expanding laboratory promotional arrangements may be anticipated but in a contracting service it will be unusual apart from vacancies.

Equipment

A decision must be made on the method of maintenance for each item of equipment in a laboratory. This may be preventive maintenance by a contract made with the supplier or by an in-house *ad hoc* system. The latter may be more economical for a laboratory within an institution with access to a department of biomedical engineering.

Health and safety

Most hospitals have a department of occupational health who will review the health of staff from time to time. Internal laboratory safety is always the responsibility of the manager, who must prepare a safety code. This must be drawn to the attention of all staff and be readily available. Model codes of practice have been prepared in the UK by the Department of Health and Social Security (9, 10) the Advisory Committee on Dangerous Pathogens (1, 2) and by the Health Services Advisory Committee (17, 18) Areas of particular hazard, e.g. biological containment, radiation, should also be subject to a permanent notice on the door. Accident prevention should be taught during in-service training periods. An accident book must be kept and examined by the manager from time to time. Each department should have a safety officer who has direct access, if necessary, to both the manager and the head of department. It is also their responsibility to report injuries, dangerous occurrences and occupational illness to the appropriate authority (15, 16).

Discipline

In a well-run laboratory this will be handled by example of senior staff, but a disciplinary procedure is essential to deal with deviants. Most hospitals have a code of procedure which lays down the officer responsible for each group of staff and the degree of discipline available before reference to a higher authority. Most codes include such grades of discipline as early warning, final warning and dismissal. It is essential for these codes of disciplinary practice to be agreed and understood by the appropriate Trades Union or Works Council.

Labour relations

Most laboratory staff belong to Trade Union or similar professional organization. The head of department and the manager must have a knowledge of the organizations involved and of the officially appointed officers in the laboratory. Arrangements for meetings of staff either within or without the confines of the building must be agreed. The Trade Union or professional representative should have direct access to the manager or, if necessary, the head of department.

Quality assurance

Both internal quality control and external quality assessment must be an integral part of good laboratory management. To this end, each haematology laboratory should have a quality control officer or officers who have direct access to the manager. The frequency of the reporting should be agreed.

Laboratory accreditation, licensing and regulation

With the increase of bureaucratic control and litigation, degrees of laboratory accreditation have been introduced with the provision in some countries of regulatory licensing (23). Accreditation for training purposes is almost universal but license to operate mainly applies to private laboratories. Such a licence will be issued for varying numbers of tests and will indicate recognition of professional or technical competence. An important part of any inspection will be evidence of good quality assurance procedures.

Legal liability

These vary from one country to another. Private laboratories are always liable directly for correct procedures and reporting but national institutions are usually covered by their employing authority. Medical staff are always responsible in any circumstance for opinion given on reports. In a specific legal case any member of a laboratory may be called as a witness.

Confidentiality

Laboratory reports on patients are confidential documents, the contents of which should only be disclosed to the doctor making the request (19). Where information is stored on computer, the data may also be available to the specific patient concerned. Inappropriate disclosure of information is a disciplinary matter.

Research and development

Even with a contracting laboratory service, research and development must be an integral part of a haematology laboratory. If there is no increase in revenue, research and development must be an item in the budget to enable these functions to continue. It is also essential to maintain staff interest in their work and to maintain morale. Revenue for research is available and it is the duty of the manager to become aware of the sources to which he can apply. Again, staff time must be allowed within the organization of the laboratory.

Evaluation of management

Quality assurance

Internal quality control is a continuing in-built form of management control, external quality assessment an intermittent form of the same which is best carried out by regional or national surveys (see Chapters 5 and 7). In addition, slide seminars are organized by colleges and societies of haematology. All methods should be educative but a mandatory requirement has been incorporated in some countries (3).

Performance indicators

These compare workload with staff numbers in laboratories of the same discipline within a region or country (11). They are dependent upon the method of measuring workload and are at best a crude guide and can only be used to indicate extremes of performance which require explanation. They must never be used to fix budgets.

Budgetary control

An annual target is set which can be compared with expenditure either monthly or quarterly so that adjustments to expenditure on staff and consumables can be made easily (12). It does not, however, offer any means of controlling workload.

Inventory control

The inventory should be checked at irregular intervals to detect both correctness of invoicing and claimed use of materials.

Cost utility

Cost benefit analysis is a management technique in which a systematic study is made of the benefits derived from a particular form of investment in resources (21). It is claimed to help decision-making in laboratory development. Cost effectiveness is another technique whereby the cost of alternative methods of practice are compared and can be applied to employment of staff as well as to choice of methods or instruments.

Conclusions

Management is becoming an increasingly necessary function of laboratory work. New tools of management are being introduced and new methods adopted. It is also subject to many differences of opinion. Those expressed here are those of the author but conform to general practice in haematology laboratories over the past 10 years. They are, therefore, those broadly agreed by British haematologists and many of their European colleagues. Marked differences will be found in the USA and countries following their procedures. This particularly applies to staff and their training. Current changes in Europe may result in an increasing similarity of management approach which must be kept under review.

References

1. ACDP (Advisory Committee on Dangerous Pathogens) (1984). Categorization of Pathogens according to Hazard and Categories of Containment. London: HMSO.
2. ACDP (Advisory Committee on Dangerous Pathogens) (1986).LAV/HTLVIII – The Causative Agents of AIDS and Related Conditions – Revised Guidelines. London: DHSS.

3. Bartels, R. A. (1983). The Peer Standard Review Organization Process – an effective tool for quality assurance. In Snyder, J. R. and Larson, A. L. (eds) *Administration and Supervision of Laboratory Medicine*, pp. 411–437. Philadelphia: Harper & Row.
4. Bradbeer, R., de Bono, P. and Lawrie, P. (1982). *The Computer Book: An Introduction to Computers and Computing*, p. 208. London: BBC.
5. BSH (1986). Guidelines for Hospital Blood Bank Computing. London: British Society for Heamatology.
6. BSH (1987) Guidelines on Computing for General Haematology. London: British Society for Haematology.
7. CAP (1981). Laboratory Workload Recording Method. Skokie, Illinois: College of American Pathologists.
8. Council of Professions Supplementary to Medicine (1979). Laboratories and Laboratory based Training. London: Council of Professions Supplementary Medicine.
9. DHSS (1980). Code of Practice for the Prevention of Infection in Clinical Laboratories and Post-mortem Rooms. London: HMSO.
10. DHSS (1981). Code of Practice for Prevention of Infection in Clinical Laboratories and Post-mortem Rooms, pp. 1–16. London: HMSO.
11. DHSS (1985). Performance Indicators for the NHS. Guidance for Users, p. 47. London: HMSO.
12. DHSS (1985) Management Budgeting in the National Health Service, p. 41. London: HMSO.
13. Eilers, R. J. (1975). Principles of total quality control. In Lewis, S. M. and Carter, J. F. (eds) *Quality Control in Haematology*, pp. 1–12. London: Academic Press.
14. Fabray, C. E. (1983). Methods of Measuring Work and Costing Activity in Pathology Departments. Financial Information Project Working Paper No. 83/01, p. 34. London: DHSS.
15. Health and Safety Executive (1985). Reporting an Injury or a Dangerous Occurrence. London: HMSO.
16. Health and Safety Executive (1985). Reporting a Case of Disease. London: HMSO.
17. Health Services Advisory Committee (1985). Safety in Health Service Laboratories: Hepatitis B. London: HMSO.
18. Health Services Advisory Committee (1986). Safety in Health Service Laboratories: The Labelling Transport and Reception of Specimens. London: HMSO.
19. Knox, E. G. (1984). The Confidentiality of Medical Records. The Principles and Practice of Protection in a Research–dependent Environment, p. 176. Luxembourg: Commission of the European Communities.
20. Lawrence, A. C. K. and Tovey, L. A. D. (1985). Model Training Programme – Haematology and Blood Transfusion. London: Association of Clinical Pathologists.
21. Pearce, D. N. (1983). *Cost–Benefit Analysis* (2nd edn), pp. 1–112. London: Macmillan.
22. Royal College of Pathologists (1982). Medical and Scientific Staffing of National Health Service Pathology Departments, p. 20. London: Royal College of Pathologists.
23. Schenken, J. R. (1983). Laboratory accreditation, licensure and regulation. In Snyder, J. R. and Larsen, A. L. (eds) *Administration and Supervision in Laboratory Medicine*, pp. 360–370. Philadelphia: Harper & Row.
24. Shinton, N. K. and Szczepura, A. (1988). Economies of automation in haematology. In J. P. Ashby (ed) Current developments for improving laboratory economics and working practise, pp. 65–87. European Committee for Clinical Laboratory Standards, Lund, Sweden.
25. Sibilia, R. A. (1983). Motivation – managerial assumptions and effects. In Snyder, J. R. and Larsen, A. L. (eds) *Administration and Supervision in Laboratory Medicine*, pp. 59–70. Philadelphia: Harper & Row.
26. Snyder, J. R. (1983). The nature of management in the clinical laboratory. In Snyder, J. R. and Larsen, A. L. (eds) *Administration and Supervision in Laboratory Medicine*, pp. 3–15. Philadelphia: Harper & Row.
27. Snyder, J. R., Padgett, W. G. and Newland, J. R. (1983). Laboratory planning, organization and control. In Snyder, J. R. and Larsen, A. L. (eds) *Administration and Supervision in Laboratory Medicine*, pp. 16–39. Philadelphia: Harper & Row.

11

Health and Safety in Laboratories

R M Rowan

Introduction

The emergence of health and safety legislation reflects growing concern over hazards in the workplace. The clinical laboratory is no exception. Perusal of medical literature suggests that the major problems are transmission of infection by hepatitis B and HIV viruses. However, although these are serious, numerically they comprise only a small fraction of potential laboratory hazards.

A laboratory health and safety programme has three main objectives: prevention of injury or sickness in laboratory personnel; protection of patients requiring to visit the laboratory for investigative purposes; and protection of third parties who for service purposes require right of entry (hospital tradesmen, service engineers, etc.). Because of the health, environmental, legal and monetary implications, the development of a comprehensive health and safety programme is in the best interests of all laboratory workers. Equally, laboratory personnel have a responsibility to adhere to the policy once it has been defined.

Accidents do not happen in the laboratory every day and the occurrence of laboratory-induced disease is infrequent. These facts give rise to a sense of complacency. Except in the highly emotive areas of hepatitis B and acquired immune deficiency syndrome (AIDS), safety measures are often considered to be inconvenient and are thus ignored. It is a prime responsibility of laboratory directors and supervisory staff to enforce health and safety regulations. Every person in the laboratory must be convinced from the start of their career of the need for safety practices and must appreciate that transgression from defined policy may result in hazard to health. Such hazards may affect not only the transgressor but equally a colleague, a patient or some other party. Safety in the laboratory must never be relegated to a position of secondary importance.

The development of an effective safety programme requires effort not only by laboratory staff but by architects and engineers who design laboratories and by manufacturers of instruments and other materials used in them. Health and safety problems must be reduced to manageable units, otherwise there arises a confusion of detail which ultimately stifles productive laboratory work and paradoxically undermines interest and effort in developing safe practices.

The vast majority of laboratory-induced injury and illness results from bad laboratory design, overcrowding, poorly maintained equipment, careless 'housekeeping', thoughtlessness and inexperience. Any approach to health and safety in laboratories has two major components: the design of premises and the environment, and the definition of standard operating procedures to deal with known hazards. Management objectives thereafter are:

(1) improvement of personnel safety attitudes and skills;
(2) development of a surveillance programme to identify hazards promptly;
(3) formulation of plans to remove these new hazards;
(4) co-ordination of laboratory safety into the hospital safety programme.

Legislation exists in many countries to achieve these objectives. This affects all persons at work, both employers and employees, and covers patients and the general public who may be affected by work activities.

Inevitably safety regulations will differ in detail from one country to another. The regulations described here are those in force in the UK. It is assumed that while legal detail differs in other countries, the principles and practices embodied in the UK legislation are applicable anywhere in the world. The aims of health and safety legislation are four-fold:

(1) to secure the health, safety and welfare of persons at work;
(2) to protect other individuals against risks to health or safety arising out of, or in connection with, the activities of persons at work;
(3) to control the storage and use of explosive or highly flammable or other dangerous substances;
(4) to control the emission into the atmosphere of noxious or offensive substances.

This chapter is designed primarily for haematologists, but the topics covered are applicable to other laboratory disciplines in hospitals. Safety programmes are equally important in decentralized sites. In the latter they may require to be even more explicit since trained laboratory staff may not be present.

Responsibility for health and safety

One of the aims of a health and safety policy is to apportion responsibility to all persons working under it, both management and workforce. While the definition and promotion of health and safety procedures is a function of management, primary responsibility for prevention of accidents and occupational illnesses rests with those persons who create the risks during their work, i.e. the workforce. The responsibilities of management and workforce are therefore complementary. Legislation is designed to re-inforce this relationship by establishing statutory duties (13).

Responsibility of the head of department

In the UK the head of a laboratory in a National Health Service hospital is an 'employee' under the Health and Safety at Work Act 1974. However, his legal responsibility arises from two sources. While these two areas of legal liability may overlap it is convenient to consider them separately.

Common law

Liability in common law relates to the 'duty of care' owed by every professional health-care worker to his patients. This 'duty of care' is assessed not only on the relationship between the health-care worker, his staff, clients (other doctors) and patients but also on his position in the hierarchy of his profession. If 'duty of care' is not fulfilled and damage follows, the individual is liable for negligence. In assessing 'duty of care' required of a head of laboratory department, a law court would have regard to the normal practice of other practitioners of similar position and standing. Secondly, under common law of contract a head of laboratory has specified duties which the employers expect and require him to carry out. In the event of failure to perform these duties there can be liability for breach of contract. In this case liability is owed solely to the employer.

Health and Safety at Work Act

Under the terms of this Act the person controlled is the employer and only incidentally the employee. The employer cannot delegate his responsibility to an employee. However, under another section of the Act 'every employee' must 'while at work' 'take reasonable care for the health and safety of himself and of other persons who may be affected by his acts or omissions at work'. The view has been taken that the more responsible the post held by a senior employee, the higher is the legal responsibility to fellow employees. Thus, the head of a laboratory department, although an employee, must carry out his duties of control and direction under this section of the Act.

Duties of employer to employee

The employer has the responsibility to provide, as far as is practicable, premises, environment, plant and work practices which will ensure the health, safety and welfare of all employees. The term 'plant' includes all machinery, equipment and appliances used at work. In addition, the employer must ensure that the use, handling, storage and transportation of articles and substances is, again so far as is reasonably practicable, safe and free from risk to health. The term 'substance' is defined as any natural or artificial substance, be that solid, liquid, gas or vapour, used at work. The employer also has an obligation to provide sufficient information, training and supervision to ensure health and safety at work and additionally to provide written statements regarding general and specific policies. The last must be updated regularly.

Duties of employers to other persons

These duties of the employer are covered by the statements in the preceding paragraph. Provision of adequate supervision supercedes information, instruction and training in this case.

Duties of employees

It is the duty of all employees 'whilst at work' to take reasonable care not only of their personal health but that of other persons who may be affected by any acts of omission. The employee also has a duty to co-operate with his employer in all matters affecting health and safety.

Duties of manufacturers and suppliers

Duties under health and safety legislation extend to those persons who design, manufacture, import, erect or install any plant, machinery, equipment or appliances or who manufacture, import or supply any substance for use at work. All plant must be designed and constructed to be safe and without risk to health. It should be delivered with adequate information about its intended use and any conditions necessary to ensure safe operation.

Staff welfare

Employee health programme

All persons working in a laboratory are deemed 'at risk' to occupational illness and injury. Pre-employment physical examination is necessary, supplemented by chest X-ray, full blood count and ESR, sickle test (if indicated by ethnic origin), screening test for tuberculosis and BCG if indicated. Vaccination should be offered against diphtheria, poliomyelitis and tetanus. Depending on local circumstances vaccination against hepatitis Bs Ag may be offered. All staff should be offered an annual chest X-ray and full blood count. Should any abnormality be detected the results should be sent to the employee's general practitioner.

These examinations will often be carried out by a hospital staff physician at the request of the laboratory director. The development of hospital occupational health services should be encouraged to assume this role and to maintain occupational health records for all employees, undertake environmental investigations, be responsible for health education, keep routine daily records of accidents at work and sickness and give advice to management on occupational health matters.

Safety officer

Every laboratory must have a safety officer (and deputy) trained in general laboratory safety and any specific hazards occurring in that laboratory. The safety officer should participate in the day-to-day work of the laboratory. A notice should be prominently displayed in the laboratory indicating the name of the safety officer (and deputy) and where he or she can be contacted at all reasonable times. Safety officers are appointed by management and are responsible to management. They must not be confused with safety representatives, elected by the laboratory staff, whose duty it is to liaise on behalf of staff on safety matters with laboratory management, health authority or trade union.

Reporting of accidents

Accidents and incidents affecting the health of laboratory employees must be recorded in a book kept solely for that purpose. Laboratory management must review the accident book regularly and take whatever action is necessary to prevent recurrence.

Provision of first-aid

There are two complementary requirements (14). First a number of persons on the staff must be trained to render first-aid in the event of an accident. A list of individuals so trained must be displayed, together with telephone numbers of the emergency services. Secondly, a first-aid box must be provided. The first-aid box must be constructed from materials which will keep the contents dust and damp-free and be easily identified (usually a white cross on a green background). The contents of the first-aid box should be restricted to the following:

(1) instruction sheet giving general guidance;
(2) individually wrapped sterile adhesive dressings in a variety of sizes;
(3) sterile eye pads, with attachment bandages;
(4) triangular bandages;
(5) sterile coverings for serious wounds;
(6) safety pins;
(7) selection of sterile but unmedicated wound dressings.

Eye-irrigation equipment must also be readily available, either of the wash-bottle type (the contents of which must be changed regularly), or a system connected to the mains water supply. Where tap water is not available, sterile water or sterile normal saline in disposable containers must be available. The correct use of eye-irrigation methods must be demonstrated.

Antidotes to poisonous chemicals used in the laboratory must be available with protocols for their use.

Finally, protective clothing and safety equipment must be provided for the person rendering first-aid.

All items must be correctly stored and regularly checked to ensure that they are in satisfactory condition. The contents of the first-aid box must be replenished immediately after use.

Safety training

Standards of laboratory safety are determined largely by the quality of training. Ideally new staff should not be allowed to start work until they have received training in the basic principles of laboratory safety. Certainly they must not be allowed to use equipment until they have received training and demonstrated their proficiency. Periodic re-training and confirmation of competence helps to re-inforce safety principles and procedures. The following must be incorporated into the preliminary safety training programme.

Personal hygiene

A commonsense approach to basic hygiene must be stressed. Regular washing of hands is perhaps the single most important safety procedure in the laboratory. Cuts and abrasions on hands and forearms must be covered by waterproof dressings. Eczema on hands should be covered by disposable protective gloves. Smoking, eating and the application of cosmetics within the laboratory must be expressly forbidden (Fig. 11.1).

Protective clothing

Protective clothing of an approved design must be worn in the laboratory and must always be fastened. This clothing must not be worn outside the laboratory. These rules are facilitated by provision of lockers for outdoor clothes and coat pegs near the exits of laboratory areas for protective clothing. Protective clothing should be sent to the laundry in special bags and laundered without being removed from the bags. Where this is not possible, disposable protective clothing should be worn and disposed of, after use, with other contaminated waste. Disposable gloves and aprons must be worn when handling specimen containers, when presenting specimens to instruments for analysis and when disinfecting surfaces and centrifuges. Gloves should be discarded when the activity ceases and must not be worn outside the laboratory area. The need to wear safety spectacles or visors when stipulated must be stressed and instructions on the correct manner of wearing these given.

Safety at work practices

Instruction on the correct use of centrifuges, electrical appliances and mechanical devices which might trap the operator's fingers, clothing or hair, must be given. Staff should be advised not to wear jewellery, watches or rings in laboratory areas. Wearing pendant necklaces must be forbidden. Since lifting equipment often causes back injury, instruction in this procedure must be provided.

Pipetting

This is a frequent procedure in hospital laboratories. Mouth pipetting must be totally

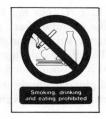

Fig. 11.1 Smoking, drinking and eating prohibited; red circle and red background to caption.

prohibited. Staff require training in the use of bulb pipettes and other hand pipetting devices.

Waste disposal

Various categories of clinical waste exist. Written procedures must describe disposal of each. Staff must be trained in methods of waste disposal.

Infected solid waste should be placed in containers or autoclavable bags. These must be autoclaved before disposal (containers and bags must be open before autoclaving) or else incinerated. If autoclaving cannot be done on the premises, a specialist disposal company should be employed and extra care taken to ensure that waste packages are well sealed. Different categories of waste are placed in colour-coded bags. Needles and other sharps must be placed in rigid containers before disposal.

Use of centrifuges

Centrifuges must have interlocks to ensure that they cannot be opened during operation (4). Centrifugation is a frequent laboratory procedure and new entrants to the laboratory must receive instruction in the correct use of centrifuges at the earliest opportunity. Tubes containing blood or other body fluids should be stoppered before being placed in the centrifuge. The risk of breakage within the centrifuge is minimized by careful balancing. The interior of the centrifuge should be cleaned daily with a suitable disinfectant such as glutaraldehyde. Gloves must be worn for this procedure. Ease of cleaning is a prime consideration when selecting a centrifuge for purchase.

Decontamination procedures

Training must be provided in decontamination procedures (6). In the event of major spillage of dangerous substances the safety officer must be informed immediately. Four main situations require decontamination procedures.

1. Breakage/spillage of specimens. The area of spillage including the broken specimen container should be flooded with appropriate disinfectant.

For most organic matter and bacteria, but not for blood or viruses, clear soluble phenol derivatives are suitable. The manufacturer's instructions for dilution should be followed. For minimal organic matter, small volumes of blood and viruses, hypochlorites are used. For general use 1 g/l available chlorine (1000 ppm) is satisfactory, but for blood spillage 10 g/l (10,000 ppm) is recommended. Hypochlorite solution should not be used for centrifuges. Activated glutaraldehyde at 30 g/l is used on surfaces for viral decontamination. Surfaces selected for bench tops should withstand this concentration of activated glutaraldehyde.

Following application of disinfectant the area is left undisturbed for 10 min prior to mopping up the fluid with an excess of cotton wool or absorbent paper. Disposable gloves, apron and goggles should be worn during the procedure. If a dustpan and brush or forceps are used these will require disinfection.

2. Breakages within centrifuge. If breakage is suspected whilst the centrifuge is running, the motor must be switched off and the equipment remain closed for 30 min. If breakage is discovered on opening the centrifuge, the lid should be replaced immediately and left for 30 min. Disposable gloves must be worn. Forceps or cotton wool held in forceps should be used to pick up glass debris. All broken tubes, glass fragments, buckets, trunnions and the rotor must be placed overnight in disinfectant. The centrifuge bowl must then be swabbed with disinfectant, left for 30 min, re-swabbed, washed with water and dried. Swabs must be treated as infected waste and disposed of accordingly.

3. Chemical spillage. A wall chart illustrating the management principles following chemical spillage should be prominently displayed. Gloves, aprons and safety goggles should be worn when dealing with spills. If the amount spilled is small, dilution with water or a detergent will suffice. With large volumes, however, spill control bags or absorbent granules should be available. These are effective for most chemicals including corrosive agents and can be swept into a container for disposal. Any spillage of carcinogenic material should be dealt with as a major spill. Water must never be used to wash down such spills until the bulk of the chemical has been treated with spill control bags or absorbent granules and swept up.

4. Decontamination of automated cell counters. During the servicing or repair of automated blood cell counters there is a small risk of the transmission of HIV (the causative agent of AIDS) and other infections unless decontamination is performed beforehand. Instrument manufacturers market cleansing materials containing sodium hypochlorite. Care should be taken not to mix instrument diluents with sodium hypochlorite since they react together and produce chlorine gas. This reaction inactivates the disinfectant making it useless for decontamination. If preparing in-house cleaning material, bleach must be laboratory-reagent sodium hypochlorite solution with no detergent, diluted in distilled or deionized water to give a final concentration of 4% available chlorine.

Fire prevention

Fire is a constant hazard in the laboratory. Advice on fire risks and their prevention must form an important part of laboratory training. All staff must know what to do in the event of an outbreak of fire. Training must include the correct use of fire extinguishers, fire blankets and fire evacuation procedures (see also p. 240).

Health and safety signs

A variety of safety signs is available to national and international standards. These are divided into four categories: mandatory, prohibition, caution and safe condition. The basic formats are illustrated in Fig. 11.2. A number of these signs are illustrated under specific subjects.

Standard operating procedures

Standard operating procedures written in the language of common use in the laboratory should describe all procedures. These must be enforced. Included in these are details of safety measures and the action to be taken following accidents. General safety protocols should also be available. Such documents are the basis of training in health and safety for the laboratory's employees. Staff should sign to indicate that they have read and understood them. It is a responsibility of the head of department to revise these documents as necessary.

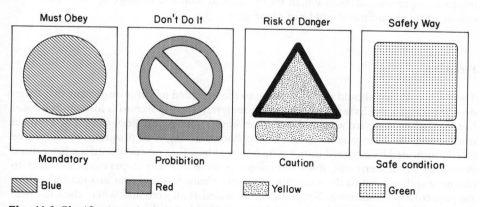

Fig. 11.2 Classification of safety signs. Mandatory has blue circle with blue notice rectangle; prohibition has red circle and bar with red notice rectangle; caution has yellow triangle enclosed by black line with yellow notice rectangle; safe condition has green square with green notice rectangle.

Premises

Laboratory design contributes to health and safety (7). Good interior design contributes not only to staff morale but also to safety of the environment.

Size of premises

Overcrowding is a common cause of accidents in the laboratory. For this reason, when planning a laboratory, expert advice is required on work and circulation space and on routes of access and egress.

In determining spatial requirements, critical dimensions must be established which are mandatory for the efficient function of an activity. They consist of all components necessary for the performance of the activity, including the equipment, furnishings, fittings and ergonomic requirements. This last is a measure of the total space required by technicians to operate and conduct the activity. Having established the critical dimensions for a finite activity, in the interests of safety no other activities should be superimposed.

Fittings and finishes

These should be designed to promote safe working practice. They should be manufactured from durable materials which are easily cleaned. Furnishings should not have sharp corners or projections. Fittings should be of ergonomically correct design for reach and height. Choice of finishes will be influenced by intended use. There is need for impervious surfaces which are resistant to stain and damage by chemicals. The colour of work surfaces should not cause glare.

Flooring

The floor covering should be appropriate to the intended use. It is important that floors do not present a slip hazard. With modern materials the slip hazard is low on dry floors but high when these are wet. In the event of liquid spillage, the floor should be mopped immediately and thoroughly dried. When floor washing is in progress this should be clearly indicated by a hazard notice which should be left in position until the floor dries. A variety of modern soft floor coverings exists which are impervious, resistant to chemical spillage and to disinfectants and easily cleaned. Vinyl tiles in a neutral colour are particularly satisfactory. These should be sealed at all joins and where the tiles meet the wall. Sloping floors and steps should be avoided but if this is impossible the hazard should be indicated by a prominent notice. In areas to which patients require access floors should be suitable for trolleys. Certain floor designs may cause disorientation in the elderly patient.

Lighting

Natural lighting should be provided in all work areas occupied for any length of time. Lighting, whether natural or artificial, must be capable of providing the required levels of illumination. Task lighting requires an intensity of approximately $23 \, lm/m^2$ with low-contrast glare-free background illumination. It may be necessary to have colour-balanced light since some tests have visual colour end-points. Fluorescent ceiling lights should be mounted directly above and parallel to benches to avoid shadows.

Ventilation

Natural ventilation should be provided whenever possible, particularly in staff rooms, offices and patient accommodation. Where mechanical ventilation is unavoidable, 6–10 air changes per hour are recommended. Noxious fumes require a higher exchange rate. Use of fume cupboards prevents unpleasant odours and removes noxious and flammable fumes. They are mandatory for certain types of activity. Ventilation exhaust systems must be sited in such a way that fumes are not sucked back into the building at a different level or into adjacent buildings. Internal rooms do not provide a good working environment and hence should be used only for infrequent or intermittent activities or when a strictly controlled environment is required. As a general principle rooms which are to be occupied for any length of time should have windows.

Storage

A minimum of consumable supplies should be stored in the laboratory area. Bulk supplies should be kept in a discrete lockable laboratory store. The use of shelving maximizes storage space but where it is necessary for items to be stored on high shelves portable step-ladders must be provided. Toxic laboratory chemicals should be kept in a separate part of the bulk store. A lockable poisons cabinet should be available. Dangerous chemicals e.g. strong acids and alkalis, must not be stored on high shelves. Chemicals which react together must be stored well apart. If there is a requirement for storage of patient samples, reagents or therapeutic materials at temperatures of $-20°C$ or lower, thermal-protective gloves should be provided.

Bulk flammable liquids must never be stored in the laboratory but require an external flammable goods store. This consists of a vented brick building with metal shelving and gas-proof electrical light fittings. (Wooden shelving should only be used for storage of corrosive substances.)

Security

Security of laboratory premises is necessary for a number of reasons. Assaults on hospital staff and theft of expensive technical and office equipment are recognized problems. There is also a deeper danger that unauthorized persons will be exposed to potential biological and chemical hazards. The entire department should be designed as an integrally secure area with all entrances capable of being controlled. Both fire and security experts should be consulted since the demands of fire safety and security may conflict.

Fire hazard

Fire prevention is subject to guidelines and statutory regulations (8, 9, 11). Because of fire and explosion risk, proximity of the laboratory to patient or staff accommodation or to areas frequented by the public is inadvisable. A laboratory must not be used as a fire escape route by patients or staff (Fig. 11.3).

In planning a laboratory, safety considerations influence overall design. At the earliest planning stage the project team should liaise with the local fire authority to determine a fire safety strategy. Principles of fire safety apply also to alteration and upgrading of existing buildings. Alterations to accommodation often provide a good opportunity for eliminating pre-existing fire risks.

Fire is a particular risk because of the flammable solvents, gases and reactive chemicals located there and the large amount of electrical equipment in use. Because of this high fire risk the location of and access to the laboratory for fire fighting is important. It is also desirable to have at least two exits from the laboratory.

Flammable substances

Most fires result from accidents with flammable substances. Oxidizing agents require particular care. These will oxidize many materials following spillage or leakage and increase the risk of fire or explosion. Explosions may occur if flammable solvents or specimens treated with them are stored in domestic refrigerators. Flammable vapour can be exploded by the normal operation of the electrical circuitry. A refrigerator specially designed for flammable solvents should be used. All manipulations of flammable solvents must be performed in a fume cupboard to avoid ignition of vapour by naked lights.

Risk of fire

Fig. 11.3 Risk of fire (yellow triangle enclosed by black line with yellow notice rectangle).

Day-to-day supplies of flammable liquids can be stored on site in flameproof cabinets but bulk stocks must be kept in an external flammable store (see p. 239).

Fire detection and alarm systems

It is recommended that fire detection and alarm systems be installed in all laboratories. In some countries this is a statutory requirement. For laboratory areas heat detection systems are necessary but for office, staff room, library, records room, stores and computer suites smoke detectors are preferable. The fire detection system should be linked directly to the hospital switchboard. In addition, breakglass call points (using a small hammer to break the glass) should be installed which are capable of triggering the alarm system. Audible alarms using sufficient sounders to ensure audibility in all areas should be located throughout the laboratory suite.

Fire extinguishers

Fire extinguishers should be located close to solvent stores, fume cupboards and other critical points. These should be capable of dealing both with chemical and electrical fires. Dry powder or carbon dioxide fire extinguishers are most suitable for laboratories since they can be used against fires caused by flammable liquids or electrical malfunction. Fire extinguishers require regular maintenance. The maintenance requirements are specified on the outside of the extinguisher. Fire blankets should also be available.

Fire precautions

The laboratory must have a fire precaution policy with written instructions for dealing with an outbreak of fire. Procedures should be reviewed regularly so that changes in structure of premises, installation of new equipment, etc. which may influence fire safety can be taken into account.

There is no doubt that the likelihood of fires starting can be reduced significantly by suitable preventive measures. The following items are of importance:

(1) good standards of electrical, chemical and general 'housekeeping';
(2) correct disposal of waste;
(3) correct incineration procedures;
(4) cigarette smoking policy;
(5) awareness of deliberate fire raising.

Fire notices which should be prominently displayed should state concisely the action to be taken on discovering a fire and on hearing an alarm.

Electrical safety

All hospital laboratories use mains voltage electrical supply. Only clinical chemistry laboratories require a high–voltage supply. Electrical hazards arise from carelessness or improper use of electrical equipment, incorrect or poorly maintained fittings and connections, and from the existence of long trailing leads (Fig. 11.4). Avoidance of electrical hazard can be achieved at two levels: (a) insistence on manufacturer certification of equipment and (b) expert installation and maintenance.

Manufacturer certification

Only equipment certified by its manufacturer as conforming to a national or international electrical safety standard (10) should be used. The manufacturer should obtain a certificate of compliance with this standard from an independent approved test house. Such equipment must not interfere with electrical devices attached to patients who may visit the laboratory, e.g. cardiac pace-maker.

Installation and maintenance

Basic hospital electrical services include lighting, power, environmental control, earth bonding of extraneous metal work and extensions for telephones, fire alarms and staff call systems. All should conform with current national regulations. Internal electrical installations must be concealed using PVC insulated cable in screwed steel conduit or trunking. Outside, the insulated cable must be enclosed in galvanized screwed steel conduit with fittings to weatherproof standards.

Mains–borne and radiofrequency interference must be eliminated as they affect computers and other electronic equipment.

Sufficient switched, shuttered socket–outlets from ring or spur circuits must be provided to ensure that all portable appliances likely to be used simultaneously are supplied individually. Fixed appliances rated up to 13 A (in UK) should be permanently connected to double-pole switched spur boxes and fused appropriately. Appliances rated greater than this or those requiring three-phase supply, should be connected permanently to individual final circuits from fuse-boards and be independently switched. Switched single sockets, usually located in corridors, should be provided for domestic cleaning appliances.

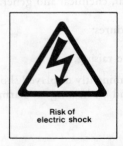

Fig. 11.4 Risks of electric shock (yellow triangle enclosed by black line with yellow notice rectangle).

All plant and equipment should be provided with local switches or other means of electrical isolation to ensure the safety of operators and maintenance staff. Automatically operating equipment should be provided with indicator lights to show when equipment is energized.

Before any new equipment is installed in the laboratory it must be examined by electrical engineers to ensure that earth continuity and the correct plugs and fuses are fitted.

Emergency electrical supply

Provision must be made for emergency electricity supplies and for stand-by lighting. Safety lighting should be available on primary escape routes. This should be a self-contained battery-operated system with integral change-over relay and charger suitable for non-maintained operation in the event of mains failure.

Mechanical and other physical hazards

Instruments

Equipment used in the laboratory should not present mechanical hazard to the user. Such hazards arise from poorly designed instruments whose casings present sharp edges and corners. Hinged protruding doors or covers should be avoided but if this is not possible they should close automatically. All mechanical moving parts should be shielded to prevent trapping of hair, fingers or clothes in the mechanism.

Accidents

Accidents and injuries may be caused by sharp instruments, needles and broken or badly chipped glassware. An untidy cluttered bench increases the risk of accidents.

Storage of reagent and waste containers in corridors creates a significant hazard. Moving heavy loads alone or without proper equipment can result in foot or back injuries.

Gases

When natural or manufactured gas is used to heat a fixed item of equipment it should be connected via a safety cock of the drop-level type to permanent pipework using screwed union connectors. Bunsen burners used only intermittently or in fume cupboards must be controlled by a safety cock. If gas supply is necessary inside a microbiological safety cabinet it must be via a solenoid valve which allows the gas to pass only when the fan is switched on and which requires manual resetting after any interruption in the current.

The use of compressed gases, be they flammable or not, presents a variety of hazards and their use should be avoided if at all possible. The smallest available cylinder should be used. In all instances prior inspection and approval by the Health and Safety Authority must be obtained. Standard operating procedures should cover the use and disposal of non-exchangeable gas cylinders. At no time should they be incinerated. Compressed gas cylinders must be kept in an external weatherproof store. If piped compressed air, specific gases or vacuum are required, the installation must be undertaken by a specialist contractor. Plugged outlets in anticipation of future change of use should not be provided. The system, however, should be readily accessible to modification by vertical or horizontal service ducts and bench spines.

Vacuum at minus 0.5–0.6 bar is sufficient for most laboratory work. The laboratory director should be consulted to establish that no substance likely to cause explosion will be drawn into the piped vacuum system.

Noise and vibration

The amount of noise and vibration produced by equipment must be controlled. Excessive noise in the laboratory, whether generated internally or transmitted from an external source, impairs the operational efficiency of the department and can cause discomfort. Noise levels should not exceed 70 dBa.

Microbiological safety

In a series of surveys published between 1949 and 1976 American workers summarized a cumulative total of 3921 cases of presumed laboratory-acquired infection (19, 21, 24, 25). The most commonly reported infections were brucellosis, typhoid, tularaemia, tuberculosis, hepatitis and Venezuelan equine encephalitis. Less than 20% of these were associated with a recognized accident (mouth pipetting or needle-stick injury). However, in more than 80% the infected individual had been exposed at work to the agent and it was presumed, although not confirmed, that infectious aerosols and minor cuts and abrasions in the hands accounted for most. Laboratory personnel are at higher risk of contracting such infections as tuberculosis, shigellosis and hepatitis than the general population (12, 22). In general, laboratory-acquired infections do not pose a threat to the community although there are some exceptions (viral haemorrhagic fevers, smallpox and Q fever).

All blood specimens should be considered potentially infective and should be handled according to established infection-control precautions. Pike (20) in a review of laboratory-acquired infection concluded that 'the knowledge, the techniques and the equipment to prevent most laboratory infections are available'. In recent years a number of authoritative publications have classified micro-organisms according to hazard and risk (1) and defined codes of practice for preventing laboratory-acquired infection (1, 2, 5, 6, 17).

Categories of pathogen

The UK Advisory Committee on Dangerous Pathogens (ACDP) has classified pathogens (1) according to inherent hazard of the organism and the risk of its transmission; the more serious the disease, the greater the hazard; the more likely infection will occur, the higher the risk. Micro-organisms are classified into four hazard groups on the basis of: (i) pathogenicity for man; (ii) hazard to laboratory personnel; (iii) transmissibility in the community; and (iv) availability of effective prophylaxis and treatment.

This categorization describes risk only to healthy laboratory workers. Persons with pre-existing disease, compromised immunity or who are pregnant may be at additional risk.

The four hazard groups defined by ACDP (1) are as follows:

Group 1 An organism that is most unlikely to cause human disease.

Group 2 An organism that may cause human disease and which might be a hazard to laboratory workers but is unlikely to spread in the community. Laboratory exposure rarely produces infection and effective prophylaxis or treatment are usually available.

Group 3 An organism that may cause severe human disease and present a serious hazard to laboratory workers. It may present a risk of spread in the community but there is usually effective prophylaxis or treatment available.

Group 4 An organism that causes severe human disease and is a serious hazard to laboratory workers. It may present a high risk of spread in the community and there is usually no effective prophylaxis or treatment.

The hazard category of a particular pathogen (an organism in group 2, 3 or 4) matches the containment level under which it must be handled. The term 'containment' describes safe methods for handling infectious agents in the laboratory environment (see below). Variations have been recommended to the codes of practices at the various levels of containment for certain organisms. This is necessary because of the immune status of the individual or the community and on the dose, route and site of infection.

Categories of containment

ACDP (1) describes four codes of practice to ensure microbiological safety, numbered according to the hazard group of the micro-organisms being handled. Reference must always be made to specific pathogens to identify variations to their containment requirements. Equivalent US biosafety levels are described by CDC/NIH (5).

General microbiological safety measures

Many of these have already been described but it is useful to summarize them. The following comprise minimum general requirements for preventing infection in the laboratory:

(1) all surfaces should be impervious to water, resistant to chemicals and easily cleaned;

(2) mechanical ventilation should ensure inward air flow by extraction;

(3) adequate hand–washing facilities (elbow or foot operating taps) must be present located near the exit;

(4) doors must be closed when work is in progress;

(5) approved protective clothing (side or back fastening) must be worn and removed on leaving;

(6) eating, drinking, smoking, storing of food and applying cosmetics must be prohibited;

(7) mouth pipetting must be prohibited;

(8) hands must be washed and disinfected immediately whenever contamination by chemical or potentially infectious material occurs and also before leaving; all persons processing blood specimens should wear gloves;

(9) masks and protective eyewear should be worn when there is any risk of mucous–membrane contact with blood;

(10) effective disinfectants must be available;

(11) bench surfaces must be cleaned after use;

(12) glassware for disinfection must be stored safely;

(13) all potentially infectious waste, not incinerated, must be rendered safe before disposal;

(14) materials for disposal must be transported safely in robust containers; and

(15) all laboratory accidents and incidents must be reported to and recorded by a responsible person.

Laboratory-acquired infection in haematology

The haematologist faces particular problems when presented with specimens which may be contaminated with the viruses causing hepatitis B or AIDS. With modern air travel sporadic cases of viral haemorrhagic fever (Lassa, Ebola and Marburg viruses) are possible. With these clinical conditions the major worry is the infected specimen from the clinically unrecognized patient. General high standards are necessary to minimize this risk. Haemorrhagic fever specimens require containment level 4.

Use of analytical equipment

The following policy has been defined by ACDP (2). Wherever possible only instruments operating on a closed system should be used, having first assessed the way in which the equipment is liable to contaminate the immediate work area. If there is a risk of droplet dispersion this should be limited by the provision of appropriate shields. Any orifice subject to splashing must be disinfected immediately after the specimens have been processed. At the end of each day's work the equipment should be thoroughly disinfected. Effluent must either be trapped in bottles containing a suitable disinfectant or discharged directly into the waste-water plumbing system. The discharge tube from the instrument must project at least 25 cm into the drain pipe. Water must flow through the waste pipe while the instrument is working. At the end of the day the drain should be flushed with disinfectant so that the trap retains an effective concentration overnight. Hepatitis and HIV risk specimens can be handled in this way. Following completion of this work all personnel must immediately remove their gloves, change their protective clothing and wash their hands before moving on to other activities.

Procedures for hepatitis and AIDS risk specimens

All routine clinical laboratory work (except that involving propagation or concentration of hepatitis or HIV) must be conducted under not less than containment level 2 supplemented by a series of conditions which are specified below. The upgraded specifications required are:

(1) limited access to laboratory;
(2) each staff member requires 24 m³ space;
(3) an autoclave for waste sterilization must be readily available, normally in the same building;
(4) bench tops must be disinfected after use;
(5) work may be conducted on the open bench.

The area in which this work is undertaken must be identified (Fig. 11.5). Where there is risk of droplet spread (vigorous shaking, mixing, ultrasonic disruption) a microbiology safety cabinet (Class I; BS 5726, 1979 or equivalent) must be used. The cabinet must exhaust to the outside atmosphere directly or via the laboratory air extraction system. A high efficiency particulate air (HEPA) filter must be incorporated.

The following modifications to containment level 2 requirements are mandatory for handling hepatitis and AIDS risk samples: work must be performed at a delineated and secluded work station previously cleared of all unnecessary equipment; the specimen must be received by a trained experienced individual who is the only person to unpack and handle it; the person performing the test must work alone, free from risk of disturbance or accidental contact with others; glass pipettes must not be used and sharp instruments should be avoided. If parenteral inoculation occurs, the wound must be

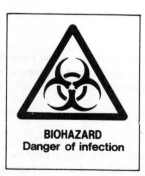

BIOHAZARD
Danger of infection

Fig. 11.5 Biohazard–Danger of infection (yellow triangle enclosed by black line with yellow notice rectangle).

treated immediately by encouraging bleeding and liberally washing with soap and water.

When centrifugation is necessary, sealed buckets must be used. These should be treated with a non-corrosive disinfectant at the end of the working day.

Testing of quality assurance materials

Whilst it is conceded that the risk of laboratory-acquired HIV infection is of a very low order and clearly much lower than that of hepatitis B, nevertheless, it is prudent to take all reasonable steps to minimize even this small risk. This involves the possible risks attached to preparation and handling of biological materials of human origin used in quality assurance procedures. In this context all materials, both commercial and in-house, used for internal quality control and for external quality assessment must be considered.

This raises the important ethical issue of testing patients for HIV without clinical indication, even with consent. The finding of a positive result has serious social, employment and financial implications. This difficulty can be circumvented if appropriate donations of blood, plasma or serum are received from a blood transfusion service where all donors are tested, knowing that their blood will be screened, and a system for counselling already exists.

It must be appreciated that no test procedure offers complete assurance that HIV infectivity is absent. In view of that the following recommendations are advisable: (i) as much information as possible be given on donor acceptance criteria; (ii) the supplier should state specifically whether or not the material has been tested at source for HIV antibody and hepatitis Bs Ag and the result of the tests; (iii) suppliers should indicate that all materials of human origin should be treated as though capable of transmitting infection and should therefore be handled in the same way as patient's samples. This warning statement should appear as part of each package insert.

Chemical hazards

A number of classes of chemical substance cause hazard in the laboratory (Fig. 11.6). Many of these may have been in the laboratory stores for years. In some instances this may render them particularly hazardous.

Carcinogens

The following may be found most frequently in research rather than routine laboratories: benzidine, *ortho*-toluidine diamino-benzidine, benzpyrene, a variety of immunosuppressive drugs, benzene. In addition formaldehyde is widely used as a fixative/preservative in the laboratory. Hydrochloric acid is also kept in these laborator-

Fig. 11.6 Toxic hazard (yellow triangle enclosed by black line with yellow notice rectangle).

ies. Formaldehyde vapour interacts with hydrogen chloride in air to form bis-chloromethyl ether which is a carcinogen. It may also be formed by reaction with certain disinfectants, e.g. hypochlorite which may have been used to wipe down benches prior to fumigation with formaldehyde.

Explosive substances

These include perchloric acid, picric acid, silver solutions and sodium azide (Fig. 11.7). Picric acid is explosive when dry. With silver solutions, both ammoniacal silver and silver nitrate, the risk arises when explosive crystals precipitate out from solution. The explosion risk associated with sodium azide has been alleviated as azide-free diluents are now provided for automated blood cell counters.

Dusts

Asbestos has, in the past, been widely used as an outer insulation (i.e. lagging) of steam, hot water plant and pipework. Abrasion of the paintwork covering this lagging leads to release of asbestos into the atmosphere. This hazard is greatest in service ducts where space is limited and environmental conditions poor.

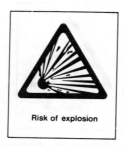

Fig. 11.7 Risk of explosion (yellow triangle enclosed by black line with yellow notice rectangle).

Solvents

A wide range of solvents is used in hospital laboratories and research departments including industrial methylated spirit, ethyl alcohol, isopropyl alcohol, acetone, diethyl-ether-dioxane, petroleum ether, toluene and xylene. Dangerous concentrations of vapour are most likely to arise in solvent distillation rooms and the chromatographic and steroid analysis sections of chemical pathology, in areas where automatic tissue-processing media are used (cytology and histopathology) but not to any great extent in haematology (see Flammable substances, p. 240). Organic solvents should not be discharged into drains but disposed of to specialist disposal companies for recycling.

Acids/corrosives

Many acids and other corrosive liquids are used in clinical laboratories including hydrochloric, nitric, sulphuric, glacial acetic, trichloroacetic and chromic acids, sodium hydroxide and potassium hydroxide. The risks involved are common to all biology laboratories (Fig. 11.8).

Cyanide solutions

Cyanide solutions are used most commonly in haematology usually as potassium cyanide for haemoglobin estimation. Cyanide is also used, but to a lesser extent, in chemical pathology and histology. However, the most likely contact with acid is when cyanide is used in automated cell counters. The effluent from these counters is usually drained into a laboratory sink where it can mix with acidic effluents to produce hydrocyanic acid.

As a safety measure a shower-head in a lobby or corridor should be provided adjacent to any work area where there is a risk of severe chemical contamination.

Fig. 11.8 Risk of chemical burn (yellow triangle enclosed by black line with yellow notice rectangle).

Radiation hazard

Although only small amounts of radionuclides are employed in diagnostic haematology, their use is governed by stringent codes of practice which in many ways resemble the codes of practice ensuring microbiological safety. An important recommendation is that radionuclides should only be used in designated laboratories. In the UK there is a statutory requirement that radionuclides only be used under the direction of an authorized person and that the doses administered must not exceed limits defined by the International Commission on Radiological Protection (18).

Safe handling of radionuclides by laboratory personnel requires both knowledge and skill. The hazard due to external radiation is negligible in view of the small quantities of isotope used. The greatest danger arises from accidental contamination of persons, work areas or equipment. To obviate the danger of undetected radiation, the radionuclide laboratory should be equipped with suitable monitoring devices capable of detecting contamination of work areas, including sinks and drains.

Advice and supervision of procedures

A radiation protection adviser (RPA) is an individual appropriately trained and duly qualified in radiation practices appointed by an employer. The RPA should be available for consultation whenever required and should receive sufficient information and facilities from his employer to enable his work to be performed effectively. Advice from the RPA *inter alia* involves identification and planning of controlled and supervised areas; dosimetry and monitoring systems, hazard assessment and contingency arrangements; drawing up standard operating procedures and arranging staff training; and finally selection of radiation protection supervisors (RPS).

The RPS plays a supervisory role in assisting the employer to comply with radiation protection requirements and should be directly involved with the work with ionizing radiation, preferably in a line-management position. Although the RPS does not require the training and expertise of the RPA, nevertheless there are certain requirements:

(1) knowledge and understanding of the statutory regulations and local rules;
(2) sufficient seniority in the establishment to command respect from the persons doing the work;
(3) knowledge and understanding of the necessary precautions to be taken.

Premises

Full consultation must take place at the planning stage by the user with the designer and the RPA. The maximum activity which can be handled in a laboratory depends on the procedures which are carried out; a greater activity is permitted where only simple wet operations are performed as opposed to procedures in which the radioactive material is handled in powder form. Haematology radionuclide work falls into the former category. If the haematological use of isotopes involves the use of γ-emitters only, then Grade C laboratory facilities are sufficient. These are as follows:

(1) Walls and ceilings should be painted with good quality, high gloss paint.
(2) Woodwork should be sealed and varnished with a suitably durable material.
(3) Floors should be covered with vinyl or linoleum sheet (not tiles) with joins sealed or welded. Linoleum must be polished.
(4) Bench tops should be constructed from resin plastic laminates carried over on to the front edge of the bench with a small upstand; the rear edge must be curved and properly sealed to the wall; there must be no gaps or overhangs around sinks.
(5) Working facilities: a wash-hand basin must be provided, fitted with arm, knee or foot operated taps. A separate laboratory sink with similar taps for disposing of liquid radioactive waste and for decontaminating apparatus is necessary. This sink must be clearly marked with radioactive warning symbol (Fig. 11.9). An integrated sink and drainer unit with an upstand all round is recommended. A second laboratory sink for non-active work must also be provided.
(6) Fume cupboard: a fume cupboard is essential for a Grade B laboratory but is only necessary in Grade C laboratories where a radioactive gas is being used, or where radioactive material may give off vapour (e.g. radio-iodine) or where particulate matter is being handled.
(7) Good ventilation is necessary. In Grade C laboratories where there is no fume cupboard, an extraction fan should be provided in the working area.
(8) Storage: A simple lockable cupboard is sufficient for Grade C laboratories. The internal finish should be high gloss paint.

Personnel monitoring policy

All staff working in designated areas must be provided with personal dosimeters, usually of the film type, which should be worn on the trunk at chest or waist level underneath any protective clothing. Dosimeters are usually worn for a monitoring period of 4 weeks. The results of personnel monitoring should be kept for the current and preceding year. Dose limits are shown in Table 11.1.

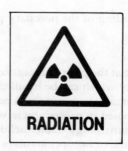

Fig. 11.9 Radiation hazard (yellow triangle enclosed by black line with yellow notice rectangle).

Table 11.1 Radiation dose limits (23)

Person	Site	Dose[a] (mSv)	Period
Employee > 18 years	Whole body	50	1 year
	Organ	500	1 year
Trainee < 18 years	Whole body	15	1 year
	Organ	150	1 year
Other Persons	Whole body	5	1 year
	Organ	50	1 year
Women of child-bearing age	Abdomen	13	3 months
Pregnant women	Abdomen	10	9 months

[a] The unit for describing biological effect is the sievert (Sv) or rem (1 rem = 0.01 Sv).

Systems of work

When working with unsealed sources of radioactivity only those persons whose presence is essential should work in the controlled area. The radiation source must be shielded until use and exposure of personnel kept as brief as possible. Persons in the controlled area must wear monitor film badges. Other persons may only work in the controlled area after radioactive sources have been removed and contamination monitoring procedures indicate that it is safe.

Operational procedures

Radioactive work should be carried out in an area of the laboratory set aside for the purpose. A washable non-absorbent working surface is necessary. The work itself must be carried out in a drip tray which should be lined with absorbent disposable material. An ample supply of paper tissues should always be available. Working vessels, whenever possible, should be contained in another vessel; cracked or chipped equipment must never be used. A laboratory coat and surgical gloves should be worn. Gloves should only be worn once and should be discarded along with and as part of the solid waste.

Non-inflammable liquid waste may be disposed of via the designated disposal sink. No more than the permitted activity can be disposed of per month from each establishment. Solid waste may be disposed of via the incinerator provided that the permitted daily activity is not exceeded. A record of the radioactive waste disposal must be kept. Careful records of receipt and usage of radionuclides must also be kept.

Accidents and spills

The radiation protection supervisor must be informed immediately. The order of priorities is as follows:

(1) protection of other personnel;
(2) confinement of contamination;
(3) decontamination of personnel;
(4) decontamination of the area involved.

All non-contaminated staff must be evacuated and re-entry forbidden.

Decontamination of skin. Wash the area thoroughly with soap and water. Do **not** use detergents or abrasive materials and take great care not to damage the skin.

Decontamination of cuts/eyes. Irrigate with water but take great care to prevent spread of contamination from one area to another.

Decontamination of clothing. Contaminated garments should be removed immediately and placed in a container. They should not be removed from the room until the contamination has been monitored.

Decontamination of work surfaces. Any surplus liquid should be mopped up with absorbent tissues, then the area washed with detergent and water. Place all contaminated materials in a separate container and retain till monitored.

Entry to the area must be restricted until contamination monitoring has been carried out and the radiation level has been measured.

Summary

Hazards to health and safety abound in the laboratory. Increasingly legislation is being passed to reduce risks in the workplace and thus maintain the health, safety and welfare of both employees and third parties who have right of access. Throughout this legislation the phrase 'as far as is reasonably practicable' appears with regularity. This is not merely a convenient escape clause for the employer; it is an important qualification on which legal judgement will be made. It implies that a computation must be made in which the quantum of risk must be placed in one scale and the sacrifice involved in the measures necessary to avert the risk (time, cost, trouble) in the other. Only when there is gross disproportion between them – the risk being insignificant in relation to the sacrifice – can there be justification for not taking every step to eliminate the risk.

Many types of document follow in the wake of legislation to assist in its interpretation, namely regulations, codes of practice and guidance notes. These are all important but have different weighting in terms of law. Regulations are law and if broken can result in prosecution. Codes of practice are intermediate, being partly legal and partly advisory. While they are admissible in evidence, they do not represent the law. Guidance notes are purely advisory with no legal backing.

A simple method of dealing with hazards in the workplace in a systematic way involves three stages:

(1) identify the hazard;
(2) find a standard for dealing with the hazard;
(3) implement the standard at work.

Management must always seek to apply the standard which solves the health and safety problem of their staff.

References

1. ACDP (Advisory Committee on Dangerous Pathogens) (1984). Categorisation of Pathogens According to Hazard and Categories of Containment. London: HMSO.
2. ACDP (Advisory Committee on Dangerous Pathogens) (1986). LAV/HTLVIII – The Causative Agent of AIDS and Related Conditions – Revised Guidelines. London: HMSO.
3. British Standards Institution (1979). BS5726 Specifications for Microbiological Safety Cabinets. London: HMSO.
4. British Standards Institution (1982). BS4402 Specifications for Safety Requirements for Laboratory Centrifuges. London: HMSO.
5. CDC/NIH (1984). *Biosafety in Microbiological and Biomedical Laboratories* Richardson, J. H. and Emmett Barkley, W. (eds). HHS Publication (CDC) 86–8395. Washington, D.C.: US Government Printing Office.
6. DHSS (1978). Code of Practice for the Prevention of Infection in Clinical Laboratories and Post-mortem Rooms. (The 'Howie Code of Practice'). London: HMSO.
7. DHSS (1981). Hospital Building Note 15. Accommodation of Pathology Services. London: HMSO.
8. DHSS/Welsh Office (1982). Fire Safety in Health Care Premises – Fire alarms and Detection Systems (HTM82). London: HMSO.
9. DHSS/Welsh Office (1982). Fire Safety in Health Care Premises – General Fire Precautions (HTM83). London: HMSO.
10. DHSS (1986). Electrical Safety Code for Hospital Laboratory Equipment (ESCHLE) (2nd edn). Health Equipment Information No. 158.
11. DHSS/Welsh Office (1987). Fire Precautions in New Hospitals (HTM 81). London: HMSO.
12. Harrington, J. M. and Shannon, H. S. (1976). Incidence of tuberculosis, hepatitis, brucellosis and shigellosis in British medical laboratory workers. *British Medical Journal* 1: 759–762.
13. Health and Safety Commission (1975). Health and Safety at Work etc. Act 1974. Advice to Employers (HSC 3). London: HMSO.
14. Health and Safety Commission (1981). Health and Safety (First Aid) Regulations. Approved Code of Practice (Guidance Notes) (CoP4). London: HMSO.
15. Health and Safety Commission (1985). The Protection of Persons Against Ionising Radiation Arising from any Work Practice: Approved Code of Practice. London: HMSO.
16. Health and Safety at Work Act (1974). London: HMSO.
17. Health and Safety Advisory Committee (1985). Safety in Health Service Laboratories: Hepatitis B. London: HMSO.
18. ICRP (International Commission on Radiological Protection) (1977). Recommendations of ICRP – A summary (Publication No. 26). Oxford: Pergamon.
19. Pike, R. M. (1976). Laboratory-associated infections; Summary and analysis of 3921 cases. *Health Laboratory Science* 13: 105–114.
20. Pike, R. M. (1979). Laboratory-associated infections; incidence, fatalities, causes and prevention. *Annual Reviews of Microbiology* 33: 44–66.

21. Pike, R. M., Sulkin, S. E. and Schulze, M. L. (1965). Continuing importance of laboratory-acquired infections. *American Journal of Public Health* **55**: 190–199.
22. Skinholj, P. (1974). Occupational risks in Danish clinical chemical laboratories. *Scandinavian Journal of Clinical Laboratory Investigation* **38**: 27–29.
23. Statutory Instruments (1985). Health and Safety: The Ionising Radiations Regulations. London: HMSO.
24. Sulkin, S. E. and Pike, R. M. (1949). Viral infections contracted in the laboratory. *New England Journal of Medicine* **241**: 205–213.
25. Sulkin, S. E. and Pike, R. M. (1951). Survey of laboratory-acquired infections. *American Journal of Public Health* **41**: 709–781.

12

Training Course in Quality Assurance

S M Lewis

Introduction

It is essential that all the staff of a haematology laboratory, both medical and technical, be familiar with the practice of quality assurance. The World Health Organization with the co-operation of ICSH has run international workshops on this topic and it also features regularly in the educational programmes of congresses of the International Society of Haematology. WHO and ICSH have collaborated in preparing a manual which provides an introduction to the principles and methods of quality assurance as applied to haematology.* The manual also includes a series of exercises to illustrate the principles, using tests which are commonly performed in the haematology laboratory.

The purpose of this chapter is to encourage the organization of comprehensive training courses similar to those of WHO. It includes a suggested programme of discussions and lectures based on the text of this book, and this is followed by a protocol for practical exercises. They are reproduced from the WHO manual with permission.

Programme of discussions and lectures

1. General principles of quality assurance

1.1 Objectives
1.2 Importance
1.3 Terminology used:
    Internal quality control
    External quality assessment
    Quality assurance
    Proficiency surveillance

*S. M. Lewis (1986). Quality Assurance in Haematology, WHO Broadsheet LAB 86.5. Geneva: World Health Organization.

Inter-laboratory trials
Quality assurance programme
Accuracy
Precision
Specificity
Sensitivity
Reference standard
Calibrator
Control material
Definitive method
Reference method
Reference reagent
Selected method
Specimen
Sample

2. Internal quality control

2.1   Principles of elementary statistics
2.2   Choice and use of calculators
2.3   Specimen collection, preservation, transport and storage
2.4   Specifications of control materials
2.5   Accuracy, precision and bias
2.6   Duplicate tests on patients' specimens
2.7   Random check test
2.8   Tests on control material
2.9   Quality control charts
2.10 CUSUM chart
2.11 Youden plots
2.12 Use of patients' data (mean indices)
2.13 Correlation assessment:
        Sequential results
        Interrelated tests
        Blood film
        Clinical state

3. External quality assessment

3.1 Organization of external quality assessment schemes (EQAS)
3.2 Preparation of material
3.3 Analysis of quantitative data
3.4 Deviation index
3.5 Youden plot and identification of bias
3.6 Analysis of qualitative results
3.7 Identification of unsatisfactory performance

3.8 Persistent poor performance
3.9 Interrelationship of local, national and international EQAS

4. Uses of EQAS

4.1 State of art
4.2 Evaluation of kits, reagents, instruments, controls and calibrators
4.3 Inter-laboratory comparability
4.4 Establishing 'truth' by consensus, reference laboratories and definitive methods
4.5 EQAS as base for training programmes and laboratory improvement

5. Identification of causes of problems in individual laboratories

5.1 Technique
5.2 Samples
5.3 Equipment
5.4 Methods
5.5 Environment
5.6 Staffing
5.7 Working space
5.8 Limits of accuracy and precision in practice

6. Elucidation of causes of error

6.1 Specimen collection
6.2 Specimen tube and anticoagulant
6.3 Transit time and environment
6.4 Specimen mix-up
6.5 Unrepresentative sampling
6.6 Faulty pipettes and pipetting errors
6.7 Instrument faults
6.8 Incorrect instrument setting/filter
6.9 Inadequate use of calibrators and control preparation
6.10 Lack of quality control
6.11 Errors of calculation
6.12 Reporting and recording errors
6.13 Inaccurate or inappropriate dilution
6.14 Incorrect method (e.g. wrong diluent, inadequate reaction)
6.15 Wrong interpretation of observation

7. Standardization

7.1 Characteristics of reference preparations for different test principles
7.2 Specifications for reference standards

Practical exercises for training course

Introduction

In the exercises which follow, haemoglobinometry and other fundamental haematological tests have been used as the model by means of which the principles and practical application of quality assurance are demonstrated. In addition, the participants will have been introduced to the use of standards and methods for standardization.

It is recommended that in order to put the exercises into perspective every participant should be regarded as an 'individual laboratory' and his or her result should be analysed individually in terms of internal quality control; at the same time all results should be analysed communally for external quality assessment. When the principles have been mastered with fundamental haematological tests, the practice of quality assurance can be extended into other tests, especially those which have a particular importance in diagnosis or health screening surveys in the area where the participants work.

For a description of the statistical principles used in the exercises, see Chapter 4.

Exercise 1: Calculation of standard deviation, variance and coefficient of variation

The following data were obtained in ten consecutive haemoglobin measurements on two haemoglobinometers, identified as A and B, respectively.

Test	A Hb g/l	B Hb g/l
1	155	150
2	148	135
3	152	145
4	147	137
5	150	153
6	156	163
7	157	155
8	153	149
9	150	144
10	150	137

Calculate for each series of readings:

(a) Mean ($\bar{x}$)

(b) $\Sigma(x - \bar{x})^2$

(c) Variance $(s^2) = \dfrac{\Sigma(x - \bar{x})^2}{n - 1}$

(d) Standard deviation (SD) $= \sqrt{s^2}$

(e) Coefficient of variation (CV) as a percentage $= \dfrac{SD}{\bar{x}} \times 100\%$

(f) Standard error of mean (SEM) $= \dfrac{SD}{\sqrt{n}}$ (or $\sqrt{\dfrac{s^2}{n}}$)

Where x represents the individual data, $\bar{x}$ is the mean, and n the number of data items in the sets.

Exercise 2: Differences between means

The simplest method for assessing whether two sets of data are similar to or different from each other is to calculate their means and SDs. If the ranges, i.e. means $\pm$ SDs do not overlap, the sets are significantly different. Thus, for example, if the mean and SD are 40 ± 3 and 50 ± 3 respectively, their 1 SD range would be 37–43 and 47–53; clearly separate sets. Conversely, if their values were 40 ± 10 and 50 ± 10 their 1 SD range would be 30–50 and 40–60; with this overlapping the sets cannot be regarded as being separate entities.

If there are differences between the two sets, the extent of difference depends on whether they can be separated at 3 SD when there is a 99% probability, or at 2 SD when there is a 95% probability, or at 1SD when there is only a 66% probability that the difference is really significant. In other words, when the sets appear separate at 1 SD range, this does not necessarily mean that they will remain separated at the 3 SD range.

A more reliable method is to analyse the standard error of the difference between the means (SE diff). In this procedure the difference between two sets of data is regarded as significant only if their means differ from each other by an amount greater than the SE diff. This is obtained by the following calculation:

$$\sqrt{\left[\frac{(SD_1)^2}{n_1} + \frac{(SD_2)^2}{n_2} \right]}$$

where SD_1 and SD_2 are the SDs of set 1 and 2 respectively, n_1 and n_2 are the number of data items in the sets.

Using both the above methods (i.e. SD of means and SE diff) determine whether there is significant difference between the measurements by the two instruments in Exercise 1.

This will indicate the extent of a systematic discrepancy (bias). Variations due to random factors which are not constant can be demonstrated by analysis of variance, as described in Exercise 3.

Exercise 3: Analysis of variance

There are several ways in which the SDs of two sets of data can be compared statistically to determine whether there are significant differences between them. One convenient way is with the 'F-ratio', which compares the variances (s^2) of the two sets.

$$F\text{-ratio} = \frac{s^2 \text{ of set A}}{s^2 \text{ of set B}}$$

The ratio must not be less than 1; accordingly, select the set with the greater variance as the numerator (i.e. set A). To determine the significance of the F-ratio as calculated, compare the figure obtained with the figures in the table in Appendix I (p. 282–285) at the appropriate degrees of freedom for the two sets of data (degree of freedom = number of measurements − 1). To be significant, the calculated ratio must be greater than the figure in the table, using the appropriate table for 99% or 95% probability, respectively.

(a) Using the data in Exercise 1, calculate the F-ratio of the two sets A and B.
(b) Is there a significant difference in the reliability of the two colorimeters?

Analysis of differences by t-test

This is another method for comparing two sets of data, using one of the following calculations:

(a) Difference in means

$$t = \frac{\bar{x} \text{ of set A} - \bar{x} \text{ of set B}}{SE \text{ diff}}$$

(b) Difference in paired results

Difference between pairs $= d$

Sum of differences $= \Sigma d$

Mean of differences $= \dfrac{\Sigma d}{n} = \bar{d}$

Variance $(s^2) = \dfrac{\Sigma(d - \bar{d})^2}{n - 1}$

SE mean of differences $= \sqrt{\dfrac{s^2}{n}}$

$$t = \frac{\bar{d}}{\sqrt{(s^2/n)}}$$

Interpretation: From Appendix II (p. 286) find t distribution for appropriate degree of freedom $(n-1)$. Express results as level of probability (P) that there is *no* significant difference between means or sets of pairs. E.g. with d.f. = 19:

$t=0$	1.25	1.65	5.65	
$P=100\%$	20–30%	10–20%	1–0.05%	0%
i.e. $P=1$	$0.3>P>0.2$	$0.2>P>0.1$	$0.001>P>0.0005$	$P=0$

As a rough guide, when $t>4$ there is a significant difference both for means and for paired results.

Exercise 4: Calculation of median

Median (m) is another measure of the midpoint of distribution. It is the point on the scale that has equal numbers of observations above and below it. Its advantage is that it is not dependent on the shape of distribution and it is less affected by outliers. The spread of distribution is based on the '50 percentile' which includes the central 50% of the values. This range is taken as the SD.

The following data were obtained from 21 different laboratories in a trial of a new method for platelet counting (results are expressed in $N \times 10^9$ per litre).

70　76　110　90　116　113　97　95　85　64　120

117　101　98　73　120　75　90　115　100　80

Calculate m and its SD. Compare with $\bar{x}$ and SD. Recalculate truncated mean and SD (x' and SD$'$) after excluding results outside 2SD.

Median (m)	
SD range (50 percentile)	
Mean ($\bar{x}$)	
SD and 2 SD range	
Truncated mean ($\bar{x}'$) SD$'$ and 2SD$'$ range	

Exercise 5: Evaluation of new method

Haemoglobin was measured on a set of specimens (A) with the ICSH reference method and (B) with a new method using undiluted blood. Evaluate the new method by t-test

	(A) Reference method (g/1)	(B) New method (g/1)	d	$(d-\bar{d})$	$(d-\bar{d})^2$
1.	70	65			
2.	76	75			
3.	110	120			
4.	90	75			
5.	116	110			
6.	113	105			
7.	97	80			
8.	95	105			
9.	85	65			
10.	64	50			
11.	120	115			
12.	116	115			
13.	101	100			
14.	98	90			
15.	73	60			
			Σ		Σ
			$\bar{d}$		

$$s^2 = \frac{\Sigma (d-\bar{d})^2}{n-1}$$

$$\text{SE diff} = \sqrt{\frac{s^2}{n}} \qquad t = \bar{d} \div \text{SE diff} =$$

on paired results and by demonstrating the extent of correlation or lack thereof by plotting the data on arithmetic graph paper.

Also assess whether there is significant difference between the means by the F-ratio (see Exercise 3).

Exercise 6

In a trial of a new method of serum iron the results given below were obtained using five control sera whose iron concentration has also been determined with a reference method. Results are given in $\mu g/dl$.

Calculate standard deviation and CV (%) at the five levels. Plot the means of the results obtained with the new method against the reference results on arithmetic graph paper. Comment on the suitability of using the new method as the selected method in your laboratory.

Control serum	Reference method	New method
A	40	51–58–67–61–63–59 60–58–61–64–59–59
B	100	126–118–226–121–123–117 114–120–122–125–118–120
C	160	184–180–177–185–181–174 179–178–180–182–183–177
D	220	244–242–237–240–236–239 244–238–240–241–235–244
E	280	278–272–264–270–266–274 264–268–270–272–274–268

	A	B	C	D	E
n					
$\bar{x}$					
SD					
CV%					

Exercise 7: Precision of pipetting

Fill one 20 µl pipette from the sample of lysate provided and dilute the measured volume in 4 ml of cyanide–ferricyanide reagent. Repeat ten times. Read each in a spectrophotometer or photoelectric colorimeter at a wavelength of 540 nm or with an appropriate filter (e.g. Ilford 625). For convenience in calculation, present the figures of the readings as whole numbers.

Test no.	Galvo reading (x)	$(x - \bar{x})$	$(x - \bar{x})^2$
1			
2			
3			
4			
5			
6			
7			
8			
9			
10			

(a) Calculate mean of series $(= \bar{x})$

(b) Calculate standard deviation $(SD) = \sqrt{\dfrac{\Sigma(x - \bar{x})^2}{n-1}}$

(c) Calculate CV $(\%) = \dfrac{SD}{\bar{x}} \times 100$

(d) Calculate $SEM = \dfrac{SD}{\sqrt{n}}$

Exercise 8: Assessment of linearity and reproducibility

Prepare the material for this exercise as follows:

(a) From one donor collect approximately 20 ml of venous blood in EDTA. Mix well and transfer approximately 8 ml, 8 ml and 4 ml into three centrifuge tubes, labelled, 1, 2 and 3, respectively.

(b) Centrifuge tubes 1 and 2; take 2 ml of plasma from each and add to tube 3. Mix the contents of tube 3 and re-label as A.

(c) Mix the contents of tubes 1 and 2, pool together and re-label as E.

(d) Make five samples as follows:

> Tube A—as above
> Tube B—2 ml of A + 1 ml of E
> Tube C—2 ml of A + 2 ml of E
> Tube D—1 ml of A + 2 ml of E
> Tube E—as above

Carry out the exercise as follows:

(a) Using a 20 μl pipette make a 1:201 dilution (in duplicate) of each of the samples

A–E in cyanide–ferricyanide reagent. Read the adsorbance (A) of each in a photometer at 540 nm (or using an appropriate yellow-green filter). By means of a haemiglobin-cyanide reference preparation convert the readings into Hb concentration (g/l).

(b) Measure the microhaematocrit of each sample in duplicate.

Record the results on the chart below:

	A^{540}	Hb (g/l)	PCV
A $\frac{1}{2}$			
B $\frac{1}{2}$			
C $\frac{1}{2}$			
D $\frac{1}{2}$			
E $\frac{1}{2}$			
HiCN ref. prep.			

(c) On arithmetic graph paper mark an arbitrary scale of 100–400 units on the horizontal axis. On the vertical axis mark one scale for A^{540} readings and another one for PCV. Plot all the measurements obtained with samples A–E—plot A at 100, B at 200, C at 250, D at 300 and E at 400. Draw a line of best fit for A^{540} measurements and another line for the PCV measurements. Note the following:

(1) Is any part of the line non-linear?
(2) Do any of the duplicate measurements not fall close to the line?
(3) To what extent does the PCV parallel the A^{540} readings?
(4) Convert the A^{540} readings to Hb concentrations and calculate the SD of the difference between duplicate measurements by the formula $SD = \sqrt{(\Sigma d^2/2n)}$, where $d =$ the differences between paired measurements, and $n =$ number of paired readings.

Have there been any significant errors in any of the duplicate measurements? This will be the case when the difference in the duplicate measurements is greater than the SD.

5. Identify the reliable range of A^{540} in the photometer, and express this in terms of Hb concentration at the dilution used.

Exercise 9: Measurement of haemoglobin

Carry out haemoglobin estimation by the haemiglobincyanide method on whole-blood samples A and B; lysed samples C and D; and diluted sample E (as HiCN). A and C should have high haemoglobin concentration, B and D low concentration.

A reference standard is provided.

	HiCN by photometer	HiCN spectrophotometric[a]
Reference preparation Absorbance (A^{540}) Hb value (g/l)		
Sample A Absorbance (A^{540}) Hb (g/l)		
Sample B Absorbance (A^{540}) Hb (g/l)		
Sample C Absorbance (A^{540}) Hb (g/l)		
Sample D Absorbance (A^{540}) Hb (g/l)		
Sample E Absorbance (A^{540}) Hb (g/l)		

[a]From formula: Hb (g/l) $= \dfrac{A^{540} \times 64{,}500 \times \text{dilution}}{44.0 \times 1000 \times d}$

where d = layer thickness of solution in cm (usually 1.000 cm).

Using all the class results, calculate $\bar{x}$, s^2, SD and CV for each specimen.

	HiCN			
	$\bar{x}$	s^2	SD	CV
Reference preparation				
Sample A				
Sample B				
Sample C				
Sample D				
Sample E				

Calculate F-ratios of various sets. Compare the following and note whether there are significant differences in reliability of measurement of Hb:

(1) High concentration (A) versus low concentration (B)
(2) High concentration (C) versus low concentration (D)
(3) Whole blood (A) versus lysate (C)
(4) Whole blood (B) versus lysate (D)
(5) Pre-diluted (E) versus self-diluted. For this, one of the samples A–D should be used to provide sample E.

Exercise 10: Haemoglobinometry

Repeat Exercise 9 on samples A, B, C, and D using another method, e.g. oxyhaemoglobin or whole-blood haemoglobinometer. Using all class results, calculate $\bar{x}$, s^2, SD and CV for each:

	$\bar{x}$	s^2	SD	CV
Reference preparation				
Sample A				
Sample B				
Sample C				
Sample D				

Calculate F-ratios and determine whether there is a significant difference in reliability in comparison with the HiCN method.

Exercise 11: Preparation of calibration graph

A calibration graph (or table) should be prepared whenever a new photometer is put into use in the laboratory and again every 6 months. Prepare a graph which relates Hb concentration to absorbance (A^{540}) by the following method:

Set up a series of five tubes and with a 10 ml graduated pipette add the following volumes of ICSH haemiglobincyanide reference standard or traceable calibrator:

Tube 1 6 ml approximately
Tube 2 4.5 ml accurately measured
Tube 3 3.0 ml accurately measured
Tube 4 1.5 ml accurately measured
Tube 5 None

Rinse the pipette well with haemiglobincyanide *reagent* and add reagent to the tubes:

Tube 1 None ($= 100\%$)
Tube 2 1.5 ml accurately measured ($= 75\%$)
Tube 3 3.0 ml accurately measured ($= 50\%$)
Tube 4 4.5 ml accurately measured ($= 25\%$)
Tube 5 6 ml approximately ($= \ 0\%$)

Mix the contents of each tube well, transfer to cuvettes and read the absorbance of each in the photometer, setting the solution from Tube 5 at zero (blank).

From the stated value of the HiCN reference preparation calculate the concentrations of the intermediate solutions. Plot the Hb concentrations on the horizontal axis and A^{540}

on the vertical axis of metric (arithmetic) graph paper. The points should fall on a line passing through zero. Extend the line beyond the last plotted point if the instrument is known to be linear beyond that (see Exercise 8).

Exercise 12: Control chart method for quality control

(A) Make a series of at least ten measurements of the control material provided and calculate the mean and standard deviation (SD) of the results. Prepare a control chart calibrating the vertical scale in appropriate units (e.g. Hb g/l), and indicate the levels of $+2\,SD$ and $-2\,SD$.

(B) The results obtained from a series of measurements on another control material are given below.

The control was preserved blood from one donor. Initially, ten replicate measurements of haemoglobin were obtained (Column A). Then haemoglobin was measured on a sample each day. Results over 20 days are shown in Columns B and C. All measurements are expressed in g/l.

A	Day	B	Day	C
142	1	142	11	145
141	2	144	12	148
146	3	143	13	148
144	4	143	14	149
143	5	141	15	151
145	6	143	16	151
140	7	145	17	152
143	8	143	18	154
142	9	144	19	154
144	10	142	20	154

Plot these measurements on a control chart and comment.

(C) Present the data obtained for the control chart (above) using a CUSUM procedure as described on p. 77.

Exercise 13: Normal range and reference values

Results given below are the measurements of haemoglobin (in 5 g/l intervals) obtained from a group of apparently normal people in a population. Plot the data as a frequency histogram on arithmetical graph paper and by eye determine the best-fit curve. Is the distribution 'normal' (i.e. Gaussian)? What is the mode and what is the median?

(a) Calculate mean ($\bar{x}$) and SD.
(b) Set a range of $\bar{x} \pm 2$ SD.
(c) Eliminate from the original data any values which are outside ± 2 SD.
(d) Re-calculate $\bar{x}$ and SD of the remaining values. Calculate the range which should include 95% of a normal population (i.e. 2 SD). Does this differ from the original group?

Hb (g/l)	No. of times
100	1
105	0
110	1
115	1
120	2
125	1
130	3
135	3
140	7
145	10
150	3
155	4
160	2
165	2
170	0

Exercise 14

Serum bilirubin was determined in a group of men students, aged 20–24 years. The results (in mg/dl) are given below. Present the figures as a histogram and comment on the distribution. Identify the mode and the median.

(a) Assuming Gaussian distribution, calculate the means, and the ranges of ± 2 SD.
(b) Comment on the validity of this method for the data provided.

0.5	0.5	0.4	0.6	0.4	2.2	1.3	0.4
0.4	0.4	0.5	0.5	1.1	0.5	2.9	0.4
0.6	0.8	0.7	0.9	0.5	0.4	0.4	0.5
0.4	0.5	1.4	0.5	0.3	0.3	0.5	0.6
0.3	0.5	1.0	0.6	0.9	0.5	0.4	1.0
0.7	0.4	0.6	0.5	0.4	0.6	1.5	1.6

Exercise 15: Red cell counts

Although in many laboratories red cell counting by counting chamber is obsolete, the following exercise has been included in order to demonstrate the principle of counting statistics.

(a) Carry out a red cell count by counting chamber and electronic counter on the provided blood in EDTA (A) and preserved blood in ACD (B), using appropriate dilution.
(b) Establish mean, count variance (σ), SD and CV.

σ represents the theoretical variation with which the cells can be expected to settle in a counting chamber (or pass through the sensing zone of an electronic counter) in consecutive similar measurements. It conforms to Poisson distribution; the variance is given by $\sqrt{\lambda}$, where λ is the total number of cells counted in the defined area/volume. This contrasts with SD, which is a measure of the variation which actually occurs between results when the test is repeated consecutively.

	Specimen	Dilution	No. of squares counted	No. of cells counted (λ)	Red cell count ($\times 10^{12}$ per litre)	σ of cells counted ($\sqrt{\lambda}$)	Range $c \pm 2\sigma$	Count CV (%)
Counting chamber counts	A							
	B							
Total class counts	A							
	B							

From these results calculate the following:

RBC ($\times 10^{12}$ per litre)		A	B
By total class count (All results pooled)	λ σ CV		
By participant counts (For EQA)	$\bar{x}$ SD CV m		
By electronic counter			

Note that 'Class count' = total number of cells counted by entire class ($=\lambda$). For 'Participant count' each member of class provides a result which is used to calculate $\bar{x}$ and SD. The count variance (σ) is $\sqrt{\lambda}$.

Keep results for Exercise 20.

Exercise 16: Total leucocyte counts

By counting chamber and electronic methods:

(a) Estimate the total leucocyte count in diluted (1:20) blood A provided.
(b) Estimate the total leucocyte count in blood samples B and C, making suitable dilutions of the blood. B is a fresh blood; C is a control preparation.

	Blood dilutions	No. of 1 mm^2 areas counted	No. of cells counted (λ)	Calculated leucocyte count ($\times 10^{12}$ per litre)	Count variance $\sigma = (\sqrt{\lambda})$	Count CV (%)
Self counts	A 1:20					
	B					
	C					
Total class counts	A					
	B					
	C					
Electronic counter	A					
	B					
	C					

Calculate the following:

WBC ($\times 10^9$ per litre)		A	B	C
By class count (pooled results)	λ			
	σ			
	CV			
By participant counts (for EQA; see note on p. 275)	$\bar{x}$			
	SD			
	CV			
	m			
By electronic counter	$\bar{x}$			
	SD			
	CV			
	m			

Keep results for Exercise 20.

Exercise 17: Differential counts

Stain film provided with a Romanowsky stain, and carry out a differential count.

Total WBC ($\times 10^9$ per litre)

Total No. cells counted		Neutrophils	Eosinophils	Basophils	Lymphocytes	Monocytes
100	As total no. As % σ ($\sqrt{\lambda}$) 2σ range					
200	As total no. As % σ ($\sqrt{\lambda}$) 2σ range					
Total class results	As total no. As % σ ($\sqrt{\lambda}$) 2σ range					

Exercise 18: Platelet count

Carry out platelet counts on fresh blood sample (A) and control preparation (B) by haemocytometer method, using ammonium oxalate diluent. Examine under phase-contrast, if this is available.

Specimen	No. of squares counted	No. of cells counted (λ)	σ ($\sqrt{\lambda}$)	Platelet count ($\times 10^9$ per litre)	CV (%)
A					
B					

Platelet count ($\times 10^9$ per litre)

From the above results calculate the following:

		A	B
By class count (pooled results)	λ		
	σ		
	CV		
By participant counts (for EQA; see note on p. 275)	$\bar{x}$		
	SD		
	CV		
	m		

Keep results for Exercise 20.

Exercise 19: Reticulocyte count

Make reticulocyte preparations from the blood provided and carry out a reticulocyte count. The total RBC will be given. Report your results as a percentage and as an absolute count.

Number of fields examined		
Average number of red cells per field (Determined from 10–15 fields)		
Approximate total number of red cells surveyed		
Total number of reticulocytes counted		
Reticulocyte percentage		
RBC ($\times 10^{12}$ per litre)		
Absolute reticulocyte count		

Calculate the following:

Individual participant
      Retic. %
      Range of 2σ	

Class count (pooled)
      Retic. %
      Range of 2σ	

Participant counts (for EQA; see note on p. 275)
      Retic. %
      Range of 2 SD
      CV of test	

Exercise 20: Inter-laboratory quality control (external quality assessment)

For this exercise, each student will be regarded as an independent laboratory.

Using the data from Exercises 15, 16, 18 and/or 19, calculate mean ($\bar{x}$) and SD, and also median (m) and 50 percentile SD. Recalculate $\bar{x}'$ and SD' after excluding results >3 SD.

Then calculate deviation index from formulae:

$$DI = \frac{x - \bar{x}'}{SD'} \text{ or } \frac{x - m}{SD'}$$

Assess performance as follows:

DI < 0.5   Excellent
DI   0.5–1.0   Good
DI   1.0–2.0   Satisfactory
DI > 2.0   Requires check

Appendix I: *F*-Distribution tables

Upper 1%

V_2 \ V_1 1	2	3	4	5	6	7	8	9
1	4052	4999·5	5403	5625	5764	5859	5928	5981	6022
2	98·50	99·00	99·17	99·25	99·30	99·33	99·36	99·37	99·39
3	34·12	30·82	29·46	28·71	28·24	27·91	27·67	27·49	27·35
4	21·20	18·00	16·69	15·98	15·52	15·21	14·98	14·80	14·66
5	16·26	13·27	12·06	11·39	10·97	10·67	10·46	10·29	10·16
6	13·75	10·92	9·78	9·15	8·75	8·47	8·26	8·10	7·98
7	12·25	9·55	8·45	7·85	7·46	7·19	6·99	6·84	6·72
8	11·26	8·65	7·59	7·01	6·63	6·37	6·18	6·03	5·91
9	10·56	8·02	6·99	6·42	6·06	5·80	5·61	5·47	5·35
10	10·04	7·56	6·55	5·99	5·64	5·39	5·20	5·06	4·94
11	9·65	7·21	6·22	5·67	5·32	5·07	4·89	4·74	4·63
12	9·33	6·93	5·95	5·41	5·06	4·82	4·64	4·50	4·39
13	9·07	6·70	5·74	5·21	4·86	4·62	4·44	4·30	4·19
14	8·86	6·51	5·56	5·04	4·69	4·46	4·28	4·14	4·03
15	8·68	6·36	5·42	4·89	4·56	4·32	4·14	4·00	3·89
16	8·53	6·23	5·29	4·77	4·44	4·20	4·03	3·89	3·78
17	8·40	6·11	5·18	4·67	4·34	4·10	3·93	3·79	3·68
18	8·29	6·01	5·09	4·58	4·25	4·01	3·84	3·71	3·60
19	8·18	5·93	5·01	4·50	4·17	3·94	3·77	3·63	3·52
20	8·10	5·85	4·94	4·43	4·10	3·87	3·70	3·56	3·46
21	8·02	5·78	4·87	4·37	4·04	3·81	3·64	3·51	3·40
22	7·95	5·72	4·82	4·31	3·99	3·76	3·59	3·45	3·35
23	7·88	5·66	4·76	4·26	3·94	3·71	3·54	3·41	3·30
24	7·82	5·61	4·72	4·22	3·90	3·67	3·50	3·36	3·26
25	7·77	5·57	4·68	4·18	3·85	3·63	3·46	3·32	3·22
26	7·72	5·53	4·64	4·14	3·82	3·59	3·42	3·29	3·18
27	7·68	5·49	4·60	4·11	3·78	3·56	3·39	3·26	3·15
28	7·64	5·45	4·57	4·07	3·75	3·53	3·36	3·23	3·12
29	7·60	5·42	4·54	4·04	3·73	3·50	3·33	3·20	3·09
30	7·56	5·39	4·51	4·02	3·70	3·47	3·30	3·17	3·07
40	7·31	5·18	4·31	3·83	3·51	3·29	3·12	2·99	2·89
60	7·08	4·98	4·13	3·65	3·34	3·12	2·95	2·82	2·72
120	6·85	4·79	3·95	3·48	3·17	2·96	2·79	2·66	2·56
∞	6·63	4·61	3·78	3·32	3·02	2·80	2·64	2·51	2·41

points

10	12	15	20	24	30	40	60	120	∞
6056	6106	6157	6209	6235	6261	6287	6313	6339	6366
99·40	99·42	99·43	99·45	99·46	99·47	99·47	99·48	99·49	99·50
27·23	27·05	26·87	26·69	26·60	26·50	26·41	26·32	26·22	26·13
14·55	14·37	14·20	14·02	13·93	13·84	13·75	13·65	13·56	13·46
10·05	9·89	9.72	9·55	9·47	9·38	9·29	9·20	9·11	9·02
7·87	7·72	7·56	7·40	7·31	7·23	7·14	7·06	6·97	6·88
6·62	6·47	6·31	6·16	6·07	5·99	5·91	5·82	5·74	5·65
5·81	5·67	5·52	5·36	5·28	5·20	5·12	5·03	4·95	4·86
5·26	5·11	4·96	4·81	4·73	4·65	4·57	4·48	4·40	4·31
4·85	4·71	4·56	4·41	4·33	4·25	4·17	4·08	4·00	3·91
4·54	4·40	4·25	4·10	4·02	3·94	3·86	3·78	3·69	3·60
4·30	4·16	4·01	3·86	3·78	3·70	3·62	3·54	3·45	3·36
4·10	3·96	3·82	3·66	3·59	3·51	3·43	3·34	3·25	3·17
3·94	3·80	3·66	3·51	3·43	3·35	3·27	3·18	3·09	3·00
3·80	3·67	3·52	3·37	3·29	3·21	3·13	3·05	2·96	2·87
3·69	3·55	3·41	3·26	3·18	3·10	3·02	2·93	2·84	2·75
3·59	3·46	3·31	3·16	3·08	3·00	2·92	2·83	2·75	2·65
3·51	3·37	3·23	3·08	3·00	2·92	2·84	2·75	2·66	2·57
3·43	3·30	3·15	3·00	2·92	2·84	2·76	2·67	2·58	2·49
3·37	3·23	3·09	2·94	2·86	2·78	2·69	2·61	2·52	2·42
3·31	3·17	3·03	2·88	2·80	2·72	2·64	2·55	2·46	2·36
3·26	3·12	2·98	2·83	2·75	2·67	2·58	2·50	2·40	2·31
3·21	3·07	2·93	2·78	2·70	2·62	2·54	2·45	2·35	2·26
3·17	3·03	2·89	2·74	2·66	2·58	2·49	2·40	2·31	2·21
3·13	2·99	2·85	2·70	2·62	2·54	2·45	2·36	2·27	2·17
3·09	2·96	2·81	2·66	2·85	2·50	2·42	2·33	2·23	2·13
3·06	2·93	2·78	2·63	2·55	2·47	2·38	2·29	2·20	2·10
3·03	2·90	2·75	2·60	2·52	2·44	2·35	2·26	2·17	2·06
3·00	2·87	2·73	2·57	2·49	2·41	2·33	2·23	2·14	2·03
2·98	2·84	2·70	2·55	2·47	2·39	2·30	2·21	2·11	2·01
2·80	2·66	2·52	2·37	2·29	2·20	2·11	2·02	1·92	1·80
2·63	2·50	2·35	2·20	2·12	2·03	1·94	1·84	1·73	1·60
2·47	2·34	2·19	2·03	1·95	1·86	1·76	1·66	1·53	1·38
2·32	2·18	2·04	1·88	1·79	1·70	1·59	1·47	1·32	1·00

V_2	V_1 1	2	3	4	5	6	7	8	9
1	161·4	199·5	215·7	224·6	230·2	234·0	236·8	238·9	240·5
2	18·51	19·00	19·16	19·25	19·30	19·33	19·35	19·37	19·38
3	10·13	9·55	9·28	9·12	9·01	8·94	8·89	8·85	8·81
4	7·71	6·94	6·59	6·39	6·26	6·16	6·09	6·04	6·00
5	6·61	5·79	5·41	5·19	5·05	4·95	4·88	4·82	4·77
6	5·99	5·14	4·76	4·53	4·39	4·28	4·21	4·15	4·10
7	5·59	4·74	4·35	4·12	3·97	3·87	3·79	3·73	3·68
8	5·32	4·46	4·07	3·84	3·69	3·58	3·50	3·44	3·39
9	5·12	4·26	3·86	3·63	3·48	3·37	3·29	3·23	3·18
10	4·96	4·10	3·71	3·48	3·33	3·22	3·14	3·07	3·02
11	4·84	3·98	3·59	3·36	3·20	3·09	3·01	2·95	2·90
12	4·75	3·89	3·49	3·26	3·11	3·00	2·91	2·85	2·80
13	4·67	3·81	3·41	3·18	3·03	2·92	2·83	2·77	2·71
14	4·60	3·74	3·34	3·11	2·96	2·85	2·76	2·70	2·65
15	4·54	3·68	3·29	3·06	2·90	2·79	2·71	2·64	2·59
16	4·49	3·63	3·24	3·01	2·85	2·74	2·66	2·59	2·54
17	4·45	3·59	3·20	2·96	2·81	2·70	2·61	2·55	2·49
18	4·41	3·55	3·16	2·93	2·77	2·66	2·58	2·51	2·46
19	4·38	3·52	3·13	2·90	2·74	2·63	2·54	2·48	2·42
20	4·35	3·49	3·10	2·87	2·71	2·60	2·51	2·45	2·39
21	4·32	3·47	3·07	2·84	2·68	2·57	2·49	2·42	2·37
22	4·30	3·44	3·05	2·82	2·66	2·55	2·46	2·40	2·34
23	4·28	3·42	3·03	2·80	2·64	2·53	2·44	2·37	2·32
24	4·26	3·40	3·01	2·78	2·62	2·51	2·42	2·36	2·30
25	4·24	3·39	2·99	2·76	2·60	2·49	2·40	2·34	2·28
26	4·23	3·37	2·98	2·74	2·59	2·47	2·39	2·32	2·27
27	4·21	3·35	2·96	2·73	2·57	2·46	2·37	2·31	2·25
28	4·20	3·34	2·95	2·71	2·56	2·45	2·36	2·29	2·24
29	4·18	3·33	2·93	2·70	2·55	2·43	2·35	2·28	2·22
30	4·17	3·32	2·92	2·69	2·53	2·42	2·33	2·27	2·21
40	4·08	3·23	2·84	2·61	2·45	2·34	2·25	2·18	2·12
60	4·00	3·15	2·76	2·53	2·37	2·25	2·17	2·10	2·04
120	3·92	3·07	2·68	2·45	2·29	2·17	2·09	2·02	1·96
∞	3·84	3·00	2·60	2·37	2·21	2·10	2·01	1·94	1·88

From Pearson, E. S. and Hartley, H. O. (eds) *Biometrika Tables for Statisticians* (3rd edn),
  Vol. I. London: Biometrika Trust, University College London. With permission.
V_1 = Degrees of freedom for numerator.
V_2 = Degrees of freedom for denominator.

points

10	12	15	20	24	30	40	60	120	∞
241·9	243·9	245·9	248·0	249·1	250·1	251·1	252·2	253·3	254·3
19·40	19·41	19·43	19·45	19·45	19·46	19·47	19·48	19·49	19·50
8·79	8·74	8·70	8·66	8·64	8·62	8·59	8·57	8·55	8·53
5·96	5·91	5·86	5·80	5·77	5·75	5·72	5·69	5·66	5·63
4·74	4·68	4·62	4·56	4·53	4·50	4·46	4·43	4·40	4·36
4·06	4·00	3·94	3·87	3·84	3·81	3·77	3·74	3·70	3·67
3·64	3·57	3·51	3·44	3·41	3·38	3·34	3·30	3·27	3·23
3·35	3·28	3·22	3·15	3·12	3·08	3·04	3·01	2·97	2·93
3·14	3·07	3·01	2·94	2·90	2·86	2·83	2·79	2·75	2·71
2·98	2·91	2·85	2·77	2·74	2·70	2·66	2·62	2·58	2·54
2·85	2·79	2·72	2·65	2·61	2·57	2·53	2·49	2·45	2·40
2·75	2·69	2·62	2·54	2·51	2·47	2·43	2·38	2·34	2·30
2·67	2·60	2·53	2·46	2·42	2·38	2·34	2·30	2·25	2·21
2·60	2·53	2·46	2·39	2·35	2·31	2·27	2·22	2·18	2·13
2·54	2·48	2·40	2·33	2·29	2·25	2·20	2·16	2·11	2·07
2·49	2·42	2·35	2·28	2·24	2·19	2·15	2·11	2·06	2·01
2·45	2·38	2·31	2·23	2·19	2·15	2·10	2·06	2·01	1·96
2·41	2·34	2·27	2·19	2·15	2·11	2·06	2·02	1·97	1·92
2·38	2·31	2·23	2·16	2·11	2·07	2·03	1·98	1·93	1·88
2·35	2·28	2·20	2·12	2·08	2·04	1·99	1·95	1·90	1·84
2·32	2·25	2·18	2·10	2·05	2·01	1·96	1·92	1·87	1·81
2·30	2·23	2·15	2·07	2·03	1·98	1·94	1·89	1·84	1·78
2·27	2·20	2·13	2·05	2·01	1·96	1·91	1·86	1·81	1·76
2·25	2·18	2·11	2·03	1·98	1·94	1·89	1·84	1·79	1·73
2·24	2·16	2·09	2·01	1·96	1·92	1·87	1·82	1·77	1·71
2·22	2·15	2·07	1·99	1·95	1·90	1·85	1·80	1·75	1·69
2·20	2·13	2·06	1·97	1·93	1·88	1·84	1·79	1·73	1·67
2·19	2·12	2·04	1·96	1·91	1·87	1·82	1·77	1·71	1·65
2·18	2·10	2·03	1·94	1·90	1·85	1·81	1·75	1·70	1·64
2·16	2·09	2·01	1·93	1·89	1·84	1·79	1·74	1·68	1·62
2·08	2·00	1·92	1·84	1·79	1·74	1·69	1·64	1·58	1·51
1·99	1·92	1·84	1·75	1·70	1·65	1·59	1·53	1·47	1·39
1·91	1·83	1·75	1·66	1·61	1·55	1·50	1·43	1·35	1·25
1·83	1·75	1·67	1·57	1·52	1·46	1·39	1·32	1·22	1·00

Appendix II: *t*-Test table

d.f.	Probability > 0·5 <	> 0·1 <	> 0·05 <	> 0·02 <	> 0·01 <	> 0·001 <
1	1·000	6·314	12·706	31·821	63·657	636·619
2	0·816	2·920	4·303	6·965	9·925	31·598
3	0·765	2·353	3·182	4·541	5·841	12·941
4	0·741	2·132	2·776	3·747	4·604	8·610
5	0·727	2·015	2·571	3·365	4·032	6·859
6	0·718	1·943	2·447	3·143	3·707	5·959
7	0·711	1·895	2·365	2·998	3·499	5·405
8	0·706	1·860	2·306	2·896	3·355	5·041
9	0·703	1·833	2·262	2·821	3·250	4·781
10	0·700	1·812	2·228	2·764	3·169	4·587
11	0·697	1·796	2·201	2·718	3·106	4·437
12	0·695	1·782	2·179	2·681	3·055	4·318
13	0·694	1·771	2·160	2·650	3·012	4·221
14	0·692	1·761	2·145	2·624	2·977	4·140
15	0·691	1·753	2·131	2·602	2·947	4·073
16	0·690	1·746	2·120	2·583	2·921	4·015
17	0·689	1·740	2·110	2·567	2·898	3·965
18	0·688	1·734	2·101	2·552	2·878	3·922
19	0·688	1·729	2·093	2·539	2·861	3·883
20	0·687	1·725	2·086	2·528	2·845	3·850
21	0·686	1·721	2·080	2·518	2·831	3·819
22	0·686	1·717	2·074	2·508	2·819	3·792
23	0·685	1·714	2·069	2·500	2·807	3·767
24	0·685	1·711	2·064	2·492	2·797	3·745
25	0·684	1·708	2·060	2·485	2·787	3·725
26	0·684	1·706	2·056	2·479	2·779	3·707
27	0·684	1·703	2·052	2·473	2·771	3·690
28	0·683	1·701	2·048	2·467	2·763	3·674
29	0·683	1·699	2·045	2·462	2·756	3·659
30	0·683	1·697	2·042	2·457	2·750	3·646
40	0·681	1·684	2·021	2·423	2·704	3·551
60	0·679	1·671	2·000	2·390	2·660	3·460
120	0·677	1·658	1·980	2·358	2·617	3·373
∞	0·674	1·645	1·960	2·326	2·576	3·291

Index

Page numbers in *italics* refer to figures, in **bold** refer to tables.